MELANIN JOURNEY

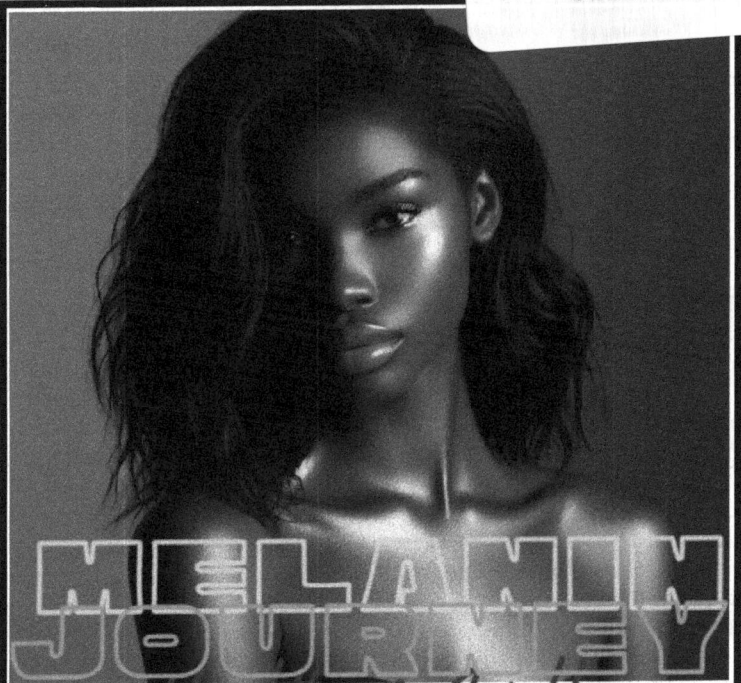

Health & Wellness

Dear Melanin Gurlll,

Your health is your wealth. Embrace your unique beauty, nourish your body with love and care, and prioritize your mental well-being. You are powerful, resilient, and deserving of the best in life. Let this guide be a source of inspiration and support on your journey to wellness. Remember, taking care of yourself is not just an act of self-love, but a revolutionary step towards a brighter, healthier future. You are worthy of happiness, health, and all the joy life has to offer. Embrace your wellness with pride and confidence. October Reign♡

The information provided in Melanin Journey: Health and Wellness is for educational and informational purposes only and should not be considered a substitute for professional medical advice, diagnosis, or treatment. Each body is unique, and what works for one person may not work for another. Always seek the advice of a licensed physician or qualified healthcare provider with any questions or concerns you may have regarding your health or a medical condition. This book offers holistic and natural insights that may complement your health journey, but it is essential to use this knowledge in conjunction with the advice of trusted professionals.

TABLE OF CONTENTS

INTRODUCTION

Melanin Journey is more than a health guide—it's an invitation for you to explore the incredible potential that lies within your melanin-rich body. Black people are not only physical beings but deeply spiritual beings, with a unique connection to the universe that is both powerful and sacred. We carry the wisdom of our ancestors in our blood, and when we learn to nurture our mind, body, and soul holistically, we unlock the true strength that resides in us.

Your melanin is more than just pigment; it is a divine gift, an anointing that connects you to the universe's energy, to the Earth's rhythms, and to each other. When you focus on reaching your full potential—through nourishing your body with whole foods, connecting with nature, practicing mindfulness, and embracing spiritual health—you awaken the full power of your being. The energy within you has the potential to heal, grow, and expand beyond the limitations imposed by societal systems.

As Black people, we have often been told that our health and wellness are not in our control. Our bodies are capable of regeneration and healing in ways that modern science has only begun to understand. From our strong immune systems to our natural resilience, there is power in our heritage, and there is power in our biology. Our melanin gives us a natural ability to thrive, endure, and adapt. It offers protection from the sun, helps us synthesize nutrients more efficiently, and connects us to the natural world in profound ways.

However, the systems we live in today do not always support this divine potential. Processed foods, environmental toxins, stress, and a disconnect from our spiritual roots can diminish this power. That's why this book encourages you to take the first steps on your Melanin Journey a journey to rediscover the ways you can heal and thrive naturally. Explore these pages, but also do your own research. Dive deeper into the practices and principles that resonate with you. Find the Melanin Journey that is right for your body, your soul, and your spirit.

The journey to health and wellness is deeply personal. It involves not only nurturing the physical body but also embracing spiritual practices, ancestral wisdom, and holistic healing methods that align with who you are at your core. You have the power to transform your life by aligning with nature and awakening the healing force within.

I encourage you to walk this path with intention and curiosity. Do the research, learn about what truly nourishes your body and spirit, and embrace the power within you. Your journey toward full health, clarity, and spiritual awakening starts here.

Let this book be your companion on the road to wellness, but remember—you are the healer, the guide, and the sacred keeper of your own body's wisdom. The power has always been yours.

With love and encouragement,

~ October Reign

Chapter 1
Journey Into Advocating for Yourself

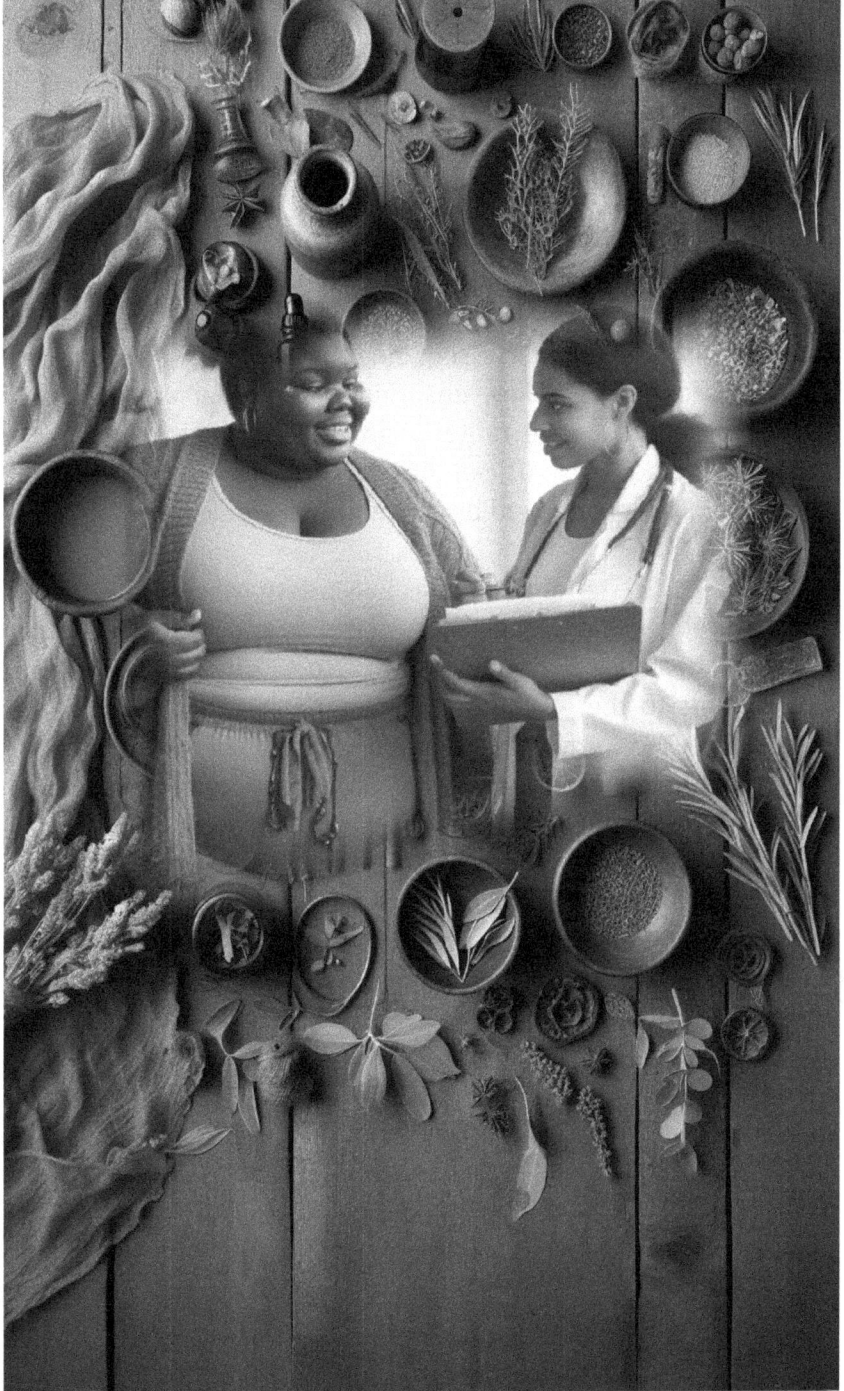

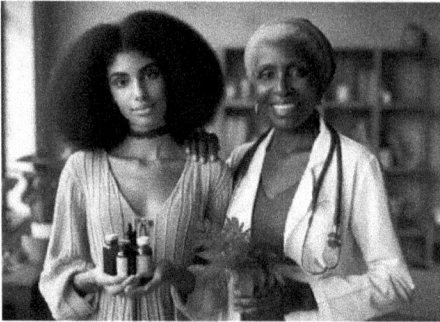

Advocating for Your Well-being in a Biased System

In today's healthcare environment, advocating for your physical and mental well-being is not just important—it's absolutely necessary, especially for African Americans. Relying solely on a single doctor's treatment plan, particularly if you feel unheard or notice no improvement, can lead to unnecessary medications and unaddressed health concerns. A proactive approach to health is key, ensuring that you are an informed participant in your care rather than a passive recipient. This is especially critical for African Americans, whose unique health needs are often overlooked by conventional medicine.

Understanding the Bias in Modern Medicine

The medical field has a long history of racism and prejudice that still impacts healthcare today. From the unethical Tuskegee experiments to the exploitation of Henrietta Lacks, Black bodies have been used in medical research without consent or care for their well-being. This legacy of injustice continues through disparities in the quality of care, misdiagnoses, and unequal access to treatments. African Americans are often subjected to inferior care, even in routine medical settings. Studies show that Black patients are less likely to be offered pain management, diagnosed later in disease progression, and given treatments not tailored to their unique physiological needs.

For African Americans, advocating for personalized healthcare means recognizing that standard medical practices may not always serve your best interests. African American bodies have distinct needs, and modern treatments or medications are frequently not designed with these differences in mind. For example, medications like certain blood pressure drugs (ACE inhibitors) are less effective for African Americans, yet they are prescribed routinely. This highlights the need for vigilance and self-advocacy.

It's important to do your own research on any prescription medications you're taking, as effectiveness and side effects can vary based on individual factors like genetics, race, and health conditions. Understanding how certain medications work for your specific needs will help you advocate for your best health outcomes. Always consult your healthcare provider and ask questions about alternative treatments if necessary.

How to Advocate for Proper Healthcare

Ask Questions and Seek Clarification: When discussing your treatment plan, don't hesitate to ask how medications will interact with your body. Inquire whether these drugs have been tested or tailored for African American patients, and ask for alternative options if you have concerns.

?QUESTIONS TO ASK HEALTHCARE PROVIDERS?

"Are these medications effective for African Americans?"
"How do these treatments interact with my body type?"
"What are the side effects specific to African American patients?"

Get a Second Opinion: If you are unsure about your diagnosis or treatment plan, seek a second opinion, preferably from a doctor who has experience treating African American patients. Don't feel obligated to stick with one doctor if they are not addressing your concerns or dismissing your symptoms.

Research and Know Your Medications: Look into the medications you're prescribed and check whether there are known disparities in their effectiveness for African American patients. For example, certain diuretics and calcium channel blockers are known to be more effective than ACE inhibitors for treating high blood pressure in Black patients. If your doctor isn't considering these alternatives, raise this concern.

Be Aware of Red Flags: If your doctor is dismissive of your pain or symptoms, prescribes medications that aren't suited for African American physiology, or doesn't seem to take your concerns seriously, these are red flags. In particular, watch out for: *Unnecessary prescriptions:* Excessive reliance on drugs rather than addressing root causes. *Dismissal of your symptoms:* Being told to "tough it out" or that your symptoms aren't serious. *Lack of cultural competency:* A healthcare provider who doesn't acknowledge the unique needs of Black patients.

Advocate for Holistic Healing

Incorporating natural and holistic healing practices into your wellness journey is a powerful way to take control of your health. Many African American ancestral practices such as herbal medicine, meditation, and nutritional healing offer ways to complement modern medicine. By blending these natural approaches with conventional treatments, you can create a balanced and personalized plan. Herbal teas, plant-based diets, and detox routines are great starting points to promote healing without relying solely on pharmaceuticals.

Tips on Affording Healthcare and Medicine

Advocating for better healthcare doesn't have to be financially draining. Here are some practical tips for managing healthcare costs and still receiving proper care: *Use Free or Low-Cost Clinics:* Many communities offer free clinics or sliding scale payment options based on your income. Research local community health centers or programs like Medicaid and Medicare that can help cover costs. *Prescription Assistance Programs:* Many pharmaceutical companies offer assistance programs that provide free or discounted medications to people who qualify. Websites like NeedyMeds and GoodRx can help you find affordable medication options.

Focus on Preventative Care: The best way to lower healthcare costs in the long run is by focusing on prevention. Regular exercise, a balanced diet, and stress management can help prevent chronic illnesses like diabetes and hypertension, which are prevalent in the African American community. Routine health screenings and early detection can also prevent more costly treatments down the line.

Natural Alternatives to Expensive Medications: Consider incorporating natural remedies into your treatment plan. Herbs such as turmeric, ginger, and garlic can be powerful anti-inflammatories, and magnesium supplements can help with conditions like hypertension. Before making any changes, consult with a healthcare provider who is open to blending natural and conventional approaches.

Be Your Own Advocate

Taking charge of your health means being informed, asking questions, and holding healthcare providers accountable for your well-being. Don't settle for substandard care or dismissive treatment. Whether through seeking second opinions, advocating for more effective treatments, or incorporating holistic and natural practices into your routine, the journey to wellness is about finding what works for your unique body and lifestyle. Your health is your power—use it wisely by demanding care that honors your melanin-rich body and supports your long-term well-being.

Find a Holistic healing, Alternative Medicine, Natural Medicine Practitioner
that's right for you!

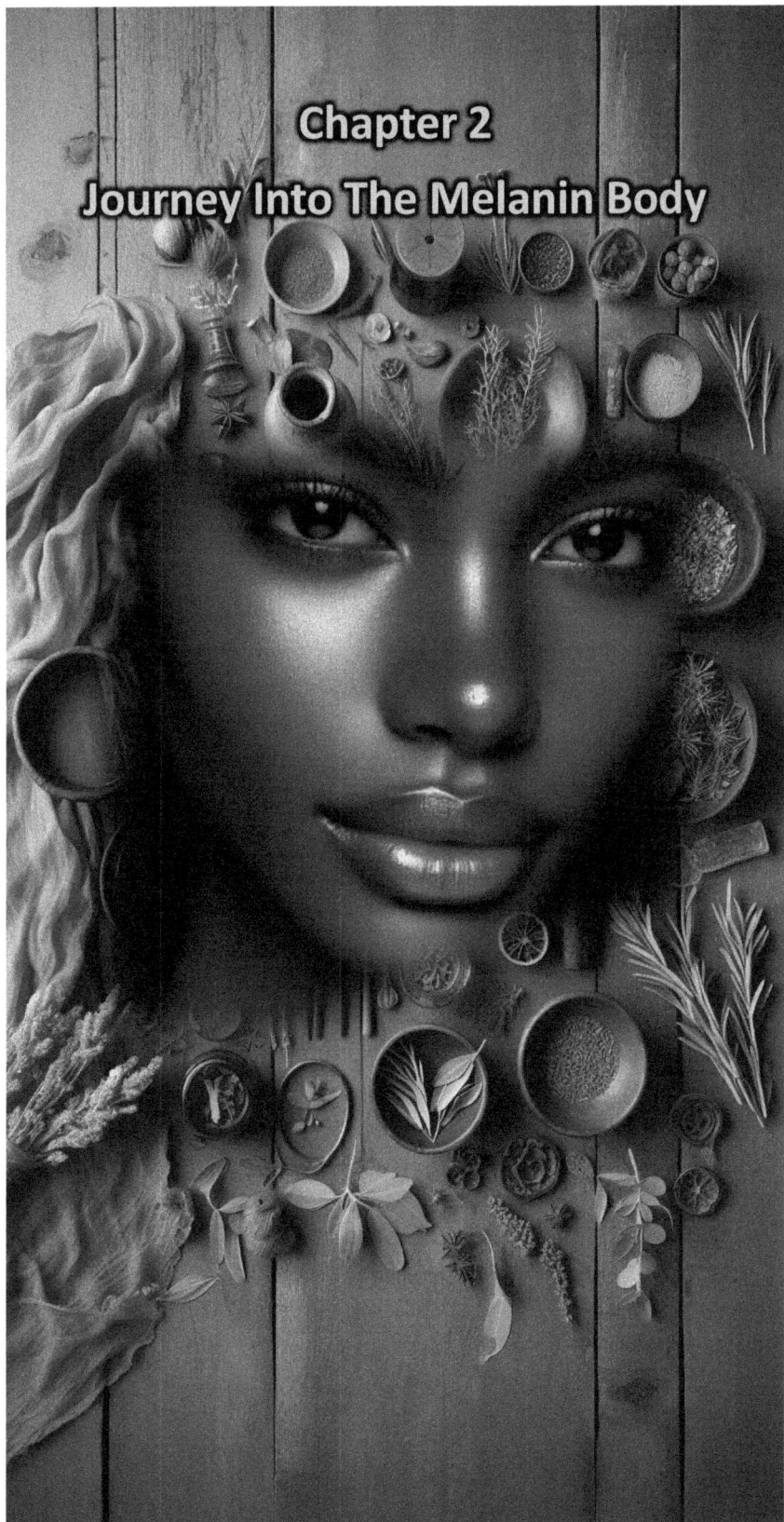

Chapter 2
Journey Into The Melanin Body

Ear Nose and Throat (ENT) System
EARS |NOSE | THROAT | SINUSES | TONSIL
Common Ailments

Ear Infections: Often seen in children, causing pain, fever, and trouble hearing. Strep Throat: A bacterial infection that causes a sore, swollen throat. Sinus Infections (Sinusitis): Inflammation of the sinuses leading to headaches, facial pain, and congestion. Why It's Important: These parts are connected, so an infection in one area can often spread to another, causing more symptoms.

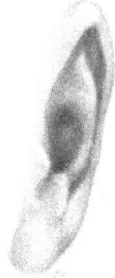

How the Ear, Nose, and Throat Are Connected

Eustachian Tube: Connects the middle ear to the back of the nose and throat. Helps equalize pressure in the ear and drains mucus from the middle ear into the throat. Nasal Passages and Sinuses: The nose is connected to the sinuses and the throat. Sinuses humidify the air and produce mucus that traps dust and germs. Throat (Pharynx): Connects the nose and mouth to the esophagus and larynx. Key for breathing, swallowing, and speaking. Tonsils and Adenoids: Lymphoid tissues in the throat and behind the nasal passages. They trap and fight infections.

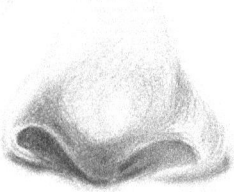

Maintaining a Healthy ENT System

Stay Hydrated: Keeps mucous membranes moist, helping trap and remove dust, allergens, and pathogens. Drink plenty of water and herbal teas. Practice Good Hygiene: Reduces the risk of infections. Wash your hands frequently, avoid touching your face, and keep your ears clean without inserting objects. Support Your Immune System: A strong immune system helps fight off infections before they become serious. Eat a balanced diet rich in vitamins C and D, zinc, and antioxidants. Incorporate immune-boosting foods like garlic, ginger, and citrus fruits. Humidify Your Environment: Prevents dry air from irritating the nasal passages and throat. Use a humidifier, especially in dry climates or during winter months. Practice Nasal Irrigation: Clears out allergens, dust, and excess mucus from the nasal passages. Use a saline nasal rinse or neti pot regularly. Get Adequate Sleep: Allows the body to repair and maintain its defense mechanisms. Aim for 7-9 hours of quality sleep each night. Practice mindfulness, meditation, or gentle exercises like yoga. Avoid Irritants: Prevents inflammation and infections in the ENT system. Stay away from smoke, pollution, and strong chemicals.

Digestive System

MOUTH |ESOPHAGUS |STOMACH|INTESTINES|LIVER |PANCREAS |GALLBLADDER

Common Ailments

Gastroesophageal Reflux Disease (GERD): Stomach acid flows back into the esophagus, causing heartburn and discomfort. Irritable Bowel Syndrome (IBS): Affects the intestines, causing cramps, bloating, diarrhea, or constipation. Gallstones: Hardened deposits in the gallbladder causing pain, especially after eating fatty foods. Why It's Important: The digestive system breaks down food into nutrients, which the body uses for energy, growth, and cell repair.

How the Digestive System Is Connected

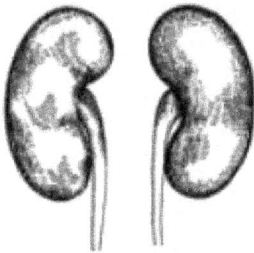

Mouth: Starts the process of digestion by chewing and mixing food with saliva. Esophagus: A muscular tube that moves food from the mouth to the stomach. Stomach: Produces acid and enzymes that digest food. Small Intestine: Absorbs nutrients from digested food. Large Intestine: Absorbs water and forms waste (stool) for elimination. Liver, Pancreas, and Gallbladder: Produce enzymes and bile to help digest food.

Mechanism of Action: How It Works

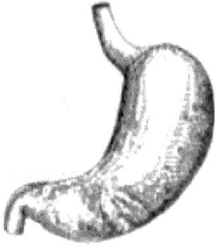

Digestion: Begins in the mouth and continues as food travels down the esophagus to the stomach, where it is broken down by stomach acid and enzymes. Nutrient Absorption: Occurs mainly in the small intestine, where nutrients pass through the intestinal walls into the bloodstream. Waste Elimination: The large intestine absorbs water and forms waste, which is then eliminated through the rectum and anus.

Maintaining Healthy Digestive System

Eat a Balanced Diet: Provides essential nutrients for the digestive process. Include a variety of fruits, vegetables, whole grains, and lean proteins in your diet. Stay Hydrated: Aids digestion and prevents constipation. Drink plenty of water throughout the day. Probiotics and Fiber: Support a healthy gut microbiome and regular bowel movements. Eat yogurt, fermented foods, and high-fiber foods like fruits, vegetables, and whole grains. Regular Exercise: Stimulates digestion and helps prevent constipation. Incorporate daily physical activity like walking, cycling, or yoga. Manage Stress: Reduces digestive problems like IBS. Practice stress-relief techniques like meditation or deep breathing exercises.

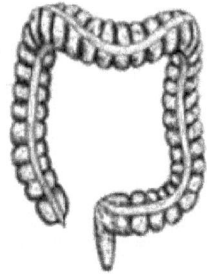

Respiratory System
LUNGS |TRACHEA (WINDPIPE) | BRONCHI | DIAPHRAGM
Common Ailments

Asthma: A condition where the airways narrow, making it hard to breathe. *Pneumonia:* An infection that inflames the air sacs in one or both lungs, causing cough, fever, and difficulty breathing. *Chronic Obstructive Pulmonary Disease (COPD):* A group of lung diseases that block airflow and make it difficult to breathe. The respiratory system supplies the blood with oxygen and removes carbon dioxide, which is essential for survival.

How the Respiratory System Is Connected

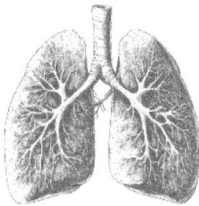

Trachea: The windpipe that carries air from the nose and mouth to the lungs. *Bronchi:* The two large tubes that branch off the trachea and carry air into each lung. *Lungs:* Main organs of the respiratory system where oxygen is exchanged for carbon dioxide in the blood. *Diaphragm:* A large muscle below the lungs that contracts and relaxes to allow breathing.

Body Maintenance for a Healthy Respiratory System

Avoid Smoking and Pollutants: Reduces the risk of respiratory diseases. Stay away from cigarette smoke, pollution, and chemicals. *Practice Deep Breathing:* Strengthens the lungs and improves oxygen exchange. Incorporate deep breathing exercises or yoga into your routine. *Stay Active:* Keeps the lungs and heart healthy. Engage in regular physical activities like walking, swimming, or cycling. *Hydrate Well:* Keeps the respiratory tract moist and helps mucus flow freely. Drink plenty of water daily. *Manage Allergies:* Prevents allergic reactions that can trigger asthma or other respiratory issues. Avoid allergens, use air purifiers, and consider natural remedies like quercetin and vitamin C.

Musculoskeletal System
BONES |MUSCLES | JOINTS |TENDONS | LIGAMENTS
Common Ailments

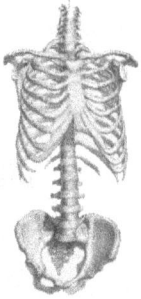

Sprains and Strains: Injuries to ligaments (sprains) or muscles/tendons (strains). *Arthritis:* Inflammation of the joints, causing pain and stiffness. *Fractures:* Broken bones due to trauma or osteoporosis. The musculoskeletal system provides structure, supports movement, and protects vital organs.

How the Musculoskeletal System Is Connected

Bones: Provide the framework for the body and protect internal organs. *Muscles:* Attach to bones and work with the skeletal system to produce movement. *Joints:* Where two or more bones meet, allowing for flexibility and movement. *Tendons and Ligaments:* Connect muscles to bones (tendons) and bones to other bones (ligaments), providing stability and strength.

Maintaining a Healthy Musculoskeletal System

Engage in Regular Exercise: Strengthens muscles and bones, improving overall mobility. Include weight-bearing exercises like walking, running, or resistance training. *Maintain a Balanced Diet:* Supports bone density and muscle health. Ensure adequate intake of calcium, vitamin D, protein, and magnesium. *Practice Good Posture:* Prevents strain on muscles and joints. Be mindful of posture when sitting, standing, and lifting objects. *Stay Hydrated:* Keeps joints lubricated and muscles functioning properly. Drink water regularly, especially during physical activities. *Manage Stress:* Reduces muscle tension and helps prevent injuries. Incorporate relaxation techniques like stretching, yoga, or deep breathing into your routine.

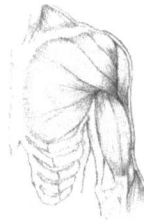

Cardiovascular System

HEART |BLOOD VESSELS |ARTERIES | VEINS | CAPILLARIES | BLOOD

Common Ailments

Hypertension (High Blood Pressure): Increases the risk of heart disease and stroke. *Heart Attack:* Occurs when blood flow to a part of the heart is blocked, damaging the heart muscle. *Stroke:* A blockage or bleed in the brain's blood vessels, causing brain damage. The cardiovascular system circulates blood throughout the body, delivering oxygen and nutrients to cells and removing waste products.

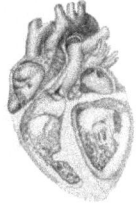

How the Cardiovascular System Is Connected

Heart: Pumps blood through the blood vessels to all parts of the body. *Arteries:* Carry oxygen-rich blood from the heart to the body. *Veins:* Return oxygen-poor blood back to the heart. *Capillaries:* Small blood vessels where oxygen and nutrients are exchanged with tissues.

Maintaining a Healthy Cardiovascular System

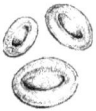

Eat a Heart-Healthy Diet: Reduces the risk of cardiovascular disease. Focus on fruits, vegetables, whole grains, lean proteins, and healthy fats like those found in olive oil and fish. *Exercise Regularly:* Strengthens the heart and improves circulation. Engage in aerobic activities like walking, running, or swimming for at least 30 minutes most days of the week. *Monitor Blood Pressure and Cholesterol:* Helps prevent heart disease and stroke. *Manage Stress:* Prevents high blood pressure and reduces the risk of heart-related issues. Incorporate stress-relief practices like meditation, deep breathing, or spending time in nature. *Avoid Smoking and Excessive Alcohol:* Protects the heart and blood vessels from damage. Quit smoking, limit alcohol consumption, and seek support if needed.

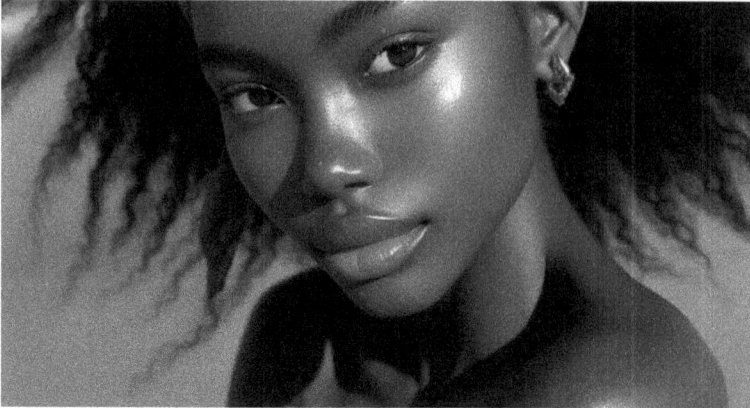

The 90-Day Cell Regeneration Cycle

The body is an incredible machine, designed to heal and regenerate itself naturally. Every 90 days, our cells undergo a renewal process, replacing old, damaged cells with new ones. For African Americans, this process is particularly significant, as we face unique health challenges influenced by genetics, environment, and lifestyle. By taking a holistic and natural approach to our health, we can harness this cycle of regeneration to promote healing, wellness, and longevity.

Cell regeneration is the process by which the body replaces old or damaged cells with new, healthy ones. This renewal is constant, but it operates in cycles, with most cells regenerating approximately every 90 days. During this period, the body works to repair tissues, organs, and systems, ensuring that we function at our best. Cells in the skin, liver, and intestines regenerate the fastest, while those in the bones and brain may take longer. For African Americans, who may be at higher risk for conditions such as hypertension, diabetes, and cardiovascular disease, supporting healthy cell regeneration is crucial for maintaining optimal health.

Preparing the Body for Regeneration

Before embarking on a 90-day regimen, it's important to prepare the body for maximum cell renewal. This preparation phase will focus on detoxification, boosting nutrition, and mental and emotional well-being.

Detoxification

Detoxifying the body helps eliminate toxins that may hinder the regeneration process., Environmental toxins and unhealthy food options in some communities may contribute to higher toxin levels.

How to detox

Start by drinking plenty of water, preferably infused with lemon or cucumber to help flush out toxins. Incorporate herbal teas like dandelion root, ginger, and burdock root, which support liver detoxification and digestion. Avoid processed foods, sugary drinks, and alcohol.

Boosting Nutrition

The body often have unique nutritional needs. For example, many people in our community are deficient in vitamin D due to darker skin, which doesn't absorb sunlight as efficiently. ***Focus on:*** Foods rich in vitamins and minerals that support cell regeneration, such as leafy greens (spinach, kale), fatty fish (salmon, sardines), nuts, seeds, and antioxidant-rich fruits (berries, citrus). Omega-3 fatty acids, vitamin D, and magnesium are particularly important for cell health.

Mental and Emotional Well-being

Health is not just about the physical body. The mind plays a crucial role in how well the body regenerates and heals itself. Mindfulness practices: Meditation, journaling, and spending time in nature are essential for stress management. African Americans often face stressors related to systemic inequalities, so it's vital to prioritize mental health. Reducing stress enhances the body's ability to regenerate by lowering cortisol levels and promoting a healthy immune response.

The 90-Day Regimen for Holistic Cell Regeneration

Once the body is properly prepared, you can follow a 90-day holistic regimen designed to optimize the natural cell regeneration cycle. This plan incorporates nutrition, movement, and spiritual practices to address the unique needs of the African American body.

PHASE 1: DAYS 1–30 – DETOXIFY AND CLEANSE

Diet: Focus on a plant-based, whole-food diet. Include plenty of raw fruits and vegetables, fiber-rich grains like quinoa and brown rice, and lean proteins such as beans and lentils. Avoid processed foods, red meats, and refined sugars, which can slow down the body's ability to regenerate cells. *Supplements:* Consider supplements like vitamin D, vitamin C, and magnesium. African Americans often have vitamin D deficiencies, which are essential for immune function and cellular health. *Physical Activity:* Gentle exercises like yoga, walking, or tai chi will promote circulation and detoxification. *Spiritual Health:* Engage in daily meditation or prayer to set intentions for healing and renewal.

PHASE 2: DAYS 31–60 – REBUILD AND STRENGTHEN

Diet: Begin incorporating more protein-rich foods to help build new cells. Opt for wild-caught fish, organic poultry, and legumes. Increase your intake of healthy fats, such as avocado, olive oil, and flaxseeds, which are essential for cellular membrane health. *Supplements:* Add omega-3 fatty acids (from fish oil or flaxseed oil) to promote brain health and reduce inflammation. *Physical Activity:* Increase intensity by incorporating strength training or resistance exercises. Muscle repair also involves cell regeneration, so keeping muscles active helps the overall process. *Spiritual Health:* Continue mindfulness practices, and begin incorporating visualization techniques, imagining your body healing and renewing itself.

PHASE 3: DAYS 61–90 – OPTIMIZE AND MAINTAIN

Diet: Maintain a balanced, nutrient-dense diet, with an emphasis on variety. Rotate your food choices to avoid nutrient deficiencies and ensure all parts of your body are receiving what they need. *Supplements:* Continue taking essential supplements, especially if dietary intake is insufficient. *Physical Activity:* Maintain a mix of cardio, strength, and flexibility exercises. Exercise boosts circulation, which helps deliver nutrients to cells and removes waste products more efficiently. *Spiritual Health:* Focus on gratitude and connection. Whether it's community involvement, spiritual practices, or self-care, continue to nurture your emotional well-being.

Melanin and Skin Cell Renewal

Melanin, the pigment that gives African Americans their rich skin tones, plays a role in protecting skin cells from damage by ultraviolet (UV) rays. However, this also means that skin cell turnover may occur at a different rate compared to lighter skin tones. Supporting skin health through proper hydration and nutrient-dense foods rich in vitamins A and E is vital.

Bone Health and Regeneration

Bone cells regenerate slowly, but weight-bearing exercises like walking or resistance training help stimulate bone density and strength. This is especially important for African Americans, who may be at higher risk for osteoporosis due to lower calcium intake.

Embrace the Cycle

The body's ability to regenerate cells is a remarkable process that can be enhanced through holistic, natural methods. For the African American body, which faces unique health challenges, a 90-day regimen focused on detoxification, nutrition, movement, and spiritual health can lead to profound physical, emotional, and mental transformation.

By embracing this natural cycle of renewal, you can optimize your health, allowing your body to heal and thrive in alignment with nature's wisdom. Remember, your health is your power—and by supporting your body through its natural regeneration process, you are taking a critical step toward living a vibrant, balanced, and empowered life.

How Cell Regeneration Works

Our cells naturally regenerate at different rates, depending on the type. For example: **Skin cells** renew every 2-3 weeks. **Red blood cells** replace themselves roughly every 120 days. **Liver cells** can regenerate over 150–500 days. **Gut lining cells** renew every 3-5 days.

During each regeneration cycle, cells divide and replicate, replacing damaged or old cells. In theory, if healthy conditions are maintained, new cells can be more resilient against damage or mutation, leading to healthier overall tissue over time. This is where lifestyle factors like diet, exercise, sleep, and stress management can play a major role in influencing the health of new cells.

Why Cell Regeneration Doesn't Automatically "Heal" Cancer

Cancer cells are different from normal cells because they have undergone genetic changes (mutations) that make them grow uncontrollably and evade normal cell death.

DNA mutations: Cancer cells often carry genetic mutations that alter their growth patterns. These mutations don't just disappear during cell division; instead, they're passed on to new cancer cells.

Lack of normal cell signaling: Cancer cells often ignore the usual signals to stop growing or die, allowing them to multiply unchecked. **Evading the immune system**: Cancer cells can disguise themselves or suppress immune responses that would otherwise recognize and destroy them.

Due to these fundamental differences, even though cells regenerate, the mutated DNA within cancer cells is passed on during cell division, meaning they often continue to grow and proliferate.

Promoting Healthier Cells During Regeneration Cycles

While cancer cells don't necessarily "heal" during cell regeneration, creating a healthy internal environment can still have a significant impact. Here's how supporting healthier cells could work: **Reducing Cellular Stress**: Minimizing exposure to carcinogens (e.g., through diet, environment, and lifestyle) can reduce oxidative stress and DNA damage, potentially preventing healthy cells from becoming cancerous. **Supporting Immune Function**: A strong immune system is better able to identify and target abnormal cells before they become cancerous. **Optimizing Nutrient Intake**: Nutrients like antioxidants, vitamins, and minerals support cellular repair and DNA health, which may reduce the likelihood of mutations. **Maintaining Balanced Hormones**: Hormonal imbalances can sometimes promote the growth of certain cancers, so balancing hormones can reduce these risks.

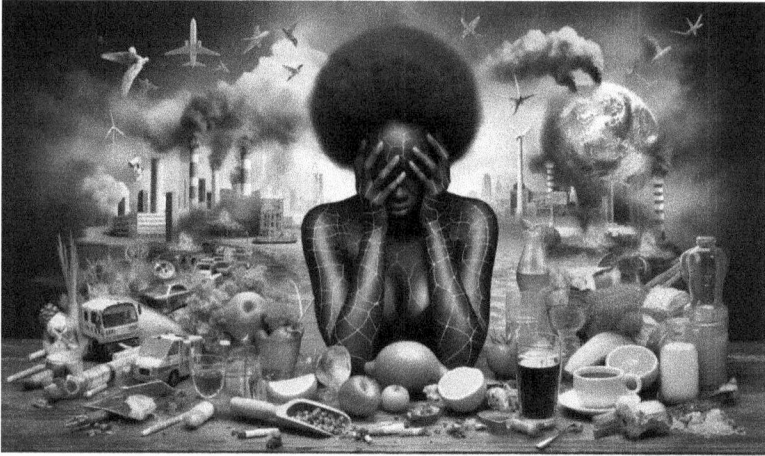

Can Cancer Cells Be "Reprogrammed"?

Research is ongoing in the field of cancer biology to explore ways of "reprogramming" cancer cells back to normal. Some promising areas include: **Epigenetics**: This field studies how lifestyle and environmental factors can influence gene expression without changing DNA. Some therapies target epigenetic mechanisms to try to "turn off" cancer-promoting genes. **Immunotherapy**: This type of therapy helps the immune system recognize and attack cancer cells. **Gene Editing**: Techniques like CRISPR are being investigated to target and correct specific mutations in cancer cells, but this research is still emerging.

While cell regeneration is a powerful mechanism for maintaining health, cancer cells' unique properties mean they don't automatically return to a healthy state with each regeneration cycle. However, creating a supportive environment through lifestyle, nutrition, and medical interventions can promote healthier cells overall and may reduce the likelihood of additional mutations or cancer development in healthy cells.

DNA Health and Oxidative Stress

DNA health refers to the condition and integrity of our genetic material, which influences how well our cells function, repair themselves, and replicate accurately. DNA contains the instructions for all cellular activities, so maintaining its health is essential for overall wellbeing and can reduce the risk of diseases, including cancer. Over time, DNA can become damaged by environmental factors, lifestyle choices, and natural aging processes. Maintaining DNA health involves protecting against this damage and supporting natural repair processes.

Oxidative Stress

Oxidative stress is a major factor in DNA damage. It occurs when there's an imbalance between free radicals—unstable molecules that can harm cells—and antioxidants, which neutralize free radicals. Free radicals are byproducts of normal metabolic processes, but they can increase due to exposure to pollutants, poor diet, smoking, radiation, and stress. Oxidative stress can damage DNA, proteins, and lipids, accelerating aging and increasing the risk of diseases, including cancer and heart disease.

How to Improve DNA Health

Improving DNA health involves reducing damage and enhancing the body's ability to repair itself. Here are ways to promote DNA health: **Diet Rich in Antioxidants** neutralize free radicals and reduce oxidative stress. Foods high in antioxidants include berries (blueberries, strawberries), leafy greens (spinach, kale), nuts, and seeds. Vitamins C and E, selenium, and flavonoids (found in fruits and vegetables) are key antioxidants that protect DNA. **Regular Physical Activity** Exercise enhances blood flow, which delivers oxygen and nutrients to cells, supporting DNA repair and reducing inflammation. However, moderation is essential; excessive exercise without recovery can increase oxidative stress.

Minimizing Exposure to Toxins Reduce exposure to environmental toxins, such as pollution, heavy metals, and radiation, which can increase oxidative stress and DNA damage. Avoid tobacco, limit alcohol consumption, and try to reduce processed foods in your diet, as these can contribute to oxidative damage.

Adequate Sleep and Stress Management Quality sleep and stress management are critical for cellular repair and regeneration, as many repair processes, including DNA repair, occur during deep sleep.

Chronic stress releases hormones like cortisol, which can increase oxidative stress, so practices like meditation, deep breathing, or yoga can help reduce its effects.

Limit Processed and Sugary Foods High sugar intake can promote inflammation and oxidative stress. Limiting added sugars and refined carbs can support DNA health by lowering the burden of oxidative stress on cells.

Consume Omega-3 Fatty Acids Omega-3s, found in fish, walnuts, and flaxseeds, are anti-inflammatory and can reduce oxidative damage. These fats help stabilize cell membranes, supporting overall cellular and DNA health.

Herbs and Supplements That May Support DNA Health Curcumin: Found in turmeric, curcumin is known for its antioxidant and anti-inflammatory properties. **Resveratrol**: Found in grapes and red wine, resveratrol supports cellular repair processes and may protect against DNA damage. Green Tea Extract: Rich in catechins, green tea provides antioxidants that protect DNA from oxidative damage.

Promote Healthy Mitochondrial Function Mitochondria, the energy-producing structures in cells, can be damaged by oxidative stress. Nutrients like CoQ10, magnesium, and B vitamins support mitochondrial health and reduce oxidative stress.

Understanding Oxidative Stress

Oxidative stress results from an imbalance between free radicals and antioxidants. While free radicals are natural byproducts of metabolism, an excess can cause cellular and DNA damage. This imbalance can occur due to: **Environmental Factors**: Pollution, UV radiation, and toxic substances. **Lifestyle Choices**: Poor diet, smoking, and excessive alcohol **Aging**: Naturally increases oxidative stress levels. The effects of oxidative stress can include premature aging, reduced cellular function, inflammation, and an increased risk of chronic diseases. DNA damage from oxidative stress can lead to mutations, which may cause cancer if repair mechanisms fail.

Key Takeaways

Protective Diet and Lifestyle: Eating a balanced diet rich in antioxidants, exercising moderately, managing stress, and getting quality sleep are fundamental for DNA protection. **Antioxidants are Crucial**: They play a central role in neutralizing free radicals, thereby reducing oxidative stress and preventing DNA damage. **Reducing Exposure to Toxins**: Avoiding pollutants and toxins in your environment can lower the impact of oxidative stress on your cells. **Support Repair and Regeneration**: Cellular repair occurs during rest, so sufficient sleep is crucial for maintaining DNA integrity.

By focusing on antioxidant-rich nutrition, managing stress, and supporting healthy lifestyle choices, you can positively influence DNA health, promote cellular resilience, and reduce the impact of oxidative stress on the body.

Drawing out Bodily Toxins and Pollutants

There are natural methods and herbal remedies that can help draw toxins and pollutants from the body. Detoxification can be supported through dietary choices, natural clays, detox baths, herbal teas, and practices that support the liver, kidneys, skin, and lymphatic system, which are the body's main pathways for eliminating toxins. Here are some effective methods:

Detoxifying Clays and Powders

Bentonite Clay (Aztec Clay): Bentonite clay is known for its ability to absorb and bind to toxins, heavy metals, and impurities. It can be used both externally (as a mask or bath) and internally (with care and under guidance). For a clay mask, mix bentonite clay with water or apple cider vinegar, apply to the skin, and rinse after it dries to draw out impurities.

Activated Charcoal: This is highly absorbent and binds to toxins in the gut. It is often used for detoxifying the digestive system but should only be used occasionally and under the advice of a healthcare provider, as it can interfere with nutrient absorption.

Detox Baths

Detox baths are a relaxing way to support toxin elimination through the skin. **Epsom Salt Bath**: Epsom salt (magnesium sulfate) helps draw out toxins, reduces inflammation, and soothes muscles. Magnesium is also absorbed through the skin, supporting relaxation and bodily functions. Add 1-2 cups of Epsom salt to a warm bath and soak for 20-30 minutes. **Baking Soda**: Baking soda alkalizes the skin and helps neutralize chemicals absorbed through the skin, like chlorine from water. Add 1 cup to a bath along with Epsom salts for enhanced detoxification. **Apple Cider Vinegar**: Vinegar baths can help restore skin pH and may assist in removing toxins. Add 1 cup of raw apple cider vinegar to a bath, soak for 15-20 minutes, and then rinse with fresh water. **Ginger**: Freshly grated ginger or ginger powder added to a warm bath induces sweating, which can help release toxins. Use sparingly (about 2-3 tablespoons), as ginger baths can be intense and increase circulation.

Herbal Teas and Supplements

Dandelion Root: Known for its liver-supporting properties, dandelion root helps the liver filter toxins from the blood. It can be consumed as a tea or supplement. **Milk Thistle**: Milk thistle contains silymarin, which protects and supports liver function, aiding in detoxification. It is available in capsule or tea form. **Burdock Root**: Traditionally used as a blood purifier, burdock root supports the liver and kidneys and is rich in antioxidants. Drinking burdock root tea can help cleanse the blood. **Nettle Leaf**: Nettle is nutrient-rich and supports kidney function, helping to filter out impurities. It is also beneficial for reducing inflammation and can be taken as a tea. **Parsley and Cilantro**: Both herbs are known for their detoxifying effects, especially for heavy metals. Cilantro is thought to bind to heavy metals, and parsley supports kidney health, which aids in flushing out toxins. Adding fresh parsley and cilantro to meals or smoothies is a simple way to incorporate them.

Natural Sweating and Skin Brushing

Sweating: Activities that promote sweating, such as exercise or using a sauna, help the body release toxins through the skin. A regular exercise routine is beneficial not only for detoxification but also for overall health. **Dry Brushing**: Dry brushing helps stimulate the lymphatic system, which plays a key role in eliminating waste. Use a natural bristle brush and gently brush your skin in circular motions, starting from the feet and working toward the heart. This helps promote circulation and remove dead skin cells, facilitating toxin release.

Probiotics and Fiber for Digestive Health

Probiotics: A healthy gut microbiome helps with detoxification, as beneficial bacteria break down toxins and prevent harmful substances from being absorbed. Probiotic-rich foods like yogurt, kefir, kimchi, and sauerkraut support gut health. **Fiber-Rich Foods**: Fiber binds to toxins in the digestive tract, aiding in their removal. Eating fiber-rich foods such as vegetables, fruits, flaxseeds, chia seeds, and whole grains can support natural detoxification.

Additional Natural Practices for Detoxification

Hydration: Drinking plenty of clean, filtered water flushes out toxins through the kidneys. Hydration also supports skin and cellular health, making it essential for any detox program. **Chlorophyll and Green Superfoods**: Foods like spirulina, chlorella, and wheatgrass are high in chlorophyll, which helps detoxify the blood and liver. These greens are also known to bind to heavy metals, assisting in their removal. **Lemon Water**: Starting the day with warm lemon water is a simple way to support liver health and digestion, aiding in detoxification. Lemon stimulates bile production in the liver, which is essential for breaking down fats and eliminating waste.

Understanding pH Balance in Detoxification

Maintaining a slightly alkaline pH can support the body's natural detoxification processes. While the body regulates blood pH tightly, a diet rich in fruits, vegetables, and greens helps maintain cellular health and supports detoxification organs like the liver and kidneys. By incorporating these natural detoxifying practices, you can support your body's natural pathways for eliminating toxins, maintaining overall health, and reducing the risk of pollutant-related health issues. Remember to listen to your body, and consult with a healthcare provider if you have specific concerns about detoxification or any new regimen.

Oxidative Stress in African Americans and Its Impact on Health

Oxidative stress is a cellular imbalance where the body produces more free radicals (unstable molecules that can damage cells) than antioxidants can neutralize. This imbalance can contribute to various health problems, including cardiovascular disease, skin health issues, and impaired vascular function. In African Americans, oxidative stress has specific implications, particularly with respect to nitric oxide (NO) function, cardiovascular health, and skin pigmentation.

Oxidation and Skin Color in African Americans

Oxidative stress can have a subtle impact on skin appearance. Though it doesn't fundamentally change the melanin-based skin color, which is genetically determined, oxidative stress can affect skin health, resulting in issues like hyperpigmentation, dullness, and uneven skin tone.

The original, naturally healthy appearance of melanated skin is vibrant and rich in even pigmentation. Oxidative stress can create an appearance of dullness or stress in the skin, but it does not alter the genetic foundation of skin color. Proper antioxidant levels help in maintaining the skin's natural radiance and healthy tone.

Young African Americans and Reduced NO-Mediated Cutaneous Vasodilation

Studies show that young African Americans tend to have reduced nitric oxide (NO)-mediated cutaneous vasodilation (expansion of blood vessels in the skin) compared to young European Americans. Nitric oxide is a molecule that aids in relaxing blood vessels, helping blood flow and regulating blood pressure. In the skin, it facilitates healthy circulation, which supports skin health, nutrient delivery, and thermoregulation. Reduced NO-mediated vasodilation in African Americans may contribute to a higher tendency for cardiovascular issues later in life, as this condition indicates lower efficiency in blood vessel relaxation.

Role of Racial Disparities in Oxidative Stress and Cardiovascular Disease (CVD)

Racial disparities can play a significant role in oxidative stress levels and cardiovascular health outcomes. Increased oxidative stress can lead to endothelial dysfunction (poor blood vessel function), inflammation, and damage to tissues. In African Americans, higher oxidative stress levels have been linked to increased cardiovascular disease risk, which is influenced by social, environmental, and genetic factors. *Socioeconomic factors*, access to quality healthcare, dietary habits, and stressors associated with racial discrimination contribute to the oxidative stress burden in African Americans, compounding health risks, particularly related to cardiovascular disease. The main symptom of *endothelial dysfunction* is chest pain, or angina, that worsens during physical activity or emotional stress.

Shortness of breath, Tiredness, Discomfort in the left arm, jaw, neck, back, or abdomen, Irregular heartbeats

In the early stages, endothelial dysfunction may not have any noticeable symptoms. As it progresses, symptoms related to other health problems may emerge. Endothelial dysfunction is a disturbance in the balance of vasoconstrictors and vasodilators, growth promotors and inhibitors, and other factors. It's a key factor in the development of atherosclerosis, which can lead to plaque formation and rupture.

If you're experiencing chest pain and other symptoms like shortness of breath, sweating, nausea, or dizziness, seek emergency medical care. If you have new or unexplained chest pain, call 911 or emergency medical assistance immediately.

eNOS Uncoupling and Cardiovascular Health

Endothelial nitric oxide synthase (eNOS) is an enzyme critical for producing nitric oxide (NO) in the blood vessels. NO helps maintain blood flow and reduces blood pressure. Oxidative stress can lead to increased levels of asymmetric dimethyl-L-arginine (ADMA), a molecule that inhibits eNOS, leading to "uncoupling." When eNOS becomes uncoupled, it produces more free radicals rather than NO, which worsens oxidative stress and damages blood vessels. eNOS uncoupling, driven by increased ADMA levels, is an essential factor in the pathogenesis (development) of cardiovascular disease, especially in populations with elevated oxidative stress, such as African Americans.

What is Asymmetric Dimethyl-L-Arginine (ADMA)?

Asymmetric Dimethyl-L-Arginine (ADMA) is a naturally occurring molecule in the body that interferes with NO production. ADMA blocks the enzyme eNOS from creating NO, reducing blood vessel relaxation and promoting oxidative stress. Higher ADMA levels are associated with increased cardiovascular risk, as they lead to endothelial dysfunction and oxidative stress, which are common in populations experiencing high oxidative stress, including African Americans.

Prevention and Remedies for Oxidative Stress

To reduce the impact of oxidative stress, particularly for African Americans, lifestyle adjustments and natural remedies can be beneficial: **Antioxidant-Rich Diet**: Consuming foods high in antioxidants helps neutralize free radicals, reducing oxidative stress. This includes fruits like berries, vegetables, nuts, and foods rich in vitamins C and E. **Nitric Oxide Support**: Foods high in nitrates, like leafy greens (spinach, arugula) and beets, can support NO production and improve blood vessel function.

L-arginine and L-citrulline supplements may help increase NO levels, promoting vascular health. **Stress Management**: Chronic stress increases oxidative stress. Incorporating stress-relieving activities like meditation, yoga, and regular exercise can help manage stress and reduce its physiological effects. **Hydration:** Proper hydration is essential for kidney function and toxin removal, which indirectly reduces oxidative stress. **Limit Exposure to Environmental Toxins:** Reducing exposure to pollutants, cigarette smoke, and heavy metals can decrease oxidative stress on the body. For individuals exposed to environmental stressors, regular detoxification practices, such as consuming antioxidant-rich foods and staying hydrated, can be beneficial. **Consistent Physical Activity:** Regular exercise promotes circulation, enhances cellular health, and helps reduce inflammation and oxidative stress in the body.

Supplements for Vascular Health

Coenzyme Q10 (CoQ10): Supports mitochondrial health, reducing oxidative stress in blood vessels. **Resveratrol:** Found in grapes and red wine, resveratrol is an antioxidant that helps reduce oxidative stress in the cardiovascular system. **Omega-3 Fatty Acids:** Found in fish oil, these acids help reduce inflammation and oxidative stress, supporting cardiovascular health. By understanding the factors that increase oxidative stress and implementing lifestyle and dietary changes, individuals, particularly African Americans, can work towards maintaining their health, particularly in reducing risks associated with cancer.

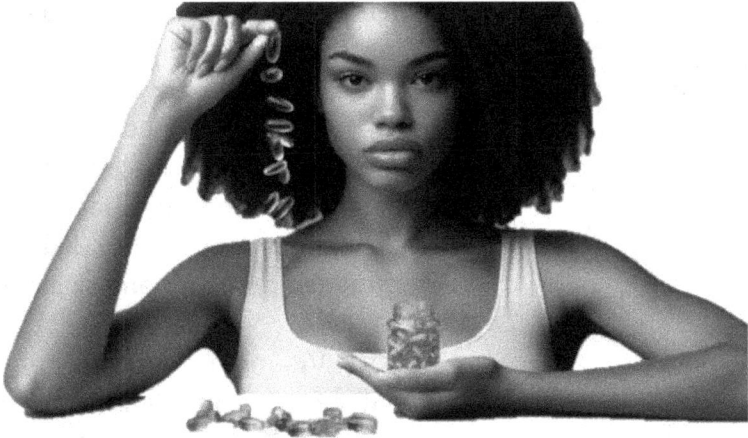

Understanding Vitamin Deficiencies

Black women often have unique body structures and compositions that distinguish them from other populations. Vitamin D plays a crucial role in overall health, influencing bone health, immune function, and the prevention of chronic diseases. Due to higher levels of melanin in the skin, Black women may experience reduced synthesis of vitamin D from sunlight, leading to a higher risk of deficiency.

Vitamin A

Vitamin A is essential for maintaining good vision, promoting healthy skin, supporting immune function, and encouraging hair growth. It plays a significant role in cell growth and development, making it crucial for maintaining healthy hair and skin. Vitamin A also has anti-inflammatory properties, helping to protect against chronic diseases like heart disease and diabetes. It is especially important for African Americans, as it supports skin health and helps prevent conditions such as dry skin or eczema, which can be exacerbated by environmental stressors. A well-balanced intake of Vitamin A promotes the production of sebum, which moisturizes the scalp and prevents hair dryness, particularly in African American hair, which tends to be more prone to dryness due to its texture. *Holistic Sources:* include carrots, sweet potatoes, spinach, kale, liver, and fish oils.

Deficiency Symptoms: may include night blindness, dry eyes, dry skin, frequent infections, and delayed wound healing. African Americans, especially those in urban environments with limited access to nutrient-rich foods, may face a higher risk of Vitamin A deficiency, leading to vision-related problems and skin issues.

Vitamin B Complex

The Vitamin B complex is a group of vitamins that work together to support energy production, brain function, and red blood cell formation. Each B vitamin plays a specific role in maintaining overall health, and they are especially beneficial for African Americans due to their roles in managing stress, supporting cardiovascular health, and promoting healthy skin and hair.

Deficiencies Symptoms

Anemia
Weakness
Tiredness
Brain Damage
Bone loss
Muscle Weakness
Fractures
Child Mental Delay
Skin issues
Dandruff
Seborrheic
Dermatitis
Night Vision Loss
Neurologic problems
Fatigue Depression
Hair Loss
Muscle Pain
Wound Healing
Frequent Illnesses
Other issues

Vitamin B1 (Thiamine)

Vitamin B1 (Thiamine) supports energy metabolism, heart function, and the nervous system. African Americans with high-carbohydrate diets may experience thiamine deficiencies, leading to fatigue, muscle weakness, and heart issues. *Holistic Sources:* Whole grains, legumes, and seeds. *Deficiency Symptoms:* Fatigue, muscle weakness, and neurological problems.

Vitamin B2 (Riboflavin)

Vitamin B2 (Riboflavin) is crucial for energy production, skin health, and eye health. Riboflavin deficiencies can lead to skin conditions like dermatitis, which may be more common among African Americans. *Holistic Sources:* Eggs, green vegetables, almonds, and dairy. *Deficiency Symptoms:* Cracked lips, sore throat, and skin disorders.

Vitamin B3 (Niacin)

Vitamin B3 (Niacin) helps metabolize fats, promotes skin health, and supports the nervous system. Although pellagra, a disease caused by niacin deficiency, is rare today, it disproportionately affected African Americans historically and can still occur in cases of severe malnutrition. *Holistic Sources:* Turkey, chicken, peanuts, and legumes. *Deficiency Symptoms:* Pellagra (diarrhea, dementia, dermatitis).

Vitamin B5 (Pantothenic Acid)

Vitamin B5 (Pantothenic Acid) supports hormone production and energy metabolism. It can help regulate the stress hormone cortisol, which is particularly beneficial for African Americans who may experience high stress levels. *Holistic Sources:* Avocados, eggs, whole grains, and broccoli. *Deficiency Symptoms:* Fatigue, irritability, and digestive issues.

Vitamin B6 (Pyridoxine)

Vitamin B6 (Pyridoxine) is essential for brain function and the production of serotonin and dopamine, the neurotransmitters responsible for mood regulation. Low B6 levels can contribute to depression and mood disorders, which are more prevalent in African American communities due to socioeconomic stressors. *Holistic Sources:* Chickpeas, tuna, bananas, and potatoes. *Deficiency Symptoms:* Mood changes, irritability, depression, and anemia.

Vitamin C

Vitamin C is a powerful antioxidant that supports immune function, promotes collagen production, and aids in wound healing. It also helps the body absorb iron from plant-based foods, which is important for preventing anemia, a condition more prevalent in African American communities. Vitamin C's role as an antioxidant makes it crucial for reducing oxidative stress, which can exacerbate skin issues like hyperpigmentation and chronic inflammation. *Holistic Sources:* include citrus fruits, strawberries, bell peppers, and broccoli. *Deficiency Symptoms:* include fatigue, bleeding gums, slow wound healing, and increased infections. African Americans, who often face higher oxidative stress due to environmental factors, can benefit from an adequate intake of Vitamin C to combat inflammation and improve overall skin health.

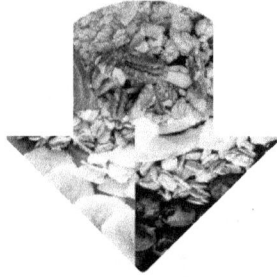

Vitamin B7 (Biotin)

Vitamin B7 (Biotin) is well-known for supporting hair, skin, and nail health, which is particularly important for African American women who experience hair thinning or breakage. *Holistic Sources:* Eggs, almonds, and sweet potatoes. *Deficiency Symptoms:* Hair loss, brittle nails, and skin rashes.

Vitamin B9 (Folate/Folic Acid)

Vitamin B9 (Folate/Folic Acid) supports DNA synthesis, red blood cell formation, and fetal development, making it essential for pregnant women. African Americans often face a higher risk of folate deficiency, which can lead to anemia and birth defects. *Holistic Sources:* Dark leafy greens, beans, peas, and fortified cereals. *Deficiency Symptoms:* Fatigue, anemia, and birth defects like neural tube defects.

Vitamin B12 (Cobalamin)

Vitamin B12 (Cobalamin) is essential for nerve health, red blood cell formation, and DNA synthesis. B12 deficiency is common in individuals who follow plant-based diets without proper supplementation, which includes many African Americans adopting vegan or vegetarian diets. *Holistic Sources:* Meat, fish, dairy, and fortified plant-based foods. *Deficiency Symptoms:* Fatigue, memory loss, and tingling sensations.

Vitamin D

Vitamin D is essential for calcium absorption, bone health, immune function, and mood regulation. African Americans are at higher risk of Vitamin D deficiency due to darker skin, which produces less Vitamin D from sunlight. This deficiency can lead to an increased risk of osteoporosis, heart disease, diabetes, and certain cancers. Vitamin D also plays a role in mental health, helping to regulate mood and reduce the risk of depression, which is particularly important for individuals facing chronic stress and systemic inequalities. *Holistic Sources:* Sunlight exposure, fortified foods, fatty fish, and egg yolks. *Deficiency Symptoms:* Bone pain, muscle weakness, depression, and increased susceptibility to infections. Ensuring adequate Vitamin D levels is crucial for African Americans, particularly for maintaining strong bones and preventing chronic diseases.

Vitamin E

Vitamin E is a powerful antioxidant that helps protect cells from oxidative damage, supports skin health, and strengthens the immune system. Its antioxidant properties are particularly important for African Americans living in environments with higher levels of pollutants, as it helps combat oxidative stress that can accelerate aging and increase the risk of chronic conditions. *Holistic Sources:* include nuts, seeds, spinach, and vegetable oils. *Deficiency Symptoms:* include muscle weakness, vision problems, and a weakened immune system. Maintaining adequate Vitamin E levels is essential for protecting against environmental pollutants and promoting healthy skin and hair.

Vitamin K

Vitamin K is important for blood clotting and bone health. It helps the body form proteins necessary for blood coagulation and bone mineralization. African Americans with diets low in green leafy vegetables may be at risk of Vitamin K deficiency, which can affect bone density and increase the risk of fractures, particularly in older adults. *Holistic Sources:* Green leafy vegetables like kale, spinach, and broccoli, as well as fermented foods. *Deficiency Symptoms:* Easy bruising, excessive bleeding, and weakened bones. Ensuring sufficient Vitamin K intake is crucial for maintaining bone strength and preventing fractures.

Choline

Choline supports brain development, liver function, and metabolism. It plays a key role in maintaining cell structure and transmitting nerve impulses. Deficiencies in choline can contribute to conditions like fatty liver disease and cognitive decline, both of which disproportionately affect African Americans. *Holistic Sources:* Eggs, meat, and soybeans. *Deficiency Symptoms:* Fatty liver disease, muscle damage, and cognitive issues.

Magnesium

Magnesium supports nerve function, muscle health, and bone structure. It also plays a critical role in regulating blood sugar and blood pressure, which is particularly important for African Americans who have higher rates of hypertension and diabetes. *Holistic Sources:* Nuts, seeds, leafy greens, and whole grains. *Deficiency Symptoms:* Muscle cramps, fatigue, high blood pressure, and heart irregularities. Magnesium deficiency is linked to conditions like hypertension and diabetes, making it an essential nutrient for African American health.

Iron Deficiency

Iron is a critical mineral necessary for the production of hemoglobin and overall health. Black women are at a higher risk of iron deficiency anemia due to various factors, including dietary habits and higher prevalence of fibroids. *Iron Importance* Iron is essential for hemoglobin production, which is necessary for transporting oxygen from the lungs to the rest of the body. It supports overall energy levels and prevents fatigue, while also playing a crucial role in cognitive function and brain health. Symptoms of iron deficiency include persistent fatigue and weakness, pale skin and nail beds due to reduced hemoglobin, shortness of breath during physical activities, and dizziness and headaches caused by poor oxygenation to the brain.

Causes of Iron Deficiency

Dietary habits that include low iron intake contribute to deficiency. Poor absorption of iron from certain foods can also exacerbate this issue. Health conditions such as fibroids, which cause heavy menstrual bleeding, lead to significant iron loss. Chronic diseases like celiac disease or Crohn's disease can impair iron absorption as well. *Prevention and Remedies for Iron Deficiency* Preventing and treating iron deficiency involves consuming iron-rich plant-based foods such as dark leafy greens, lentils, quinoa, and fortified cereals. Pairing these foods with vitamin C-rich items like citrus fruits, bell peppers, and tomatoes enhances absorption. Consulting a healthcare provider for appropriate iron supplements and regular blood tests to monitor iron levels, especially for those with heavy menstrual cycles or diagnosed conditions, is important. Ensuring a balanced diet that includes a variety of iron-rich foods and reducing consumption of calcium-rich foods and beverages, tea, and coffee around meals high in iron can avoid inhibiting absorption. Using cast iron cookware can also increase the iron content of food.

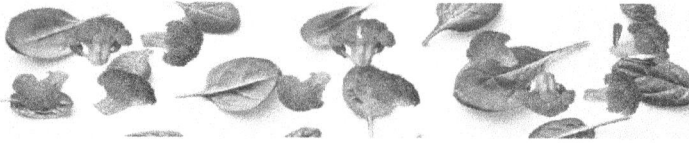

The Root Causes of Anemia and Low Iron

Anemia and low iron levels are widespread health concerns, especially among Black women, who may be more susceptible due to genetic factors, dietary habits, and socioeconomic conditions. Traditionally, when an individual is diagnosed with anemia, the immediate response is to increase iron intake through diet or supplements. However, this approach can be overly simplistic and may overlook a critical aspect of iron metabolism: absorption.

Iron is absorbed in the small intestine, particularly in the duodenum and upper jejunum, where it is taken up by specialized cells called enterocytes. These cells transport iron into the bloodstream, where it can be used by the body to form hemoglobin, the protein in red blood cells that carries oxygen. If the small intestine is compromised—due to conditions like celiac disease, Crohn's disease, or other forms of gut inflammation—the absorption process can be significantly hindered. This means that even with adequate iron intake, the body may not be able to utilize the iron effectively, leading to persistent low iron levels and anemia.

Several factors can impair the small intestine's ability to absorb iron. Chronic inflammation in the gut, often caused by an imbalanced diet, stress, or autoimmune conditions, can damage the intestinal lining. This damage reduces the number of functioning enterocytes and disrupts the absorption of not only iron but also other essential nutrients like vitamin B12, folate, and magnesium, which are all critical for the production of healthy red blood cells.

Moreover, gut flora imbalances, where harmful bacteria outnumber beneficial ones, can also play a role in poor iron absorption. The microbiome in the gut is essential for maintaining the health of the intestinal lining and aiding in the digestion and absorption of nutrients. An imbalance can lead to a condition known as "leaky gut," where the intestinal lining becomes too permeable, allowing toxins to enter the bloodstream and further exacerbating inflammation and malabsorption issues.

Another consideration is the presence of substances that inhibit iron absorption. For example, certain compounds found in foods, such as phytates in grains and legumes, calcium in dairy products, and tannins in tea and coffee, can bind to iron and prevent it from being absorbed efficiently. While these foods are healthy in moderation, consuming them in large quantities, especially alongside iron-rich meals, can contribute to low iron levels.

For many Black women, the root cause of anemia may also be linked to conditions like fibroids, heavy menstrual bleeding, and other gynecological issues that increase iron loss. However, addressing only the iron loss without considering the absorption aspect may lead to a cycle of temporary fixes rather than long-term solutions.

This understanding of the root cause of anemia underscores the importance of a holistic approach to health. Rather than simply increasing iron intake, it's crucial to assess and improve gut health, address potential sources of inflammation, and balance the diet to enhance nutrient absorption. For instance, pairing iron-rich foods with vitamin C-rich foods can enhance iron absorption, while reducing intake of inhibitors like tea and coffee around meals can make a significant difference.

The Role of Gut Health in Iron Absorption

Iron absorption occurs primarily in the small intestine, specifically in the duodenum and the upper part of the jejunum. When the gut is compromised, whether due to inflammation, an imbalance of gut flora, or other digestive issues, it can lead to poor absorption of not only iron but also other essential vitamins and minerals. This is why it is crucial to assess and address gut health when dealing with any illness or ailment, including anemia. An unhealthy gut can manifest in various ways, such as bloating, constipation, diarrhea, or even seemingly unrelated symptoms like fatigue and skin issues.

The Hidden Dangers of Ice Consumption

A common symptom of iron deficiency anemia is pica, a condition that drives the compulsive eating of non-food items, such as ice. While it might seem harmless, excessive ice consumption can be detrimental to your health. Chewing ice can lead to dental issues, including enamel erosion and tooth fractures. Additionally, the constant cold exposure can reduce the efficiency of your digestive system, further impairing nutrient absorption. Consuming ice in large quantities is also a red flag that your body is not getting the nutrients it needs, signaling deeper issues related to gut health and mineral absorption.

?QUESTIONS TO ASK HEALTHCARE PROVIDERS?

When dealing with low iron or anemia, it is important to have a thorough discussion with your healthcare provider.

What is the underlying cause of my anemia?

Could there be an issue with my small intestine affecting iron absorption?

What specific tests can identify problems with nutrient absorption? How can I improve my gut health to enhance nutrient absorption?

!TESTS TO REQUEST!

Testing might include a complete blood count (CBC) to assess the severity of anemia, iron studies to check iron levels and stores, and possibly an endoscopy or a test for celiac disease to examine the health of the small intestine.

Recognizing Symptoms of Small Intestine Issues

Indications that the small intestine may not be functioning optimally include chronic fatigue, persistent bloating, unexplained weight loss, nutrient deficiencies, and gastrointestinal discomfort. If these symptoms are present, it's essential to look beyond just dietary intake and consider the health of the digestive system as a whole.

Natural Approaches to Healing

From a holistic standpoint, healing the small intestine involves dietary and lifestyle changes. Incorporating foods that promote gut health is crucial. This includes: **Probiotic-rich foods**: such as sauerkraut, kimchi, and kombucha, which help restore healthy gut bacteria. **Anti-inflammatory foods:** like turmeric, ginger, and leafy greens, which can reduce inflammation in the gut. **Iron-boosting herbs and foods:** such as nettle, burdock root, and dark leafy greens that not only provide iron but also support digestive health. In addition, practices such as mindful eating, reducing stress, and avoiding foods that irritate the gut (such as gluten and dairy for some individuals) can significantly improve nutrient absorption. For those who are prone to anemia, it is important to focus not just on iron intake but on the overall health of the gut to ensure that the body can absorb and utilize the nutrients it receives.

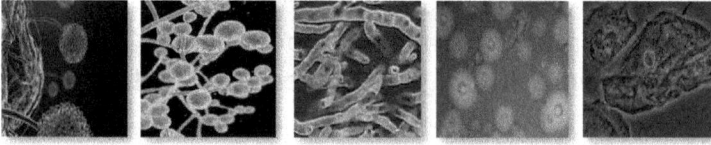

Fungal vs. Bacterial vs. Viral Infections and Ailments

Understanding the differences between fungal, bacterial, and viral infections is essential for determining the appropriate treatment approach, especially within a holistic framework. Each type of infection affects the body differently, and the body requires specific support to combat each type effectively.

Nature of Fungal Infections

Fungal infections are caused by fungi, which are parasitic organisms that thrive in warm, moist environments. Common examples include yeast infections (*Candida*), athlete's foot, and ringworm. ***Effect on the Body:*** Fungi can invade and colonize the skin, mucous membranes, and other areas of the body. They often cause persistent itching, redness, and discomfort. In more severe cases, fungi can enter the bloodstream, leading to systemic infections.

Treatment for Fungal Infection Dietary Changes

Avoid Sugar and Refined Carbs: These feed fungi like *Candida*, promoting overgrowth. ***Incorporate Antifungal Foods:*** Garlic, coconut oil, and oregano are natural antifungals. **Topical Treatments:** ***Tea Tree Oil:*** Dilute with a carrier oil and apply to affected areas for its antifungal properties. ***Apple Cider Vinegar:*** Use as a topical rinse or soak to create an inhospitable environment for fungi. **Boost Immune Function:** ***Probiotics:*** Support a healthy microbiome to prevent fungal overgrowth. ***Vitamin C:*** Enhances immune function, helping the body fight off fungal infections.

Candida Overgrowth: Common in women, leading to yeast infections, oral thrush, and digestive issues. *Athlete's Foot:* Affects the feet, causing itching, peeling, and discomfort.

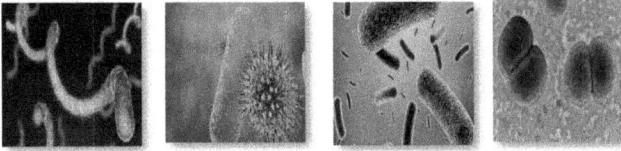

Nature of Bacterial Infections

Bacterial infections are caused by bacteria, which are single-celled organisms that can multiply rapidly within the body. Common bacterial infections include strep throat, urinary tract infections (UTIs), and bacterial pneumonia. *Effect on the Body* Bacteria can produce toxins that damage tissues and trigger immune responses, leading to inflammation, fever, and other symptoms. They can affect various parts of the body, depending on the strain.

Treatment for Bacterial Infections

Natural Antibiotics: *Garlic:* Has potent antibacterial properties; can be consumed raw or as a supplement. *Echinacea:* Boosts the immune system and helps the body fight off bacterial infections. **Hydration and Detoxification:** *Water:* Flushes out toxins produced by bacteria. *Herbal Teas:* Such as echinacea or goldenseal can support detoxification. **Support Immune Health:** *Probiotics:* Help maintain gut flora balance, especially after antibiotic use. *Zinc:* Plays a crucial role in immune function and wound healing. *Strep Throat:* Caused by *Streptococcus* bacteria, leading to sore throat and fever. *Urinary Tract Infections (UTIs): Often* caused by *E. coli* bacteria, leading to pain and frequent urination.

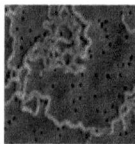

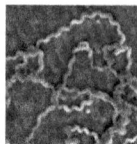

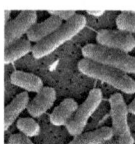

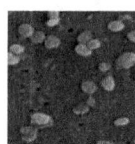

Nature of Viral Infections

Viral infections are caused by viruses, which are microscopic pathogens that invade living cells to replicate. Common viral infections include the flu, the common cold, and herpes. *Effect on the Body:* Viruses hijack the host's cells to reproduce, often leading to cell damage or death. The immune response to viral infections typically includes inflammation, fever, and fatigue.

Treatment for Viral Infections

Antiviral Herbs and Supplements: *Elderberry:* Known for its ability to shorten the duration of viral infections like the flu. *Astragalus:* Supports immune function and may help the body resist viral infections. **Immune System Support:** *Vitamin D:* Essential for immune regulation and defense against viral pathogens. *Vitamin C:* Reduces the severity and duration of viral infections by boosting immune function. **Rest and Recovery:** *Adequate Sleep:* Vital for immune function and recovery. *Hydration:* Important for maintaining mucous membranes, which act as barriers against viruses. *Influenza (Flu):* Causes fever, chills, and respiratory symptoms. *Herpes Simplex Virus (HSV):* Leads to cold sores or genital herpes, depending on the type.

How These Infections Affect the Body

Fungal Infections: Often result in localized symptoms such as itching, redness, and discomfort. The body needs antifungal agents, immune support, and a balanced microbiome to combat fungal infections. *Bacterial Infections:* Typically cause inflammation, fever, and localized pain. The body requires natural antibiotics, detoxification support, and immune boosters to fight bacterial infections. *Viral Infections:* Can lead to systemic symptoms like fever, fatigue, and respiratory issues. The body needs antiviral support, immune-enhancing nutrients, and rest to recover from viral infections.

What the Body Needs to Combat Infections

A Strong Immune System: The foundation for fighting any infection. This includes adequate nutrition, rest, hydration, and stress management. *Specific Nutrients:* Vitamins C, D, and zinc are crucial for immune function. *Probiotics:* Support gut health, which is closely linked to immune function. *Herbal Remedies:* Depending on the type of infection, herbs like garlic, elderberry, and tea tree oil can be effective.

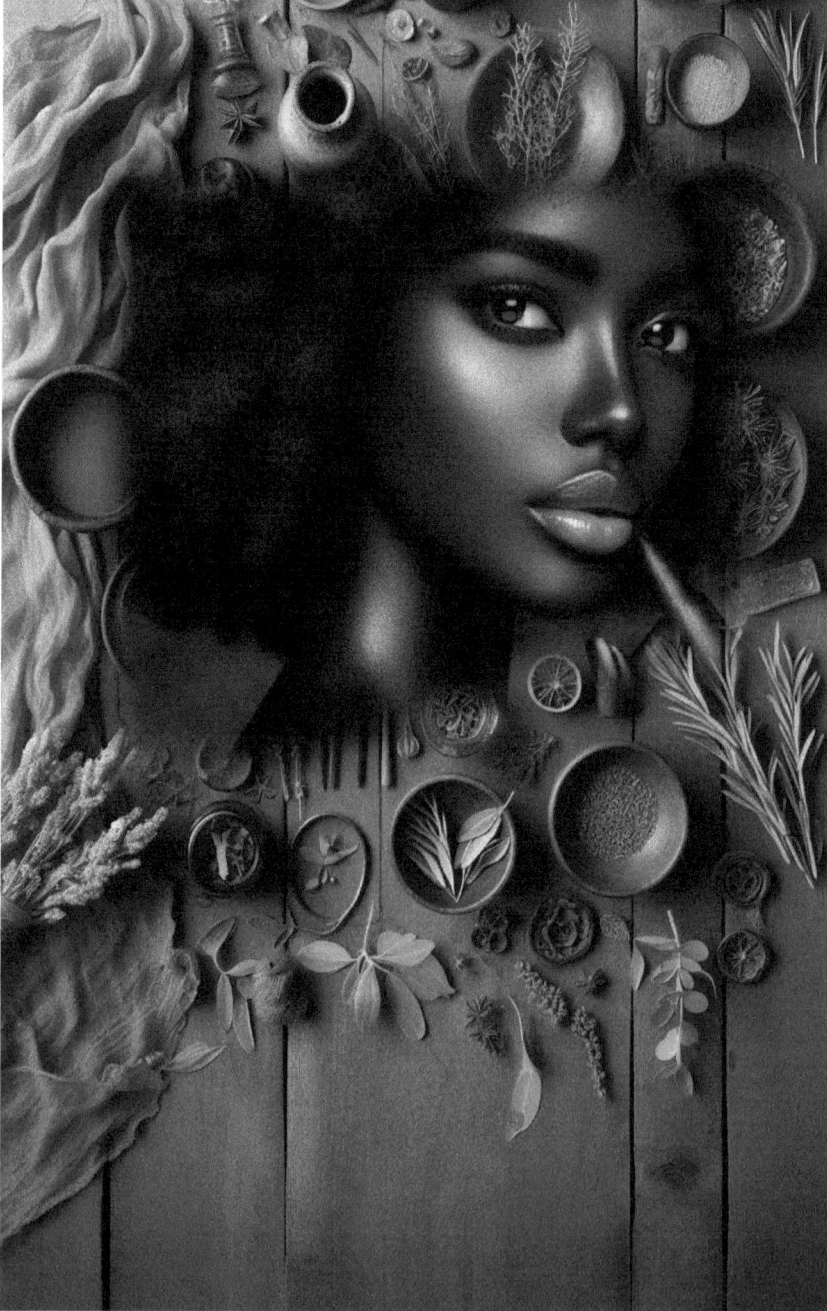

Chapter 3
Journey Into Understanding Blood Types

Endocrine System
GLANDS THAT SECRETE HORMONES INTO THE BLOOD

The endocrine system is an intricate network of glands and organs that produce and secrete hormones into the bloodstream, functioning as the body's chemical messengers to regulate numerous physiological processes. This system plays a critical role in maintaining homeostasis and influencing almost every cell, organ, and function of the body. Understanding the endocrine system from a holistic and natural standpoint can provide valuable insights into managing and optimizing hormonal health.

Hormones are natural substances that carry information and instructions from one set of cells to another. They are essential in regulating growth and development, metabolism, reproduction, sexual function, sleep, hunger, mood, energy levels, and the body's response to injury and stress. Glands, which are distributed throughout the body, including the hypothalamus, pituitary gland, pancreas, ovaries, and adrenal glands, are responsible for producing these hormones. Receptors in various organs and tissues recognize and respond to these hormones, ensuring that the body's functions are precisely regulated.

The hypothalamus, located in the brain, plays a pivotal role in controlling the endocrine system by sending signals to the pituitary gland, often referred to as the master gland. The pituitary gland, in turn, releases hormones that influence other glands throughout the body. For instance, the pancreas produces insulin, a hormone that signals muscle cells to rapidly absorb glucose, thus regulating blood sugar levels. The ovaries produce estrogen, which is crucial for uterine growth and the development of female secondary sex characteristics.

Approaches to Endocrine Health

Maintaining endocrine health requires a comprehensive approach that includes diet, lifestyle changes, and natural remedies. A nutrient-dense diet rich in whole foods can support hormonal balance. Incorporating foods such as flaxseeds, which are high in phytoestrogens, can help modulate estrogen levels. Additionally, foods rich in omega-3 fatty acids, such as chia seeds and walnuts, can support hormone production and reduce inflammation.

Regular physical activity is also essential for maintaining endocrine health. Exercise helps regulate hormones such as insulin and cortisol, enhancing overall metabolic health. For Black women, engaging in activities that reduce stress, such as yoga and meditation, can be particularly beneficial as chronic stress can lead to hormonal imbalances.

Gland/Organ Hypothalamus
Hormone Produced Various releasing hormones **Function** Controls pituitary gland **Health Tips** Stress management, meditation

Gland/Organ Pituitary Gland
Hormone Produced Growth hormone, others **Function** Regulates other glands **Health Tips** Regular exercise, balanced diet

Gland/Organ Pancreas
Hormone Produced Insulin **Function** Regulates blood sugar **Health Tips** levels Low-glycemic diet, regular meals

Gland/Organ Ovaries
Hormone Produced Estrogen, progesterone **Function** Regulates menstrual cycle, fertility **Health Tips** Phytoestrogen-rich foods, hormonal balancing herbs

Gland/Organ Adrenal Glands
Hormone Produced Cortisol, adrenaline **Function** Stress response, metabolism **Health Tips** Adaptogens like ashwagandha, adequate sleep

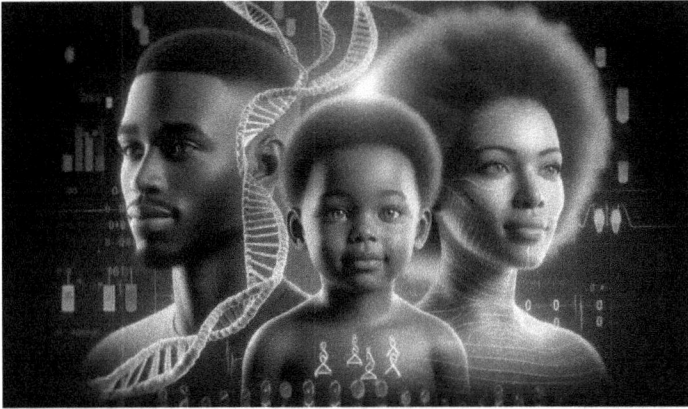

Understanding the Blood Type Inheritance Chart

O and O: Always produce children with O blood type.

O and A: Can produce children with O or A blood types.

O and B: Can produce children with O or B blood types.

O and AB: Can produce children with A or B blood types.

A and A: Can produce children with O or A blood types.

A and B: Can produce children with O, A, B, or AB blood types.

A and AB: Can produce children with A, B, or AB blood types.

B and B: Can produce children with O or B blood types.

B and AB: Can produce children with A, B, or AB blood types.

AB and AB: Can produce children with A, B, or AB blood types.

Blood Type Inheritance Chart

Parent 1 Blood Type	Parent 2 Blood Type	Possible Child Blood Types
O	O	O
O	A	O, A
O	B	O, B
O	AB	A, B
A	A	O, A
A	B	O, A, B, AB
A	AB	A, B, AB
B	B	O, B
B	AB	A, B, AB
AB	AB	A, B, AB

Rh Factor

Rh -

Rh +

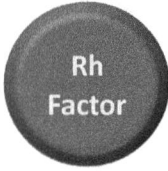

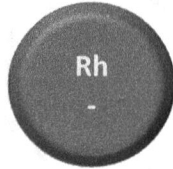

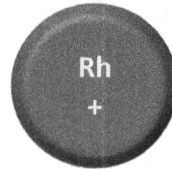

How to Use the Blood Type Inheritance Chart

Identify Parents' Blood Types: Determine the blood types of both parents. **Locate Possible Child Blood Types:** Find the intersection of the two parental blood types on the chart to see the possible blood types for their children. **Consider Rh Factor:** Check the Rh factor of both parents to determine the possible Rh factor of their children.

Rh Factor Inheritance

Parent 1 Rh Factor	Parent 2 Rh Factor	Possible Child Rh Factor
Positive	Positive	Positive, Negative
Positive	Negative	Positive, Negative
Negative	Negative	Negative

Blood Type Compatibility Chart

BLOOD TYPE	CAN GIVE TO	CAN RECEIVE FROM
O-	O-, O+, A-, A+, B-, B+, AB-, AB+	O-
O+	O+, A+, B+, AB+	O-, O+
A-	A-, A+, AB-, AB+	O-, A-
A+	A+, AB+	O-, O+, A-, A+
B-	B-, B+, AB-, AB+	O-, B-
B+	B+, AB+	O-, O+, B-, B+
AB-	AB-, AB+	O-, A-, B-, AB-
AB+	AB+	All (Universal Recipient)

Understanding the Blood Type Compatibility Chart

O-:(Universal Donor): Can donate to all blood types but can only receive from O-.

O+: Can donate to all positive blood types but can only receive from O- and O+.

A-: Can donate to A-, A+, AB-, and AB+ but can only receive from O- and A-.

A+: Can donate to A+ and AB+ but can receive from O-, O+, A-, and A+.

B-: Can donate to B-, B+, AB-, and AB+ but can only receive from O- and B-.

B+: Can donate to B+ and AB+ but can receive from O-, O+, B-, and B+.

AB-: Can donate to AB- and AB+ but can receive from O-, A-, B-, and AB-.

AB+: (Universal Recipient): Can only donate to AB+ but can receive from all blood types.

How to Use the Blood Type Compatibility Chart

Identify Your Blood Type: Determine your blood type (including Rh factor). ***Find Compatible Donors:*** Look at the "Can Receive From" column to see which blood types you can receive from. ***Find Compatible Recipients:*** Look at the "Can Give To" column to see which blood types you can donate to.

Best Practices Based on Blood Types
Blood Type O

Hair Health and Porosity Women with blood type O often have low hair porosity, meaning their hair can struggle to retain moisture. This type of hair benefits from lightweight oils like jojoba or grapeseed, which can penetrate the hair shaft more easily. **Dietary Needs** An alkaline diet rich in lean proteins, vegetables, and fruits is beneficial for blood type O. Foods such as spinach, broccoli, and seafood are highly recommended. Limiting grains and dairy can help reduce digestive issues. **Prone Conditions** Black women with blood type O are prone to conditions such as thyroid dysfunction and ulcers. Regular screening for thyroid levels and digestive health is important. **For Thyroid Health:** *Ashwagandha and bladderwrack.* **For Digestive Health:** *Ginger and peppermint.*
Maintaining a high level of physical activity can greatly benefit women with blood type O, helping to manage stress and maintain overall health.

Blood Type A

Hair Health and Porosity Blood type A women often have medium to high hair porosity, making their hair more susceptible to damage and frizz. Deep conditioning treatments and protein-rich hair masks can help maintain hair health. **Dietary Needs** A vegetarian or plant-based diet is ideal for blood type A. Foods like soy, vegetables, and whole grains should be staples. Reducing meat intake can help improve digestive health and overall well-being. **Prone Conditions** Women with blood type A may be more prone to cardiovascular diseases and diabetes. Regular monitoring of blood pressure and blood sugar levels is crucial. **For Heart Health:** *Hawthorn berry and green tea.* **For Blood Sugar Regulation:** *Cinnamon and fenugreek.* Incorporating stress-reducing practices such as yoga or meditation can greatly benefit women with blood type A, helping to maintain emotional and physical balance.

Blood Type B

Hair Health and Porosity Women with blood type B tend to have hair with variable porosity, requiring a balanced approach to hair care. Using a combination of moisture and protein treatments can keep the hair healthy. **Dietary Needs** A balanced diet that includes both animal and plant-based foods is suitable for blood type B. Foods such as eggs, leafy greens, and fortified plant-based milks, leafy greens, and sunlight exposure are beneficial. Avoiding corn, wheat, and lentils can help reduce inflammation. **Prone Conditions** Black women with blood type B may be more susceptible to autoimmune diseases and chronic fatigue. Regular health check-ups focusing on immune function are important. **For Immune Support:** *Echinacea and elderberry.* **For Energy and Vitality:** *Ginseng and maca root.* Engaging in moderate physical activities like swimming or hiking can help maintain energy levels and overall health for women with blood type B.

Blood Type AB

Hair Health and Porosity Blood type AB women often have high hair porosity, which can lead to dryness and breakage. Using heavier oils like coconut oil and shea butter can help seal in moisture and protect the hair. **Dietary Needs** A varied diet that includes a balance of plant-based and lean animal proteins is best for blood type AB. Foods such as tofu, fish, and green vegetables are recommended. Limiting processed foods and caffeine can improve overall health. **Prone Conditions** Women with blood type AB are at a higher risk for cardiovascular diseases and digestive issues. Regular cardiovascular screenings and digestive health check-ups are important. **For Heart Health:** *Hibiscus and garlic.* **For Digestive Health:** *Licorice root and chamomile.* Maintaining a balanced lifestyle with a mix of physical activity and relaxation techniques such as tai chi or qigong can benefit women with blood type AB.

TYPE O

Blood Type O

Hair Porosity Low **Dietary Needs** High-protein, alkaline **Prone Conditions** Thyroid dysfunction, ulcers **Best Herbal Regimen** Ashwagandha, bladderwrack, ginger, peppermint **Additional Tips** High physical activity

TYPE A

Blood Type A

Hair Porosity Medium to high **Dietary Needs** Vegetarian, plant-based **Prone Conditions** Cardiovascular diseases, diabetes **Best Herbal Regimen** Hawthorn berry, green tea, cinnamon, fenugreek **Additional Tips** Stress-reducing practices

TYPE B

Blood Type B

Hair Porosity Variable Dietary Needs Balanced diet **Prone Conditions** Autoimmune diseases, chronic fatigue **Best Herbal Regimen** Echinacea, elderberry, ginseng, maca root **Additional Tips** Moderate physical activities

TYPE AB

Blood Type AB

Hair Porosity High **Dietary Needs** Balanced diet **Prone Conditions** Cardiovascular diseases, digestive issues **Best Herbal Regimen** Hibiscus, garlic, licorice root, chamomile **Additional Tips** Mix of physical activity and relaxation techniques

Health Facts for Blood Type O

Blood Type O is often considered the "universal donor" due to its compatibility with all other blood types. However, individuals with Blood Type O have unique health considerations that can impact their overall well-being. This section explores the general health facts for individuals with Blood Type O and delves into specific considerations for Black women, focusing on dietary recommendations and their impact on various aspects of health, from head to toe.

High-Protein Diet

Individuals with Blood Type O often benefit from a high-protein diet. Protein is crucial for maintaining muscle mass, supporting metabolic function, and promoting overall health. *Sources of Protein:* Lean meats, fish, eggs, and legumes are excellent sources of protein. These foods support muscle strength and repair, essential for daily functioning and physical activity. *Keratin Production:* Protein is also essential for hair strength and growth. Hair is primarily made of keratin, a type of protein. Consuming adequate protein helps maintain healthy hair by providing the necessary building blocks for keratin production.

Iron-Rich Foods

Iron is vital for the formation of hemoglobin, which carries oxygen in the blood. Adequate iron intake ensures efficient circulation and oxygen delivery to tissues, including hair follicles, which supports overall hair health. *Sources of Iron:* Red meat, poultry, fish, lentils, spinach, and fortified cereals are good sources of iron. These foods help prevent iron-deficiency anemia, which can lead to fatigue and weakened immunity.

Digestive Health

Individuals with Blood Type O tend to have higher levels of stomach acid, which aids in the digestion of protein and fat. However, they may also be more prone to digestive issues if they consume too many grains or dairy products. **Recommended Foods:** Emphasize lean meats, fish, vegetables, and fruits. *Foods to Avoid:* Limit intake of grains, dairy, and processed foods to prevent digestive discomfort.

Metabolic Health

A high-protein diet can support a healthy metabolism, which is essential for weight management and energy levels. Regular physical activity is also crucial for maintaining a healthy metabolism. *Exercise Recommendations:* Engage in regular cardiovascular and strength-training exercises to support metabolic health and overall well-being.

Hair Health

Maintaining healthy hair is a significant concern for many Black women. A diet rich in protein and iron can promote hair strength and growth. *Protein Sources:* Incorporate lean meats, fish, eggs, and legumes into the diet to support keratin production and hair health. *Iron-Rich Foods:* Consume iron-rich foods like spinach, lentils, and red meat to enhance circulation and oxygen delivery to hair follicles.

Skin Health

Skin Health Black women may have unique skin health needs, including higher susceptibility to conditions like hyperpigmentation and keloids. ***Nutrient-Rich Diet:*** A diet rich in vitamins and minerals, including vitamins A, C, and E, can support skin health and repair. ***Hydration:*** Ensure adequate hydration by drinking plenty of water and consuming hydrating foods like fruits and vegetables.

Cardiovascular Health

Black women have a higher risk of hypertension and cardiovascular diseases. A balanced diet and regular exercise are crucial for managing these risks. ***Heart-Healthy Diet:*** Emphasize lean proteins, vegetables, fruits, and whole grains. Limit sodium intake and avoid processed foods. ***Exercise:*** Engage in regular cardiovascular exercise, such as walking, running, or cycling, to support heart health.

Bone Health

Black women may have a higher risk of vitamin D deficiency, which can impact bone health. Ensuring adequate intake of calcium and vitamin D is essential. ***Sources of Calcium:*** Dairy products, leafy greens, and fortified plant-based milks. ***Vitamin D:*** Spend time outdoors in sunlight and consider vitamin D supplements if needed.

Reproductive Health

Hormonal balance is crucial for reproductive health. A diet that supports hormonal regulation can benefit Black women with Blood Type O. ***Balanced Diet:*** Include a variety of nutrient-rich foods to support hormonal balance. Omega-3 fatty acids, found in fish and flaxseeds, can help regulate hormones. ***Herbal Supplements:*** Consider herbal supplements like spearmint tea, which can help balance hormones and alleviate symptoms of conditions like PCOS.

Health Facts for Blood Type A

T
Y
P≡
A

Blood Type A individuals often thrive on plant-based diets and have specific health needs and considerations that impact their overall well-being. This section provides a comprehensive exploration of health facts for individuals with Blood Type A, focusing on general dietary recommendations and specific considerations for Black women.

Plant-Based Diet

Individuals with Blood Type A generally benefit from a diet rich in plant-based foods. This includes plenty of vegetables, fruits, and whole grains, while minimizing the intake of animal products. *Vegetables and Fruits:* These are the cornerstone of a Blood Type A diet. Vegetables provide essential vitamins, minerals, and antioxidants, while fruits offer natural sugars and fiber. *Whole Grains:* Brown rice, quinoa, and oats are excellent sources of fiber and essential nutrients. *Legumes:* Beans, lentils, and peas are good plant-based protein sources that support overall health.

Protein Sources

While plant-based proteins are emphasized, some animal proteins can be beneficial in moderation. *Lean Proteins:* Include poultry and fish, which are easier to digest compared to red meat. *Plant-Based Proteins:* Tofu, tempeh, and legumes are excellent sources of protein for Blood Type A individuals. *Dairy and Eggs* Blood Type A individuals might find it beneficial to limit dairy intake due to potential digestive issues. *Dairy Alternatives:* Consider plant-based milks like almond, soy, or oat milk, which are often fortified with calcium and vitamin D.

Digestive Health

Individuals with Blood Type A often have a sensitive digestive system and may benefit from a diet that emphasizes easily digestible foods. *Recommended Foods:* Vegetables, fruits, whole grains, and lean proteins. *Foods to Avoid:* Red meat, processed foods, and high-fat dairy products, which can be hard to digest.

Immune System

Blood Type A individuals may have a predisposition to weaker immune responses, making it important to focus on immune-boosting foods. *Immune-Boosting Foods:* Garlic, ginger, green tea, and foods high in antioxidants like berries and leafy greens.

Hair Health

Maintaining healthy hair is crucial for many Black women. A diet rich in plant-based proteins, vitamins, and minerals can support hair strength and growth. *Protein Sources:* Incorporate tofu, tempeh, and legumes into the diet to support keratin production, which is essential for hair strength. *Iron-Rich Foods:* Consume iron-rich plant foods like spinach, lentils, and quinoa to enhance circulation and oxygen delivery to hair follicles, promoting healthy hair growth.

Skin Health

Black women may have unique skin health needs, including higher susceptibility to conditions like hyperpigmentation and keloids. *Nutrient-Rich Diet:* A diet rich in vitamins A, C, and E, along with adequate hydration, supports skin health and repair. *Hydration:* Ensure adequate hydration by drinking plenty of water and consuming hydrating foods like fruits and vegetables.

TYPE 3

Cardiovascular Health

Black women have a higher risk of hypertension and cardiovascular diseases. A balanced diet and regular exercise are crucial for managing these risks. *Heart-Healthy Diet:* Emphasize plant-based proteins, vegetables, fruits, and whole grains. Limit sodium intake and avoid processed foods. *Exercise:* Engage in regular cardiovascular exercise, such as walking, running, or cycling, to support heart health.

Bone Health

Black women may have a higher risk of vitamin D deficiency, which can impact bone health. Ensuring adequate intake of calcium and vitamin D is essential. *Sources of Calcium:* Leafy greens, fortified plant-based milks, and tofu. *Vitamin D:* Spend time outdoors in sunlight and consider vitamin D supplements if needed.

Reproductive Health

Hormonal balance is crucial for reproductive health. A diet that supports hormonal regulation can benefit Black women with Blood Type A. *Balanced Diet:* Include a variety of nutrient-rich foods to support hormonal balance. Omega-3 fatty acids, found in flaxseeds and walnuts, can help regulate hormones. *Herbal Supplements:* Consider herbal supplements like chasteberry, which can help balance hormones and alleviate symptoms of conditions like PMS.

Health Facts for Blood Type B

Blood Type B is known for its flexibility and adaptability to different dietary environments. However, individuals with Blood Type B also have specific health needs and considerations that impact their overall well-being. This section provides a comprehensive exploration of health facts for individuals with Blood Type B, focusing on general dietary recommendations and specific considerations for Black women.

Balanced Diet

Individuals with Blood Type B often thrive on a balanced diet that includes a variety of foods from both plant and animal sources. This flexibility can support overall health and well-being. *Protein Sources:* Incorporate lean meats, fish, dairy, and eggs into the diet. These foods provide essential amino acids necessary for muscle repair, immune function, and overall vitality. *Dairy:* Unlike some other blood types, individuals with Blood Type B typically tolerate dairy products well, which can be a good source of calcium and vitamin D for bone health.

Vegetables and Fruits

A diet rich in vegetables and fruits provides essential vitamins, minerals, and antioxidants that support various bodily functions. *Leafy Greens:* Spinach, kale, and other leafy greens are excellent sources of vitamins A, C, and K, and minerals like iron and calcium. *Fruits:* Berries, bananas, and grapes are beneficial for providing fiber, vitamins, and natural sugars that boost energy levels. *Grains and Legumes* Whole grains and legumes should be consumed in moderation. They provide essential nutrients and fiber but should not dominate the diet. *Whole Grains:* Opt for oats, rice, and millet over wheat-based products, which can sometimes cause digestive issues for individuals with Blood Type B. *Legumes:* Beans and lentils are good protein sources but should be balanced with other protein types to avoid digestive discomfort.

Digestive Health

Individuals with Blood Type B generally have a robust digestive system but should avoid certain foods that can cause bloating or discomfort. *Recommended Foods:* Lean meats, fish, vegetables, fruits, and dairy. *Foods to Avoid:* Avoid excessive consumption of corn, wheat, peanuts, and sesame seeds, which can disrupt digestive efficiency. *Immune System* Blood Type B individuals tend to have a strong immune system but should still prioritize immune-boosting foods. *Immune-Boosting Foods:* Include foods rich in vitamins C and D, zinc, and antioxidants such as citrus fruits, berries, and cruciferous vegetables.

Hair Health

Maintaining healthy hair is crucial for many Black women. A balanced diet that includes sufficient protein, vitamins, and minerals can support hair strength and growth. *Protein Sources:* Incorporate lean meats, fish, eggs, and dairy into the diet to support keratin production, which is essential for hair strength. *Iron-Rich Foods:* Consume iron-rich foods like spinach, lentils, and red meat to enhance circulation and oxygen delivery to hair follicles, promoting healthy hair growth.

Skin Health

Black women may have unique skin health needs, including higher susceptibility to conditions like hyperpigmentation and keloids. *Nutrient-Rich Diet:* A diet rich in vitamins A, C, and E, along with adequate hydration, supports skin health and repair. *Hydration:* Ensure adequate hydration by drinking plenty of water and consuming hydrating foods like fruits and vegetables.

Cardiovascular Health

Black women have a higher risk of hypertension and cardiovascular diseases. A balanced diet and regular exercise are crucial for managing these risks. *Heart-Healthy Diet:* Emphasize lean proteins, vegetables, fruits, and whole grains. Limit sodium intake and avoid processed foods. *Exercise:* Engage in regular cardiovascular exercise, such as walking, running, or cycling, to support heart health.

Bone Health

Black women may have a higher risk of vitamin D deficiency, which can impact bone health. Ensuring adequate intake of calcium and vitamin D is essential. *Sources of Calcium:* Dairy products, leafy greens, and fortified plant-based milks. *Vitamin D:* Spend time outdoors in sunlight and consider vitamin D supplements if needed.

Reproductive Health

Hormonal balance is crucial for reproductive health. A diet that supports hormonal regulation can benefit Black women with Blood Type B. *Balanced Diet:* Include a variety of nutrient-rich foods to support hormonal balance. Omega-3 fatty acids, found in fish and flaxseeds, can help regulate hormones. *Herbal Supplements:* Consider herbal supplements like chasteberry, which can help balance hormones and alleviate symptoms of conditions like PMS.

Health Facts for Blood Type AB

TYPE AB

Blood Type AB is the rarest blood type and often considered a blend of the characteristics of Blood Types A and B. Individuals with Blood Type AB have unique health needs and dietary considerations. This section provides a comprehensive exploration of health facts for individuals with Blood Type AB, focusing on general dietary recommendations and specific considerations for Black women.

Dietary Recommendations: Balanced Diet

Individuals with Blood Type AB benefit from a balanced diet that includes a mix of both plant-based and animal-based foods. This type can tolerate a wide variety of foods but must be mindful of specific dietary needs. *Vegetables and Fruits:* A diet rich in vegetables and fruits provides essential vitamins, minerals, and antioxidants. Emphasize leafy greens, berries, and citrus fruits. *Lean Proteins:* Include moderate amounts of lean proteins such as fish, poultry, tofu, and legumes. These foods support muscle health and overall bodily functions. **Dairy:** Individuals with Blood Type AB can usually tolerate dairy products, which are good sources of calcium and vitamin D for bone health. *Grains and Legumes* Whole grains and legumes should be part of the diet but balanced with other food groups. *Whole Grains:* Opt for oats, quinoa, and brown rice for fiber and essential nutrients. *Legumes:* Beans, lentils, and chickpeas provide plant-based protein and fiber.

Digestive Health

Individuals with Blood Type AB often have sensitive digestive systems and should focus on easily digestible foods. *Recommended Foods:* Vegetables, fruits, lean proteins, and dairy in moderation. *Foods to Avoid:* Avoid excessive consumption of red meat, processed foods, and high-fat dairy products, which can cause digestive discomfort.

Immune System

Blood Type AB individuals may have a variable immune response, making it important to focus on immune-boosting foods. *Immune-Boosting Foods:* Garlic, ginger, green tea, and foods high in antioxidants like berries and leafy greens. Maintaining healthy hair is crucial for many Black women. A diet rich in protein, vitamins, and minerals can support hair strength and growth. *Protein Sources:* Incorporate lean meats, fish, eggs, tofu, and legumes into the diet to support keratin production, which is essential for hair strength. *Iron-Rich Foods:* Consume iron-rich foods like spinach, lentils, and quinoa to enhance circulation and oxygen delivery to hair follicles, promoting healthy hair growth.

Skin Health

Black women may have unique skin health needs, including higher susceptibility to conditions like hyperpigmentation and keloids. *Nutrient-Rich Diet:* A diet rich in vitamins A, C, and E, along with adequate hydration, supports skin health and repair. *Hydration:* Ensure adequate hydration by drinking plenty of water and consuming hydrating foods like fruits and vegetables.

Cardiovascular Health

Black women have a higher risk of hypertension and cardiovascular diseases. A balanced diet and regular exercise are crucial for managing these risks. ***Heart-Healthy Diet:*** Emphasize lean proteins, vegetables, fruits, and whole grains. Limit sodium intake and avoid processed foods. **Exercise:** Engage in regular cardiovascular exercise, such as walking, running, or cycling, to support heart health.

Bone Health

Black women may have a higher risk of vitamin D deficiency, which can impact bone health. Ensuring adequate intake of calcium and vitamin D is essential. ***Sources of Calcium:*** Dairy products, leafy greens, and fortified plant-based milks. ***Vitamin D:*** Spend time outdoors in sunlight and consider vitamin D supplements if needed.

Reproductive Health

Hormonal balance is crucial for reproductive health. A diet that supports hormonal regulation can benefit Black women with Blood Type AB. ***Balanced Diet:*** Include a variety of nutrient-rich foods to support hormonal balance. Omega-3 fatty acids, found in fish and flaxseeds, can help regulate hormones. ***Herbal Supplements:*** Consider herbal supplements like chasteberry, which can help balance hormones and alleviate symptoms of conditions like PMS.

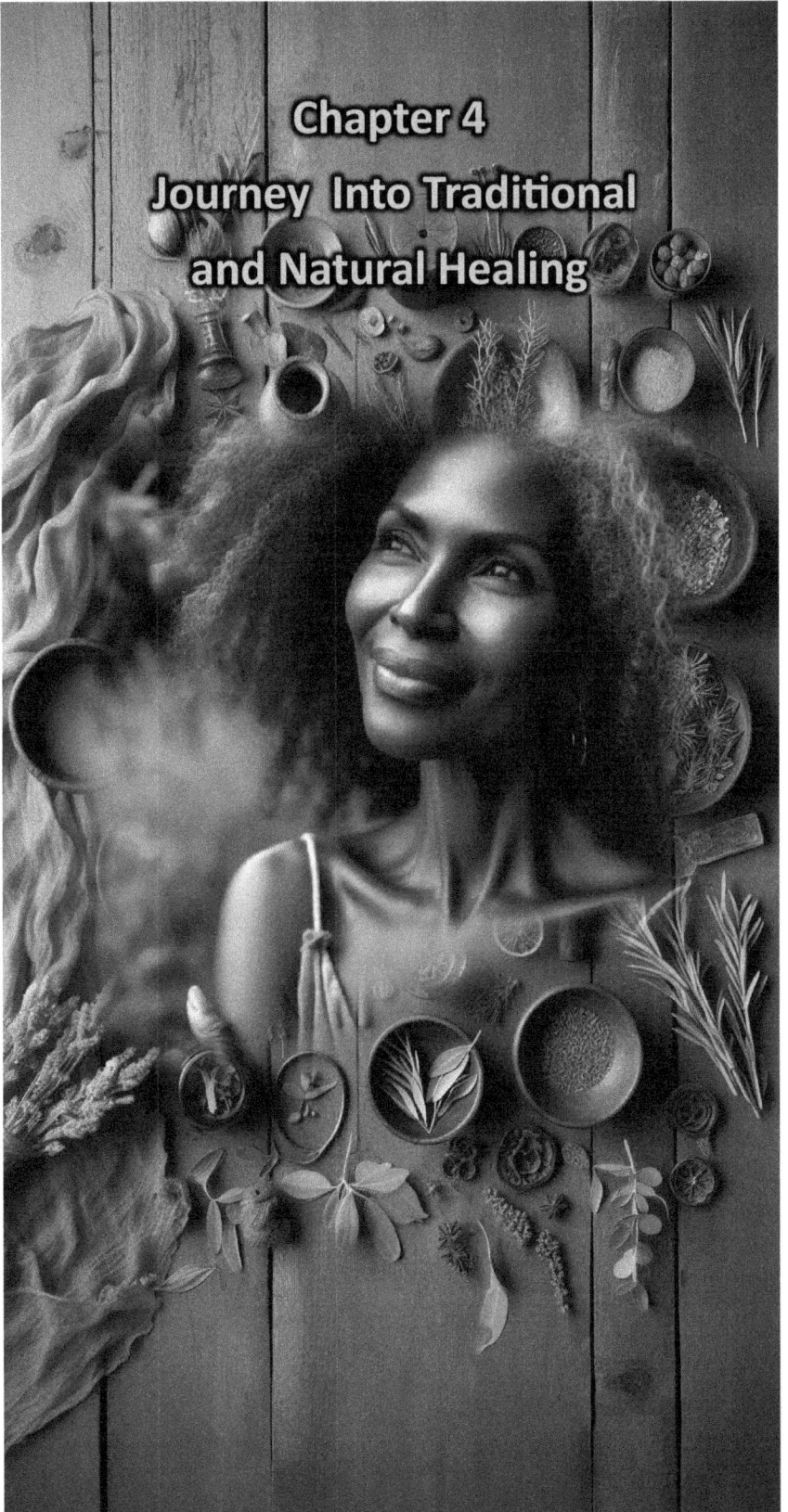

Chapter 4
Journey Into Traditional
and Natural Healing

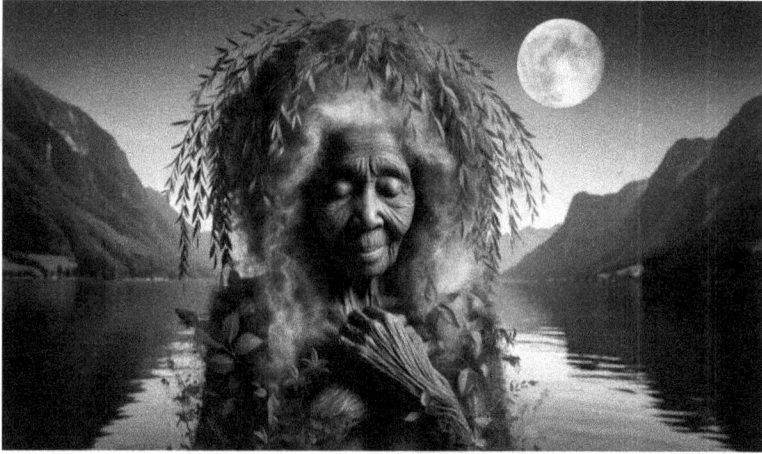

The Connection to Earth's Elements

The body is made up of the same elements found in nature: earth, water, fire, air, and ether (spirit). These elements exist within us, influencing our physical, mental, and spiritual health. Connecting the human body to Earth's natural rhythms and elements is a fundamental principle in full body natural health practices. Understanding this relationship can guide us toward aligning our full-body health with nature's cycles, helping us achieve balance, wellness, and a deeper sense of harmony.

Earth: The earth element relates to our bones, muscles, and tissues, providing structure and stability. Just as the soil nourishes plant life, grounding practices like walking barefoot on the earth (earthing) can help us absorb its energy, improve circulation, and reduce inflammation.

Water: Water represents our bodily fluids and is linked to emotions and flow. Our bodies are 60-70% water, mirroring the Earth's water content. The ocean's tides, influenced by the moon, reflect the rhythms in our bodies, such as the menstrual cycle. Staying hydrated and connecting with water through baths or swimming can enhance emotional balance and detoxification.

Fire: The fire element is associated with our metabolism and digestive system. It represents transformation, just like the sun fuels life on Earth. Eating seasonally and according to your body's needs can help balance your internal fire (agni), aiding digestion and energy.

Air: Air governs movement, breath, and the nervous system. Just as the wind moves across the Earth, the breath moves through our bodies, bringing oxygen to every cell. Deep breathing and practices like meditation help align the mind and body with the gentle flow of air, calming the nervous system.

Ether (Spirit): Ether is the space that holds all the elements. It represents our spiritual and energetic body. Connecting with ether involves tuning into our intuition and the unseen energies around us through practices like mindfulness, meditation, and spending time in nature.

The Influence of the Moon and Tides on the Body

The moon's gravitational pull influences the ocean's tides, and similarly, it affects the water within our bodies. This connection is particularly significant for women, whose menstrual cycles often align with the lunar phases.

New Moon and Full Moon: These phases are times for reflection, renewal, and manifestation. The new moon is a good time to set health goals or begin detoxification, while the full moon can be a time of increased energy, perfect for deep physical and emotional release.

Menstrual Cycle Alignment: Many women find that their cycles naturally align with the lunar phases, highlighting a deep, biological connection to the moon's rhythms. Aligning your self-care routines with these cycles can enhance hormone health and emotional well-being.

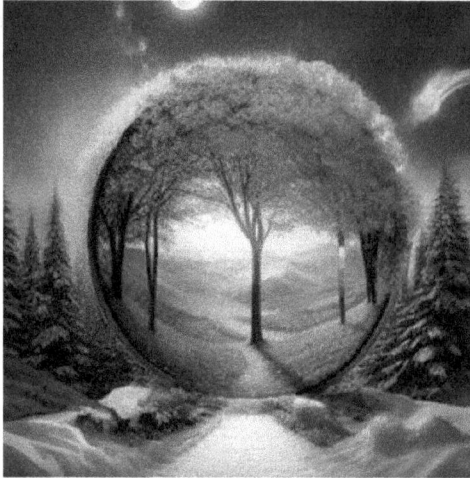

Seasonal Changes and Health Alignment

Each season brings different energies and requires our bodies to adapt.

Spring: A time of renewal and growth, perfect for detoxification and starting new health practices. Nature provides fresh greens and herbs that support liver health and cleansing.

Summer: The energy of summer is vibrant and warm. It's a time to enjoy lighter, hydrating foods like fruits and salads, and focus on outdoor activities to sync with the longer daylight hours.

Autumn: A season of grounding and preparation for rest. It's beneficial to consume warm, nourishing foods like root vegetables, which align with the earth element and help strengthen the immune system.

Winter: The colder, darker months are a time for rest and introspection. Eating warming, hearty foods like stews and focusing on self-care rituals align the body with the natural slowing down of the earth.

The Role of Ether and Connection to Spirit

The concept of ether or spirit goes beyond the physical and connects us with the universal energy. Practices like meditation, sound healing, and energy work help us tap into this element, aligning our personal vibrations with the Earth's frequency (often referred to as the Schumann resonance). This alignment can help reduce stress, enhance mental clarity, and foster a deeper sense of peace.

Bringing It All Together: A Natural Journey to Health

By aligning our lifestyle with the Earth's natural cycles and elements, we create a holistic approach to wellness. This journey involves nourishing our bodies with seasonal foods, syncing our energy with the moon's phases, and practicing grounding techniques that connect us back to the earth. It's about embracing the natural ebb and flow of life, listening to our bodies, and respecting the wisdom of nature.

This approach not only enhances physical health but also deepens our spiritual connection, guiding us on a path of natural, harmonious living.

Traditional Medicinal Practices

Before the 1920s, natural health-related findings were primarily based on traditional knowledge, herbal medicine, and holistic practices that had been passed down through generations. These practices were often rooted in cultural traditions and were used to prevent and treat various ailments long before the advent of modern medicine.

Religion and Nontraditional Medicinal Practices

Holistic medicinal practices, such as the use of crystals, frequency healing, and chakras, can align with religious beliefs like Christianity by focusing on the spiritual and energetic aspects of health that reflect God's design for the body and the universe. While some may view these practices as separate from traditional religious teachings, many find common ground in the belief that the body, mind, and spirit are interconnected, as emphasized in Christian scripture. For example, frequency healing and chakras, which involve balancing the body's energy centers, can be seen as tools to maintain the body as a "temple of the Holy Spirit" (1 Corinthians 6:19).

Similarly, crystals, often used for their energetic properties, can be viewed as part of God's creation, with the potential to bring balance and healing. Prayer, meditation, and faith-based affirmations in Christianity resonate with these practices by focusing on inner peace, spiritual growth, and divine healing, fostering a holistic approach that emphasizes well-being in mind, body, and spirit. Through this lens, both traditional and holistic methods can work in harmony, complementing faith by encouraging self-care and a deeper connection with the divine.

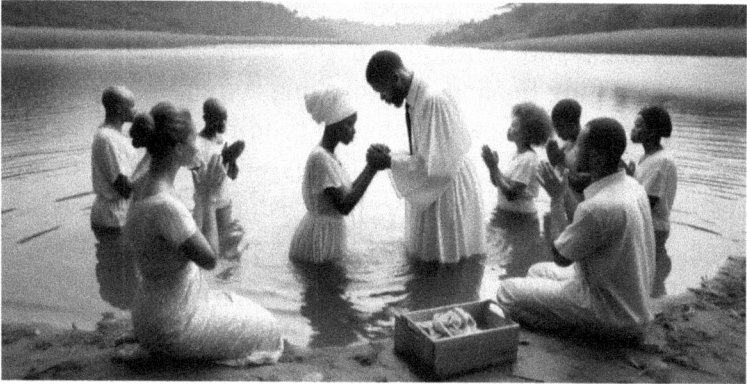

Herbal Medicine

Herbal medicine was the cornerstone of health care in many cultures. Plants like willow bark were used for pain relief (later leading to the discovery of aspirin), echinacea for immune support, and garlic for its antimicrobial properties. These remedies were used to treat everything from infections to digestive issues. *Traditional Chinese Medicine (TCM):* TCM, which has been practiced for thousands of years, includes the use of herbs, acupuncture, and dietary therapy. The principles of yin and yang, along with the concept of Qi (vital energy), were central to maintaining health.

Acupuncture

Acupuncture is a cornerstone of Traditional Chinese Medicine (TCM), with origins dating back over 2,500 years. It is a therapeutic practice that involves inserting thin, sterile needles into specific points on the body known as acupuncture points or meridians. These points are believed to correspond to different organs and systems in the body, and the stimulation of these points is thought to balance the flow of energy, or Qi (pronounced "chee"), within the body. The practice of acupuncture is rooted in the idea that health is achieved when the body's energy flows freely and is in balance. When the flow of Qi is disrupted—whether by stress, injury, poor diet, or other factors—illness and pain can occur.

By inserting needles at strategic points, acupuncture aims to restore balance and harmony to the body's energy pathways, thereby promoting healing and relieving symptoms. Acupuncture has been used to treat a wide range of conditions, including chronic pain, migraines, anxiety, digestive issues, and infertility. In addition to needle insertion, practitioners may also use techniques such as cupping, moxibustion (burning herbs near the skin), and acupressure (applying pressure to acupuncture points without needles) to enhance the therapeutic effects.

The Principles of Yin and Yang and the Concept of Qi

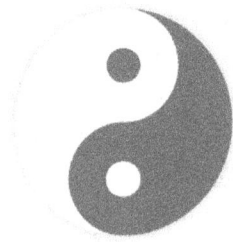

The principles of Yin and Yang and the concept of Qi are fundamental to understanding Traditional Chinese Medicine and its approach to health and healing. **Yin and Yang** represent the dualistic nature of existence. Yin is associated with qualities such as darkness, cold, passivity, and femininity, while Yang is linked to light, warmth, activity, and masculinity. These two forces are complementary and interdependent, constantly interacting to create balance in the universe and within the human body. In TCM, health is seen as a state of harmony between Yin and Yang. Imbalances—whether an excess or deficiency of Yin or Yang—are believed to lead to illness. For example, too much Yang energy might manifest as inflammation or fever, while an excess of Yin could result in coldness or lethargy. **Qi**, often translated as "vital energy" or "life force," is the energy that flows through all living things. It is the force that animates the body and sustains life. Qi flows through pathways called meridians, which connect the body's organs and systems. Good health is thought to depend on the smooth, unimpeded flow of Qi. When Qi is blocked or stagnant, disease can arise. Acupuncture, herbal medicine, and other TCM practices aim to restore the balanced flow of Qi, thus maintaining or restoring health.

Ayurveda

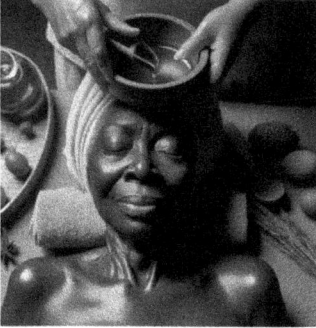

Doshas: Ayurveda, an ancient system of medicine from India, emphasized the balance of the three doshas (Vata, Pitta, Kapha) to maintain health. Imbalances in these doshas were believed to cause disease, and treatment involved diet, herbal remedies, and lifestyle adjustments. *Panchakarma:* Detoxification procedures such as Panchakarma were used to cleanse the body of toxins and restore balance. These practices included oil massages, steam baths, and the use of medicinal herbs.

Doshas

In Ayurveda, an ancient system of natural healing that originated in India more than 3,000 years ago, the concept of Doshas is fundamental. According to Ayurvedic principles, every individual is born with a unique combination of three Doshas: Vata, Pitta, and Kapha. These Doshas represent the elemental forces within the body and mind, each governing specific physiological and psychological functions. *Vata Dosha* is associated with air and space elements. It governs movement, including the circulation of blood, the breath, and the transmission of nerve impulses. Individuals with a predominant Vata are often energetic, creative, and flexible but may also be prone to anxiety, dry skin, and irregular digestion.

Pitta Dosha is related to fire and water elements. It controls digestion, metabolism, and energy production. Those with a dominant Pitta are typically driven, intelligent, and ambitious but may struggle with anger, inflammation, and overheating. *Kapha Dosha* corresponds to earth and water elements. It is responsible for structure, stability, and lubrication in the body. People with a predominant Kapha tend to be calm, strong, and loyal, but they might also experience weight gain, lethargy, and congestion.

Panchakarma

Panchakarma is a comprehensive Ayurvedic detoxification and rejuvenation program designed to restore balance to the Doshas and cleanse the body of toxins (Ama). The term "Panchakarma" translates to "five actions" or "five treatments," referring to the five therapeutic procedures that form the core of this healing practice.

The five treatments include: *Vamana (Emesis Therapy):* Induced vomiting to cleanse the upper gastrointestinal tract, mainly targeting the lungs and stomach. *Virechana (Purgation Therapy):* Use of laxatives to cleanse the lower gastrointestinal tract, primarily the intestines. *Basti (Enema Therapy):* Herbal decoctions or oils are administered through enemas to cleanse the colon and balance Vata Dosha. **Nasya (Nasal Administration):** Application of herbal oils or powders through the nostrils to cleanse the nasal passages and head region. *Raktamokshana (Bloodletting Therapy):* Removing impure blood to treat various blood-related disorders.

Panchakarma is usually preceded by preparatory treatments like Abhyanga (oil massage) and Svedana (herbal steam therapy) to loosen toxins in the body. The process is highly individualized, with specific treatments prescribed based on a person's Dosha imbalance, age, and health condition. It is considered a powerful method for detoxification, rejuvenation, and restoring the body's natural balance.

D O S H A S   O V E R V I E W

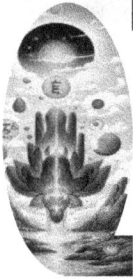

Vata Dosha: Movement & Mobility

Elements: Air + Ether
Season: Fall to Early Winter
Active Times: 2 AM - 6 AM and 2 PM - 6 PM
Primary Functions: Circulation, Breathing, Nerve Impulses
Associated Body Parts: Large Intestine, Pelvic Cavity, Bones, Ears, Thighs

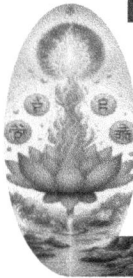

Pitta Dosha: Transformation & Heat

Elements: Fire + Water
Season: Summer
Active Times: 10 AM - 2 PM and 10 PM - 2 AM
Primary Functions: Digestion, Metabolism, Body Temperature Regulation
Associated Body Parts: Small Intestine, Stomach, Liver, Eyes, Skin

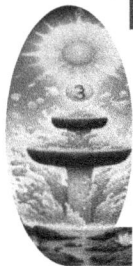

Kapha Dosha: Stability & Structure

Elements: Earth + Water
Season: Late Winter to Spring
Active Times: 6 AM - 10 AM and 6 PM - 10 PM
Primary Functions: Lubrication, Structure, Immunity
Associated Body Parts: Lungs, Stomach, Pancreas, Joints, Lymphatic System

P A N C H A K A R M A

VAMANA (THERAPEUTIC EMESIS)

Induced vomiting to eliminate toxins from the stomach and respiratory tract
To remove Kapha-related toxins, primarily from the upper body
Herbal decoctions, milk, licorice root
Stomach, respiratory tract

VIRECHANA (PURGATION)

Controlled purgation to cleanse the intestines and liver
To remove Pitta-related toxins from the body
Laxatives, herbal purgatives, medicated ghee
Small intestine, liver, gallbladder

BASTI (MEDICATED ENEMA)

Enema therapy using herbal oils or decoctions
To cleanse and rejuvenate the colon, remove Vata-related toxins
Herbal oils, decoctions, medicated milk
Colon, large intestine

NASYA (NASAL ADMINISTRATION)

Nasal administration of herbal oils or powders
To cleanse and clear toxins from the head and neck region
Herbal oils, powders, steam inhalation
Sinuses, nasal passages

RAKTAMOKSHANA (BLOODLETTING)

Controlled bloodletting to remove impurities from the blood
To remove toxins from the circulatory system and balance blood disorders
Leeches, venesection, needle pricking
Blood, circulatory system

Homeopathy

Homeopathy, developed by Samuel Hahnemann in the late 18th century, is a system of alternative medicine based on the "Law of Similars." This principle suggests that a substance that can cause symptoms in a healthy person can, in very small doses, treat similar symptoms in a sick person. This idea is encapsulated in the phrase "like cures like." For example, a substance that causes symptoms of a cold, such as a runny nose or watery eyes, when given in highly diluted forms, might be used to treat those same symptoms in someone suffering from a cold. The goal is to stimulate the body's natural healing response by introducing a substance that mimics the illness, prompting the body to combat the condition itself.

Minimal Doses

Homeopathy also operates on the principle of "minimal doses," meaning the remedies are highly diluted, sometimes to the point where no molecules of the original substance remain. This dilution process, known as potentization, involves repeatedly diluting a substance and then vigorously shaking it. Homeopaths believe that this process transfers the "essence" or "memory" of the substance to the remedy, which then exerts a therapeutic effect.

The idea behind using minimal doses is to avoid side effects and to gently stimulate the body's own healing processes. Critics argue that such extreme dilutions render the remedies ineffective, but homeopathy proponents claim that the energetic imprint left by the original substance is potent enough to promote healing.

Hydrotherapy

Hydrotherapy, or the use of water for therapeutic purposes, was a popular natural treatment. Techniques such as hot and cold baths, steam baths, and the use of mineral springs were believed to improve circulation, detoxify the body, and relieve pain. **Vincent Priessnitz:** An early proponent of hydrotherapy, Priessnitz used cold water treatments to treat injuries and illnesses, believing that water had the power to cleanse and heal the body.

Hot Baths: Immersing the body in warm water can help relax muscles, improve circulation, and alleviate pain. Hot baths are often recommended for conditions like arthritis, muscle stiffness, and stress-related disorders.

Cold Water Immersion: Also known as cold plunging or cryotherapy, involves brief exposure to cold water to reduce inflammation, boost circulation, and enhance recovery after exercise.

Steam Baths/Saunas: Exposing the body to steam or dry heat can promote sweating, which helps detoxify the body, improve circulation, and relieve respiratory conditions.

Contrast Baths: Alternating between hot and cold water baths stimulates blood flow and can reduce inflammation, improve circulation, and promote healing.

Compresses: Applying hot or cold compresses to specific areas of the body can alleviate localized pain, reduce swelling, and Hydrotherapy is often used in combination with other treatments, such as massage or physiotherapy, to enhance its effects. It's known for its ability to improve circulation, detoxify the body, and promote relaxation, and improve blood flow to the targeted area.

Noise and Frequency Healing

The concept of healing through sound is rooted in the belief that sound frequencies can influence our physical, emotional, and spiritual well-being. This ancient practice has been used in various cultures around the world, employing different instruments and techniques to achieve therapeutic effects.

Healing Through Sound

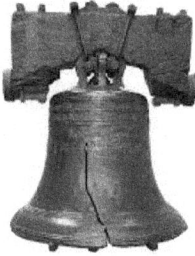

Iron Bells: The ringing of iron bells is one example of sound therapy. The vibrations produced by these bells are believed to resonate with the body's energy fields, helping to clear blockages and restore balance. The rich, deep tones of iron bells can induce a state of relaxation and meditation, aiding in stress reduction and emotional healing. *Tuning Forks:* Another tool used in sound therapy, tuning forks are calibrated to specific frequencies that correspond to different energy centers or chakras in the body. When struck, the tuning fork emits a pure tone that can help align the body's energy, promote relaxation, and alleviate physical and emotional tension. *Gongs and Singing Bowls:* These instruments produce a broad spectrum of harmonic frequencies when played. The vibrations are said to penetrate the body at a cellular level, promoting healing, reducing stress, and enhancing mental clarity. *Mantras and Chanting:* The use of vocal sounds, such as chanting mantras, is another form of sound healing. Repeating certain sounds or words can have a calming effect on the mind and body, helping to reduce stress and promote healing.

Sound therapy is based on the principle that everything in the universe, including our bodies, is in a state of vibration. By using sound frequencies, we can influence our vibrational state, promoting healing, reducing stress, and enhancing overall well-being.

Naturopathy

Holistic Healing: Naturopathy, which emerged in the late 19th century, focused on the body's ability to heal itself through natural means. This approach combined diet, exercise, herbal medicine, and lifestyle changes to promote health and prevent disease. *The Healing Power of Nature:* Naturopaths believed that the body could restore health if given the right conditions, emphasizing natural foods, pure water, sunlight, and fresh air.

Diet and Nutrition

Natural Diets: Before the 1920s, there was a focus on diets rich in whole foods, including fruits, vegetables, grains, and nuts. The connection between diet and health was recognized in various cultures, with an emphasis on consuming foods in their natural, unprocessed state. *Raw Food Movements:* Early proponents of raw food diets believed that cooking destroyed essential nutrients and enzymes necessary for health. Raw foodists advocated for a diet primarily consisting of raw fruits, vegetables, nuts, and seeds.

Chiropractic Care

Spinal Health: The chiropractic profession, founded by D.D. Palmer in the late 19th century, was based on the idea that many diseases were caused by misalignments in the spine (subluxations) that affected nerve function. Adjustments were performed to correct these misalignments and restore health.

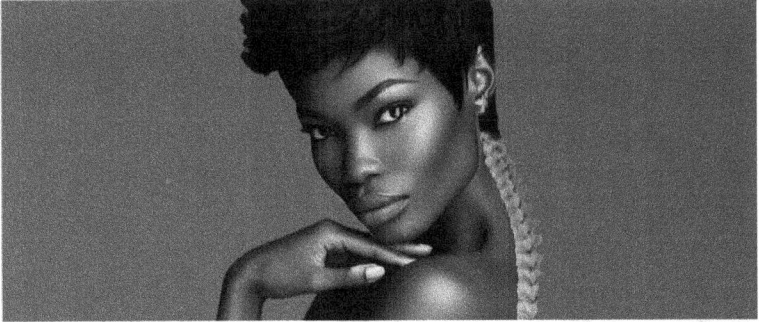

Spinal Health and Nerve Function

Chiropractic care is a form of alternative medicine that focuses on diagnosing and treating mechanical disorders of the musculoskeletal system, particularly the spine. The central concept is that proper alignment of the spine is crucial for overall health because it directly impacts the nervous system.

The spine is composed of vertebrae that protect the spinal cord, which is a major component of the central nervous system (CNS). Misalignments or subluxations in the spine can lead to nerve interference, causing pain, discomfort, and impaired function in various parts of the body. Chiropractors use manual adjustments or manipulations to correct these misalignments, thereby restoring proper nerve function and promoting the body's natural ability to heal itself.

Chiropractic adjustments are believed to help with a range of conditions, including back pain, headaches, joint pain, and even systemic issues like digestive problems. The underlying philosophy is that by maintaining spinal health, the entire body can function more effectively, reducing the need for medication or surgery.

Nitric Oxide (NO) Facts and Benefits

Nitric oxide, represented by the chemical formula NO, is a gas at room temperature with a short-lived and highly reactive nature. Despite its transient existence, nitric oxide plays a crucial role as a signaling molecule in the body, influencing various physiological and pathological processes.

Health Benefits of Nitric Oxide

Cardiovascular Health: Nitric oxide is essential for maintaining cardiovascular health due to its vasodilatory properties. It helps relax and dilate blood vessels, which improves blood flow and reduces blood pressure. By supporting overall cardiovascular function, nitric oxide can reduce the risk of heart disease, contributing to a healthier heart. **Immune Function:** In the immune system, nitric oxide acts as a defense mechanism against pathogens. It aids in the destruction of bacteria and other harmful microorganisms, enhancing the body's ability to fight infections and maintain immune health.

Exercise Performance: Nitric oxide plays a significant role in improving exercise performance. By enhancing blood flow to muscles, it facilitates better oxygen delivery and nutrient uptake, which can boost endurance and muscle efficiency during physical activities. **Cognitive Function:** As a neurotransmitter, nitric oxide supports brain function and cognitive processes. It contributes to neurotransmission, which is crucial for maintaining mental acuity and cognitive health. **Wound Healing:** Nitric oxide promotes blood flow to tissues, aiding in wound healing and recovery from injuries. Its ability to enhance tissue repair makes it a vital component in the body's natural healing processes.

HUMMM! FOR YOUR HEALTH

Natural Ways to Boost Nitric Oxide

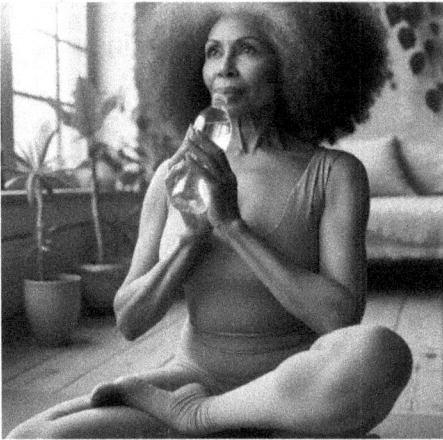

Consuming nitrate-rich foods is an effective way to boost nitric oxide levels. Leafy greens such as spinach and arugula, beets, and celery are high in nitrates that the body converts to nitric oxide. Additionally, foods rich in antioxidants like berries, citrus fruits, and nuts help protect nitric oxide from oxidative damage, ensuring its efficacy in the body.

Exercise: Regular aerobic exercise is a powerful stimulator of nitric oxide production. Engaging in consistent physical activity not only enhances nitric oxide levels but also improves overall cardiovascular health, contributing to a well-functioning circulatory system. **Supplements:** Certain amino acids, such as L-arginine and L-citrulline, are known to increase nitric oxide levels in the body. These supplements can be an effective addition to the diet to support nitric oxide production and its associated health benefits.

Humming and Nitric Oxide Production

Humming is a simple and effective technique to significantly increase the production of nitric oxide in the body. This practice stimulates the production of nitric oxide in the nasal passages by increasing airflow and vibration in the sinuses. Enhanced nitric oxide production from humming helps clear nasal passages, reduce sinus infections, and improve overall respiratory health. Additionally, nitric oxide dilates airways, which improves oxygen exchange and respiratory efficiency.

How to Incorporate Humming for Health Benefits

Daily Practice: Incorporate humming into your daily routine by spending a few minutes each day practicing it. Humming can be done while meditating or during deep breathing exercises to maximize its benefits. *Mindful Breathing*: Combine humming with slow, deep nasal breathing. Inhale deeply through the nose and hum gently on the exhale, focusing on the vibrations in your nasal passages and sinuses. *Yoga and Meditation:* Incorporate humming into yoga or meditation practices to enhance relaxation and nitric oxide production. This integration can promote a state of calm and well-being while boosting nitric oxide levels.

Example Exercise: Humming for Nitric Oxide Boost

Find a Comfortable Position: Sit or lie down in a comfortable position with your back straight. *Deep Nasal Breathing:* Inhale deeply through your nose, filling your lungs completely. *Humming Exhale:* As you exhale, hum a steady and gentle tone. Feel the vibrations in your nasal passages and sinuses. *Repeat:* Continue this process for 5-10 minutes, focusing on slow, deep breaths and steady humming.

Incorporating humming into your daily routine can be a simple and effective way to naturally boost nitric oxide levels, supporting overall health and well-being. This holistic approach, combined with dietary and exercise practices, can significantly enhance the body's nitric oxide production, contributing to improved cardiovascular, immune, cognitive, and respiratory health.

High Nitric Oxide (NO) Producers

Salads: Combine raw arugula, lettuce, spinach, and kale for a nutrient-dense salad. Add shredded carrots and thinly sliced beets for added benefits. Smoothies: Blend raw spinach, kale, or beet greens into your favorite fruit smoothie. Roasted Vegetables: Roast cauliflower, broccoli, and carrots with a little olive oil and your favorite herbs. *Stir-Fries:* Include bok choy, cabbage, and mustard greens in stir-fries for a nutritious and delicious meal. *Soups and Stews:* Add chopped kohlrabi, kale, and carrots to soups and stews for a hearty and nitrate-rich dish. Juices: Make fresh beet and carrot juice for a refreshing and NO-boosting drink. *Side Dishes:* Steam or sauté chicory, mustard greens, and bok choy as side dishes to accompany your meals.

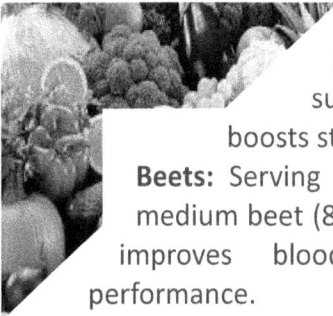

Arugula: Serving Size: 1 cup (20 grams) Benefits: Rich in nitrates, supports cardiovascular health, and boosts stamina.

Beets: Serving Size: 1 cup (136 grams) cooked or 1 medium beet (82 grams) raw Benefits: High in nitrates, improves blood flow, and enhances exercise performance.

Bok Choy: Serving Size: 1 cup (170 grams) cooked or 1 cup (70 grams) raw Benefits: Provides nitrates, vitamins, and antioxidants that support heart health.

Broccoli: Serving Size: 1 cup (156 grams) cooked or 1 cup (91 grams) raw Benefits: Contains nitrates and is rich in vitamins C and K, fiber, and antioxidants.

Cabbage: Serving Size: 1 cup (150 grams) cooked or 1 cup (89 grams) raw Benefits: High in nitrates and vitamin K, supports digestion and heart health.

Carrot: Serving Size: 1 cup (128 grams) chopped Benefits: Contains nitrates and beta-carotene, promoting eye and cardiovascular health.

Cauliflower: Serving Size: 1 cup (124 grams) cooked or 1 cup (107 grams) raw Benefits: Provides nitrates, fiber, and antioxidants, supporting heart and digestive health.

Chicory: Serving Size: 1 cup (29 grams) raw Benefits: High in nitrates and fiber, supports digestive health and blood sugar control.

Kale: Serving Size: 1 cup (67 grams) chopped, raw or 1 cup (130 grams) cooked Benefits: Rich in nitrates, vitamins A, C, and K, and antioxidants, promoting heart health.

Kohlrabi: Serving Size: 1 cup (135 grams) chopped Benefits: High in nitrates, fiber, and vitamin C, supporting cardiovascular and immune health.

Lettuce: Serving Size: 1 cup (36 grams) shredded Benefits: Provides nitrates and fiber, supporting hydration and heart health.

Mustard Greens: Serving Size: 1 cup (140 grams) cooked or 1 cup (56 grams) raw Benefits: High in nitrates, vitamins A, C, and K, and antioxidants, promoting heart health.

Spinach: Serving Size: 1 cup (180 grams) cooked or 1 cup (30 grams) raw Benefits: Rich in nitrates, iron, and vitamins A and K, supporting cardiovascular and overall health.

Medium Nitric Oxide (NO) Producers

Salads: Add watercress, celery, and tomatoes to your salads. Use coleslaw as a side dish or as part of a salad. *Smoothies:* Blend melons and strawberries into smoothies for a refreshing and NO-boosting drink. *Roasted Vegetables:* Roast artichokes, asparagus, eggplant, and potatoes with a bit of olive oil and your favorite herbs. *Soups and Stews:* Include a variety of these vegetables in soups and stews to create nutrient-dense and NO-rich meals. *Vegetable Juice:* Make your own vegetable juice at home using a mix of tomatoes, celery, and other medium NO-producing vegetables. *Stir-Fries:* Add asparagus, celery, and eggplant to stir-fries for a nutritious and delicious meal. *Snacks:* Enjoy raw celery sticks or melon slices as healthy snacks throughout the day.

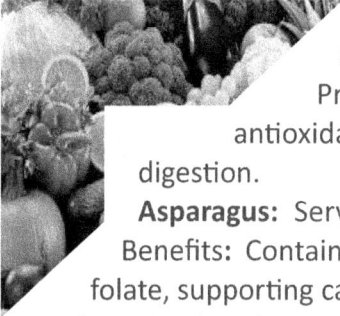

Artichoke: Serving Size: 1 medium artichoke (120 grams) cooked Benefits: Provides dietary nitrates, fiber, and antioxidants that support heart health and digestion.

Asparagus: Serving Size: 1 cup (134 grams) cooked Benefits: Contains nitrates, vitamins A, C, and K, and folate, supporting cardiovascular and overall health.

Celery: Serving Size: 1 cup (101 grams) chopped Benefits: High in nitrates, supports blood pressure regulation, and provides hydration.

Coleslaw: Serving Size: 1 cup (150 grams**) Benefits:** Made from cabbage, which is a good source of nitrates and supports digestive and heart health.

Eggplant: Serving Size: 1 cup (99 grams) cooked Benefits: Provides nitrates, fiber, and antioxidants, supporting cardiovascular and digestive health.

Garlic: Serving Size: 1 clove (3 grams) or 1 teaspoon minced Benefits: Contains allicin, which supports nitric oxide production, heart health, and immune function.

Melon (Cantaloupe, Honeydew, Watermelon): Serving Size: 1 cup (160 grams) chopped Benefits: Hydrating and provides nitrates, supporting cardiovascular health and hydration.

Potato: Serving Size: 1 medium potato (213 grams) baked Benefits: Contains nitrates, potassium, and vitamin C, supporting heart health and blood pressure regulation.

Strawberry: Serving Size: 1 cup (152 grams) whole Benefits: Provides nitrates, vitamins, and antioxidants, supporting cardiovascular and immune health.

Tomato: Serving Size: 1 cup (180 grams) chopped or 1 medium tomato (123 grams) Benefits: Rich in nitrates, lycopene, and vitamin C, supporting heart health and reducing inflammation.

Vegetable Juice: Serving Size: 1 cup (240 milliliters) Benefits: Contains a blend of nitrates from various vegetables, supporting overall health and hydration.

Vegetable Soup: Serving Size: 1 cup (245 grams) Benefits: A mixture of vegetables provides nitrates, fiber, and vitamins, supporting heart health and digestion.

Watercress: Serving Size: 1 cup (34 grams) chopped Benefits: High in nitrates, vitamins, and antioxidants, supporting cardiovascular health and immune function.

Low Nitric Oxide (NO) Producers

Salads: Add raspberries, bean sprouts, and onions to your salads for a nutritious boost. *Smoothies:* Blend bananas, cherries, and figs into smoothies for a sweet and nutrient-rich drink. *Snacks:* Enjoy prunes, raisins, and fresh figs as healthy snacks throughout the day. *Side Dishes:* Roast sweet potatoes or steam string beans to serve as side dishes with your meals. *Main Dishes:* Include chickpeas in stews, curries, or salads for a protein and fiber boost. *Desserts:* Use cherries, raspberries, and figs in desserts like parfaits, tarts, or yogurt bowls. *Beverages:* Enjoy a glass of red wine in moderation as part of a balanced diet. *Casseroles and Stir-Fries:* Add string beans and onions to casseroles or stir-fries for added flavor and nutrition.

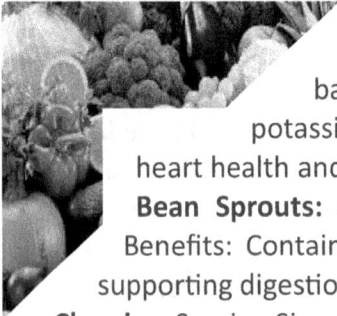

Bananas: Serving Size: 1 medium banana (118 grams) Benefits: Provides potassium, vitamins B6 and C, supporting heart health and energy metabolism.

Bean Sprouts: Serving Size: 1 cup (104 grams) raw Benefits: Contains vitamins C and K, folate, and fiber, supporting digestion and immune function.

Cherries: Serving Size: 1 cup (154 grams) pitted Benefits: Rich in antioxidants and anti-inflammatory compounds, supporting joint health and reducing oxidative stress.

Chickpeas: Serving Size: 1 cup (164 grams) cooked Benefits: High in protein, fiber, and iron, supporting muscle health, digestion, and energy levels.

Figs: Serving Size: 2 medium figs (100 grams) Benefits: Provides fiber, vitamins, and minerals, supporting digestive health and bone health.

Onions: Serving Size: 1 cup (160 grams) chopped Benefits: Contains antioxidants and sulfur compounds, supporting heart health and immune function.

Prunes: Serving Size: 1 cup (174 grams) pitted Benefits: High in fiber and antioxidants, supporting digestive health and reducing inflammation.

Raisins: Serving Size: 1/4 cup (40 grams) Benefits: Provides iron, fiber, and antioxidants, supporting energy levels and digestion.

Raspberries: Serving Size: 1 cup (123 grams) Benefits: Rich in fiber, vitamins C and K, and antioxidants, supporting immune health and reducing inflammation.

Red Wine: Serving Size: 5 ounces (148 milliliters) Benefits: Contains resveratrol and antioxidants, supporting heart health and reducing oxidative stress (consumed in moderation).

String Beans (Green Beans): Serving Size: 1 cup (125 grams) cooked Benefits: Provides vitamins A, C, and K, fiber, and antioxidants, supporting heart health and digestion.

Sweet Potato: Serving Size: 1 medium sweet potato (130 grams) baked Benefits: High in beta-carotene, fiber, and vitamins, supporting vision health and immune function.

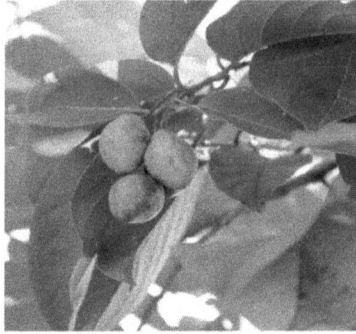

The Power of Haritaki and Its Impact on the Pineal Gland

Haritaki (Terminalia chebula) is an ancient, powerful fruit used in Ayurveda and traditional holistic healing systems, revered for its potent medicinal and healing properties. Known as the "King of Herbs," Haritaki is often referred to as the "Mother of all herbs" due to its wide range of health benefits, especially its role in detoxifying the body and mind. This miraculous herb has been a cornerstone of holistic medicine for thousands of years, especially in regions of South Asia, where it grows abundantly.

Haritaki is rich in tannins, flavonoids, and antioxidants, making it an ideal herb for cleansing, rejuvenation, and healing. In Sanskrit, Haritaki means "that which steals away diseases," and this description truly embodies the herb's profound healing capacity.

Health Benefits of Haritaki

Digestive Health Haritaki acts as a natural laxative, supporting digestion, cleansing the intestines, and aiding in the elimination of toxins. By enhancing the digestive fire, it promotes a healthy metabolism and ensures proper absorption of nutrients. Haritaki is often used to treat constipation, bloating, indigestion, and gas, making it a key herb in maintaining gut health.

Haritaki's Impact on Gut Health

Removes toxins from the digestive tract, supporting overall detoxification. Stimulates peristalsis, the natural wave-like movements in the intestines, which help with regular bowel movements. Balances the gut microbiome by reducing the harmful bacteria and promoting the growth of beneficial bacteria.

Respiratory Health Haritaki has powerful anti-inflammatory and antibacterial properties, making it effective in treating respiratory ailments such as coughs, asthma, and bronchitis. It clears mucus and congestion from the lungs, allowing for easier breathing.

Antioxidant and Anti-aging Properties As a rich source of antioxidants, Haritaki fights free radicals in the body, which are responsible for cellular damage and aging. By reducing oxidative stress, it helps slow down the aging process and promotes healthy, radiant skin.

Weight Management Haritaki supports healthy metabolism and fat burning by enhancing digestion and promoting the body's ability to break down and eliminate fats. Additionally, it suppresses hunger naturally and detoxifies the body, making it beneficial for those on weight-loss journeys.

Detoxification and Cleansing Haritaki's powerful detoxifying properties cleanse the blood and tissues by removing harmful toxins accumulated through diet, pollution, and stress. This detoxification effect extends to all organs, ensuring the body functions optimally and remains disease-free.

Brain and Cognitive Function One of Haritaki's lesser-known yet profound benefits lies in its ability to enhance brain function. It improves memory, concentration, and cognitive abilities by increasing the brain's natural capacity to function. Haritaki also balances the nervous system, making it useful in reducing stress, anxiety, and depression.

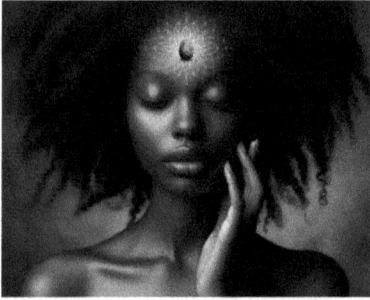

Haritaki's Connection to the Pineal Gland

The pineal gland, often referred to as the "Third Eye" in ancient spiritual practices, is a small, pea-shaped gland located in the center of the brain. It is responsible for producing melatonin, a hormone that regulates sleep-wake cycles, and is deeply linked to spiritual awakening, intuition, and consciousness. The pineal gland has long been revered as the seat of the soul, and when functioning optimally, it allows for heightened mental clarity, spiritual insight, and inner peace.

Decalcification of the Pineal Gland

In modern society, due to the consumption of processed foods, exposure to fluoride in water, and pollution, the pineal gland often becomes calcified. Calcification is the accumulation of calcium deposits, which inhibit the pineal gland's functioning and block spiritual growth. Detoxifying the pineal gland is essential for restoring balance and awakening one's true potential.

Haritaki's Role in Activating the Pineal Gland

Haritaki is one of the most powerful herbs for decalcifying and activating the pineal gland. It helps remove heavy metals, environmental toxins, and other impurities that contribute to pineal calcification. When taken regularly, Haritaki detoxifies the entire system, promoting optimal function of the pineal gland, leading to enhanced mental clarity, better sleep patterns, and increased spiritual awareness.

How Haritaki Benefits the Pineal Gland: *Detoxification:* Haritaki helps to flush out fluoride and other toxins that calcify the pineal gland, restoring its function. *Spiritual Activation:* In many ancient traditions, Haritaki is said to open the Third Eye, enhancing intuition and spiritual perception. *Improved Sleep Cycles:* By balancing melatonin production, Haritaki helps regulate sleep patterns, leading to better rest and mental clarity.

Benefits of a Healthy Pineal Gland

Enhanced Mental Clarity and Focus When the pineal gland functions optimally, it supports improved cognitive abilities, allowing for sharper mental focus, better decision-making, and a deeper understanding of complex concepts. ***Better Sleep and Circadian Rhythm*** The pineal gland is directly responsible for regulating the body's internal clock through the secretion of melatonin. A healthy pineal gland means better regulation of sleep cycles, leading to more restful sleep and increased energy throughout the day. ***Heightened Intuition and Spiritual Awareness*** A balanced pineal gland is associated with enhanced spiritual awareness and intuition. It helps individuals connect with their higher self, leading to profound insights, inner peace, and spiritual growth. ***Emotional Stability*** By balancing the release of hormones, the pineal gland helps regulate emotions and maintain emotional stability. A well-functioning pineal gland contributes to reduced stress and anxiety, promoting overall mental well-being.

Little-Known Facts About Haritaki

Haritaki is known as a "spiritual cleanser" because of its profound impact on consciousness and its ability to detoxify the mind as well as the body. Ancient texts describe Haritaki as the herb that removes not only physical toxins but also "mental toxins," helping individuals release negative thoughts, emotional blockages, and limiting beliefs. It is often used in yogic practices to enhance meditation, mindfulness, and the opening of the Third Eye.

How to Incorporate Haritaki into Daily Life

Powder Form: Haritaki powder can be mixed with warm water and consumed daily. It's best taken on an empty stomach in the morning or before bed. *Capsules:* For those who prefer not to taste the bitterness of the herb, Haritaki capsules offer a convenient way to receive its benefits. *Haritaki Oil:* Haritaki can also be applied topically as an oil, massaged into the skin to promote healing and reduce inflammation.

Haritaki is a powerful herb that goes beyond physical healing. Its ability to cleanse and activate the pineal gland makes it a critical tool in both mental and spiritual health. In a world filled with environmental toxins and stress, incorporating Haritaki into a holistic healing regimen can restore balance, enhance mental clarity, and awaken the true potential within. As a profound detoxifier and spiritual activator, Haritaki is a treasure that has been passed down through generations for a reason. Now, more than ever, it serves as a bridge between physical well-being and spiritual enlightenment.

"Mother of All Herbs" and Their Benefits

Herb Name Haritaki

Origin India, Southeast Asia **Key Benefits** Detoxifies the body, enhances digestion, improves brain function, decalcifies the pineal gland, supports spiritual clarity

Herb Name Holy Basil (Tulsi)

Origin India **Key Benefits** Reduces stress, balances hormones, supports respiratory health, boosts immunity, promotes longevity

Herb Name Gotu Kola

Origin South Asia **Key Benefits** Enhances brain function, improves circulation, reduces anxiety, supports wound healing, promotes skin health

Herb Name Ashwagandha

Origin India, Middle East **Key Benefits** Reduces stress, supports adrenal health, boosts energy, improves sleep, enhances brain function

Herb Name Moringa

Origin Africa, India **Key Benefits** Rich in vitamins and minerals, anti-inflammatory, detoxifies the body, boosts immune function, improves energy levels

Herb Name **Neem**

Origin India, Southeast Asia **Key Benefits** Purifies the blood, supports skin health, boosts immunity, combats infections, detoxifies the liver

Herb Name Shatavari

Origin India, Sri Lanka **Key Benefits** Supports reproductive health, balances hormones, enhances digestion, boosts immune system, promotes vitality

Herb Name Brahmi

Origin India **Key Benefits** Enhances cognitive function, improves memory, calms the nervous system, supports mental clarity and spiritual growth

Herb Name **Fenugreek**

Origin Mediterranean, India **Key Benefits** Improves digestion, balances blood sugar, supports lactation, enhances libido, aids in reducing inflammation

Herb Name Amalaki (Indian Gooseberry)

Origin India **Key Benefits** High in vitamin C, boosts immunity, detoxifies the body, supports liver health, improves digestion

These herbs have been revered for centuries for their profound healing properties due to their extensive range of benefits for physical, mental, and spiritual health.

Understanding and Balancing Chakras

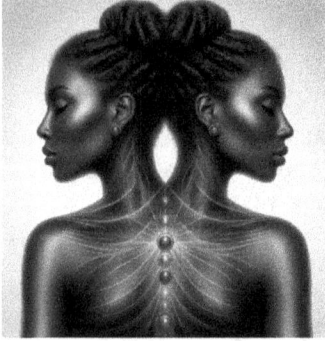

Some say that meditation, breathing exercises, yoga, and visualization can help balance chakras. These practices can help you relax, calm your thoughts, and downregulate your stress response, which can help your systems work better. Chakras are fundamental to the understanding of energy flow and spiritual well-being in various Eastern traditions. This section delves into what chakras are, the different types, their functions, and how to heal and balance them for overall wellness.

What Are Chakras? Chakras are centers of spiritual power in the human body, originating from ancient Indian traditions and prominently featured in practices such as yoga, Ayurveda, and meditation. The term "chakra" means "wheel" or "disk" in Sanskrit, representing the spinning energy centers in our bodies that correspond to different physical, emotional, and spiritual aspects.

The Concept of Energy Flow

Chakras are believed to be part of the subtle body, interacting with physical and metaphysical aspects of human existence. Proper functioning of these energy centers is crucial for maintaining health and balance in the body and mind. When chakras are blocked or out of balance, it can lead to physical, emotional, and spiritual disturbances.

Types of Chakras There are seven main chakras aligned along the spine, from the base to the crown of the head. Each chakra has its own characteristics, functions, and associated elements.

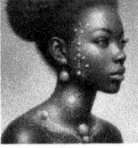

CROWN CHAKRA (SAHASRARA)

Color: Violet or white **Element:** Thought **Function:** Spiritual connection, enlightenment **Location:** Top of the head **Associated Body Parts:** Brain, nervous system, pineal gland

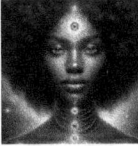

THIRD EYE CHAKRA (AJNA)

Color: Indigo **Element:** Light **Function:** Intuition, insight, wisdom **Location:** Forehead, between the eyes **Associated Body Parts:** Brain, eyes, pituitary gland

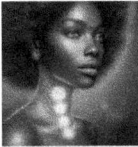

THROAT CHAKRA (VISHUDDHA)

Color: Blue **Element:** Ether **Function:** Communication, expression, truth **Location:** Throat **Associated Body Parts:** Throat, neck, thyroid

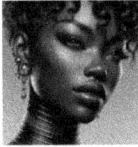

HEART CHAKRA (ANAHATA)

Color: Green **Element:** Air **Function:** Love, compassion, relationships **Location:** Center of the chest **Associated Body Parts:** Heart, lungs, thymus

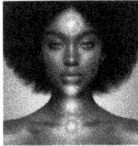

SOLAR PLEXUS CHAKRA (MANIPURA)

Color: Yellow **Element:** Fire **Function:** Personal power, will, self-esteem **Location:** Upper abdomen, above the navel **Associated Body Parts:** Digestive system, pancreas, liver

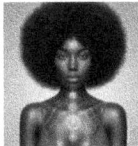

SACRAL CHAKRA (SVADHISTHANA)

Color: Orange **Element:** Water **Function:** Creativity, Sexuality, Pleasure **Location:** Lower abdomen, about 2in. below the navel **Associated Body Parts:** Reproductive organs, kidneys, bladder

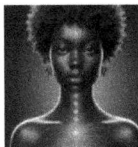

ROOT CHAKRA (MULADHARA)

Color: Red **Element:** Earth **Function:** Grounding, survival, security **Location:** Base of the spine **Associated Body Parts:** Legs, feet, bones, large intestines

Healing and Balancing Chakras

Signs of Imbalanced Chakras Imbalanced chakras can manifest in various ways, both physically and emotionally.

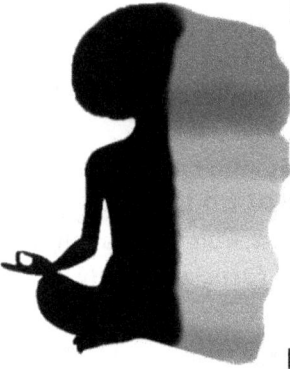

Crown Chakra
Spiritual disconnection, depression, cognitive issues

Third Eye Chakra
Lack of intuition, headaches, vision problems

Throat Chakra
Communication issues, sore throat, thyroid problems

Heart Chakra
Difficulty in relationships, jealousy, heart problems

Solar Plexus Chakra
Low self-esteem, lack of control, digestive issues

Sacral Chakra
Emotional instability, sexual dysfunction, lower back pain

Root Chakra
Anxiety, insecurity, financial problems, constipation

Meditation - Meditation is a powerful tool for balancing chakras. Focused meditation on each chakra can help clear blockages and restore energy flow. Visualizing the color and location of each chakra while meditating can enhance the process.

Yoga

Techniques for Balancing Chakras Balancing chakras involves various techniques aimed at restoring the proper flow of energy. These techniques can include meditation, yoga, affirmations, diet, and the use of crystals and essential oils.

Crown Chakra Yoga Poses (Asanas)
Headstand (Sirsasana), Corpse pose (Savasana)
Third Eye Chakra Yoga Poses (Asanas)
Child's pose (Balasana), Downward Facing Dog (Adho Mukha Svanasana)
Throat Chakra Yoga Poses (Asanas)
Shoulder Stand (Sarvangasana), Plow pose (Halasana)
Heart Chakra Yoga Poses (Asanas)
Camel pose (Ustrasana), Bridge pose (Setu Bandhasana)
Solar Plexus Chakra Yoga Poses (Asanas)
Boat pose (Navasana), Warrior pose (Virabhadrasana)
Sacral Chakra Yoga Poses (Asanas)
Bound Angle pose (Baddha Konasana), Goddess pose (Utkata Konasana)
Root Chakra Yoga Poses (Asanas)
Mountain pose (Tadasana), Tree pose (Vrikshasana)

Affirmations Positive affirmations can reinforce the qualities associated with each chakra. Repeating these affirmations regularly can help shift your energy and mindset.

Crown Chakra	"I am connected to the divine."
Third Eye Chakra	"I trust my intuition."
Throat Chakra	"I express my truth with clarity."
Heart Chakra	"I am open to love and compassion."
Solar Plexus Chakra	"I am confident and strong."
Sacral Chakra	"I embrace my creativity and sexuality."
Root Chakra	"I am safe and secure."

Diet A diet rich in specific foods can support each chakra's energy.

Crown Chakra
Fasting, light foods like fruits and vegetables
Third Eye Chakra
Dark chocolate, purple fruits and vegetables
Throat Chakra
Blueberries, herbal teas, seaweed
Heart Chakra
Leafy greens, green vegetables
Solar Plexus Chakra
Grains, legumes, yellow fruits and vegetable
Sacral Chakra
Sweet fruits, nuts, seeds
Root Chakra
Protein-rich foods, root vegetables

Crystals and Essential Oils
Crystals and essential oils can be used to enhance chakra healing.
Crown Chakra
Clear quartz, selenite; frankincense, myrrh oil
Third Eye Chakra
Amethyst, lapis lazuli; frankincense, lavender oil
Throat Chakra
Lapis lazuli, turquoise; peppermint, eucalyptus oil
Heart Chakra
Rose quartz, green aventurine; rose, bergamot oil
Solar Plexus Chakra
Citrine, tiger's eye; lemon, ginger oil
Sacral Chakra
Carnelian, orange calcite; ylang-ylang, sandalwood oil
Root Chakra
Red jasper, hematite; vetiver, cedarwood oil

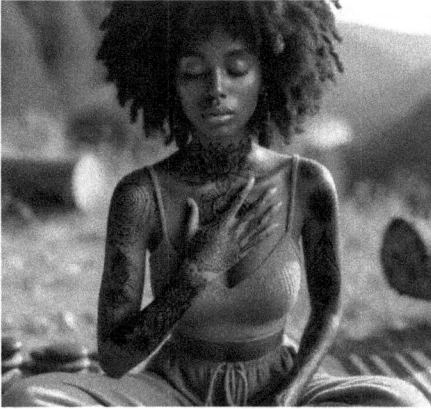

What is Reiki?

Reiki is a form of energy healing that originated in Japan in the early 20th century. The term "Reiki" is derived from two Japanese words: "Rei," meaning "universal," and "Ki," meaning "life energy." Reiki is based on the belief that there is a universal life force energy that flows through all living things. When this energy is strong and balanced, a person is more likely to experience physical, emotional, and spiritual well-being. Conversely, if the energy is weak or blocked, it can lead to illness or stress.

Reiki practitioners use a technique known as palm healing or hands-on healing to channel this life force energy into the patient's body. The aim is to promote relaxation, reduce stress, and facilitate the body's natural healing processes. Reiki is often used as a complementary therapy, alongside conventional medical treatments, to enhance overall well-being.

How to Perform Reiki

Preparation

Find a Quiet Space: Choose a peaceful environment free from distractions. This can be a dedicated room or a quiet corner where you won't be interrupted. ***Set Your Intention:*** Before beginning a Reiki session, it's important to set a clear intention for the healing. This could be for stress relief, emotional balance, physical healing, or spiritual growth. ***Ground Yourself:*** Take a few moments to center yourself. This can be done through deep breathing, meditation, or visualization. Imagine roots growing from your feet into the earth, grounding you.

Connecting to Reiki Energy

Attunement: Traditionally, Reiki practitioners receive attunements from a Reiki Master, which helps them connect to the Reiki energy. If you're new to Reiki, consider receiving an attunement to fully access this healing energy. *Invoke Reiki Energy:* Once attuned, you can invoke Reiki energy by placing your hands together in a prayer position, and silently or aloud, ask to be connected to the Reiki energy. You may feel warmth, tingling, or a sense of peace as the energy flows through you.

Performing Reiki on Yourself

Hand Positions: Start by placing your hands on or just above different parts of your body. Common hand positions include the crown of the head, the eyes, the throat, the heart, the solar plexus, the abdomen, and the lower abdomen. *Hold Each Position:* Hold your hands in each position for 3-5 minutes, or until you feel the energy has moved or you sense it's time to shift. Focus on the warmth and energy flowing from your hands into your body. *Trust Your Intuition:* Reiki is an intuitive practice. If you're drawn to place your hands on a particular area of your body, follow that instinct.

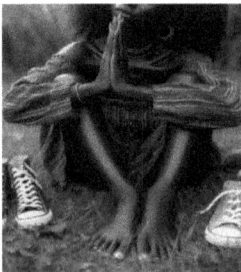

Performing Reiki on Others

Ask for Permission: Before performing Reiki on someone else, always ask for their consent. Ensure they are comfortable with the process. **Hand Positions:** Similar to self-Reiki, use a series of hand positions to channel energy into the recipient's body. You can hover your hands just above the body or lightly touch the person, depending on their comfort level. **Stay Present:** Focus on the flow of energy, keeping your mind clear and your intention strong. Stay aware of the recipient's energy and any shifts or changes that occur.

Closing the Session

Seal the Energy: Once you've completed the session, seal the energy by moving your hands over the person's body, from head to toe, as if brushing away any residual energy. **Thank the Reiki Energy:** Take a moment to express gratitude for the Reiki energy and for the healing that has taken place. **Grounding:** After the session, ground yourself again by visualizing your connection to the earth. Encourage the recipient to do the same, perhaps by having them drink water or eat something light.

Post-Session Reflection

Reflect: Take some time to reflect on the experience, either by journaling or meditating. Note any sensations, thoughts, or feelings that arose during the session. Rest and Hydrate: It's important to rest and hydrate after a Reiki session to help the body integrate the healing energy.

Benefits of Reiki

Stress Reduction: Reiki promotes relaxation and reduces stress, allowing the body to heal naturally. **Emotional Balance:** Reiki can help release emotional blockages, promoting a sense of calm and emotional well-being. **Physical Healing:** Reiki supports the body's natural healing processes, which can aid in recovery from illness or injury. **Spiritual Growth:** Reiki enhances spiritual awareness and connection, fostering personal growth and self-discovery.

Reiki is a gentle, non-invasive practice that can be used by anyone to enhance their health and well-being. Whether you choose to receive Reiki from a practitioner or learn to practice it yourself, it can be a valuable tool in your health journey.

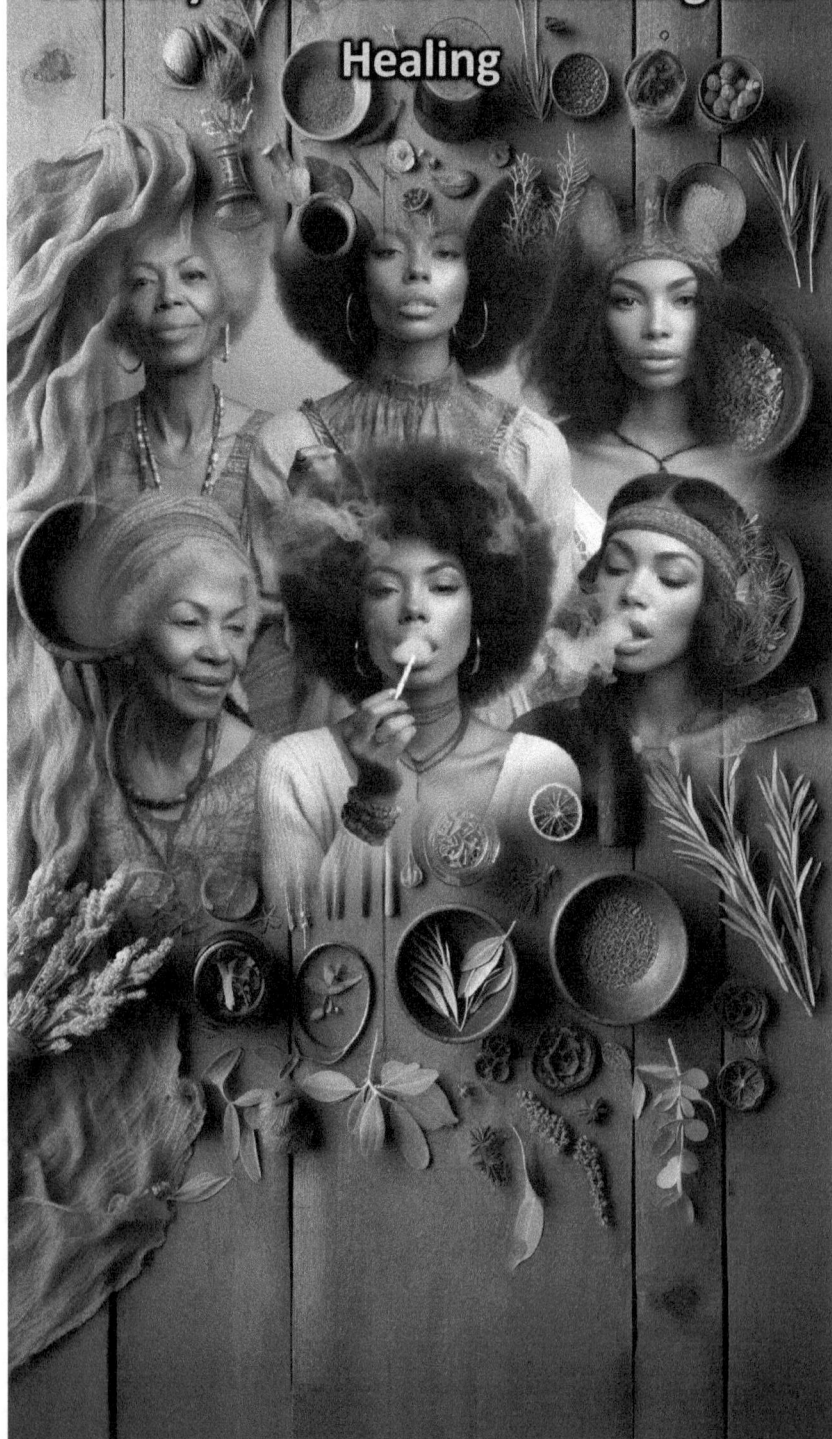

Chapter 5
Journey Into Herbs for Smoking and Healing

Herbs Smoking Traditions

Smoking herbs is a practice that dates back thousands of years and spans various cultures around the world. Traditionally, herbs were smoked for their medicinal properties, spiritual significance, and ceremonial uses. While tobacco and marijuana are the most well-known plants for smoking today, many other herbs offer therapeutic benefits when smoked. This section explores the holistic effects of smoking herbs like mugwort, raspberry leaf, and rose, among others, focusing on their health benefits, cultural significance, particularly in African American heritage, and important considerations for safe use.

Mugwort (Artemisia vulgaris)

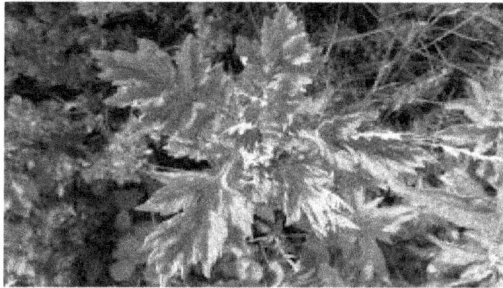

Dream Enhancement

Mugwort is known for its ability to enhance dreams and support lucid dreaming. It has a long history of use in shamanic practices and rituals for promoting vivid, memorable dreams. When smoked, mugwort can help clear the lungs and sinuses, making it beneficial for those with respiratory issues. Mugwort has mild sedative properties, making it useful for reducing anxiety and promoting relaxation.

Cultural and Historical Significance

Mugwort has been used in various folk practices within the African American community, often as a protective herb. It was believed to ward off evil spirits and negative energies, a belief that may have its roots in African spiritual traditions. Mugwort should be smoked in moderation. It is not recommended for pregnant or breastfeeding women, as it can stimulate menstruation and potentially cause uterine contractions.

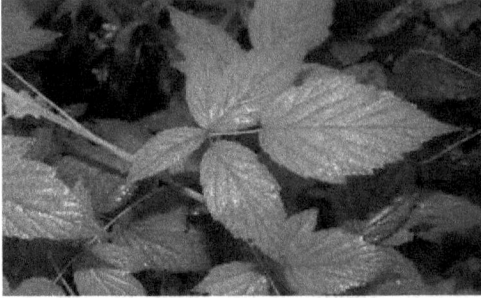

Raspberry Leaf (Rubus idaeus)

Respiratory Support

Raspberry leaf is known for its gentle effects on the respiratory system. It can soothe the throat and lungs, making it beneficial for smokers who want to reduce irritation. Raspberry leaf is traditionally used to support women's reproductive health, particularly for balancing hormones and easing menstrual cramps. When smoked, it may provide mild relaxation and relief from menstrual discomfort. Rich in antioxidants, raspberry leaf can help protect cells from oxidative stress, potentially offering benefits to the overall immune system.

Cultural and Historical Significance

Raspberry leaf has been a staple in herbal remedies used by African American herbalists, especially in the care of women's health. Its use has been passed down through generations, often in the form of teas, but it is also smoked in certain traditions. While generally safe, raspberry leaf should be used cautiously by pregnant women, as it is traditionally used to tone the uterus. Always consult with a healthcare provider if you are pregnant or breastfeeding.

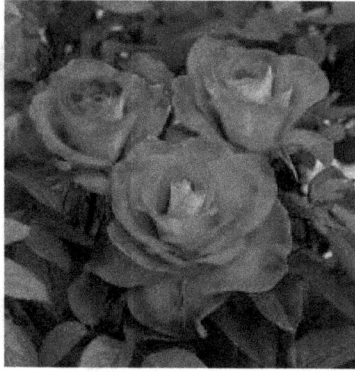

Rose (Rosa spp.)

Emotional Healing

Rose petals are known for their ability to open the heart chakra, providing emotional balance and promoting feelings of love, peace, and compassion. Smoking rose petals can help alleviate symptoms of depression and anxiety. Rose petals have mild expectorant properties, which can help clear mucus from the respiratory tract. They are also gentle on the lungs, making them a good choice for those with sensitive respiratory systems. Roses are rich in antioxidants and have anti-inflammatory properties that can help reduce inflammation in the body.

Cultural and Historical Significance

Roses have been used in various cultural rituals and remedies, including African American spiritual practices. Rose water, rose oil, and rose petals are often incorporated into healing rituals to promote love, healing, and spiritual growth. Ensure that the roses used for smoking are organic and free from pesticides. Smoking rose petals in moderation is key to avoid potential irritation to the lungs.

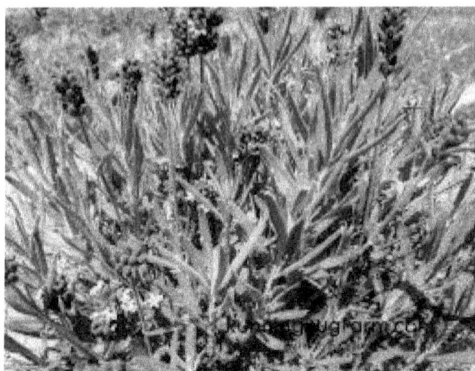

Lavender (Lavandula angustifolia)

Calming and Relaxation

Lavender is renowned for its calming effects, making it an excellent herb for reducing stress, anxiety, and promoting restful sleep. When smoked, it can quickly help ease tension and provide a sense of tranquility. Lavender has mild expectorant properties that can help clear the respiratory tract, making it useful for relieving coughs and colds.

Mood Enhancement

The soothing aroma and effects of lavender can help elevate mood and relieve symptoms of depression.

Cultural and Historical Significance

Lavender has been used in African American herbal practices, often as a calming agent in times of stress or emotional turmoil. Its calming properties have made it a staple in both spiritual and medicinal uses. Lavender is generally safe to smoke but should be used in moderation. Overuse can lead to headaches or mild dizziness. Always ensure the lavender is organic and free from chemicals.

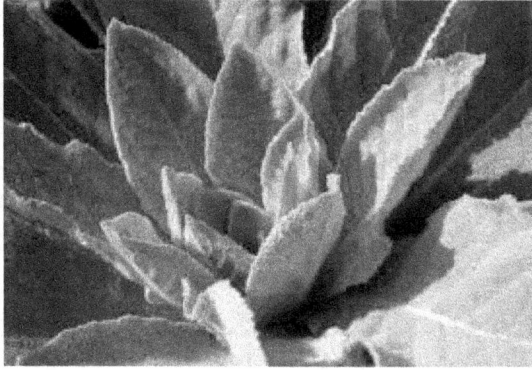

Mullein (Verbascum thapsus)

Respiratory Support

Mullein is one of the most effective herbs for respiratory health. When smoked, it helps to clear congestion, soothe the lungs, and alleviate symptoms of asthma, bronchitis, and other respiratory conditions.

Anti-inflammatory

Mullein has anti-inflammatory properties that can help reduce inflammation in the respiratory tract, making it easier to breathe.

Detoxification

Smoking mullein can help cleanse the lungs of toxins, which is particularly beneficial for former tobacco smokers.

Cultural and Historical Significance

Mullein has been used in traditional African American medicine as a remedy for respiratory issues. Its use was passed down through generations, often in the form of teas or smoked in pipes. Mullein is generally considered safe to smoke, but it should be dried properly to avoid mold. Always use organic mullein to avoid exposure to pesticides.

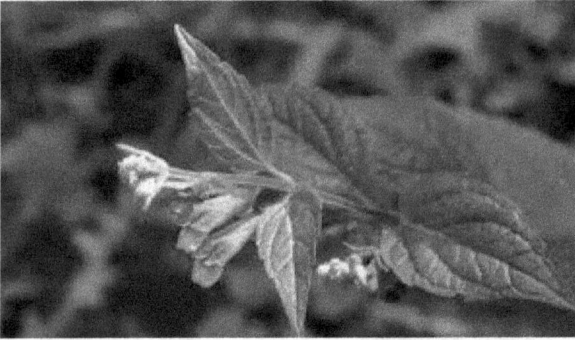

Skullcap (Scutellaria lateriflora)

Nervous System Support

Skullcap is known for its ability to calm the nervous system, making it effective for reducing anxiety, stress, and promoting relaxation. Smoking skullcap can help alleviate symptoms of insomnia and nervous tension.

Pain Relief

Skullcap has mild analgesic properties, which can help relieve pain, particularly headaches, and muscle tension.

Mood Stabilization

Skullcap is often used to stabilize mood, making it beneficial for those dealing with emotional instability or mood swings.

Cultural and Historical Significance

Skullcap has been used in African American herbalism as a calming herb, often included in blends for relaxation and emotional healing. Its use reflects a broader tradition of utilizing herbs to address mental and emotional health. Skullcap should be used with caution, as excessive use can lead to dizziness or confusion. Always start with small amounts to gauge your body's reaction.

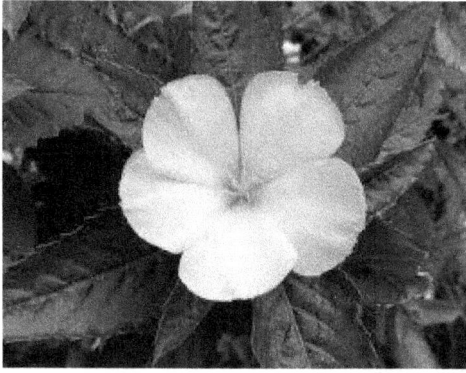
Damiana (Turnera diffusa)

Aphrodisiac
Damiana is well-known for its aphrodisiac properties, helping to enhance libido and sexual function. When smoked, it can increase energy and improve mood.

Mood Enhancement
Damiana has uplifting effects on the mind and can help alleviate symptoms of depression and anxiety. Damiana can be smoked to relieve respiratory issues, as it acts as a mild expectorant, helping to clear the lungs of mucus.

Cultural and Historical Significance
Damiana has been used in African American herbal practices as a tonic for both physical and emotional well-being. It is often included in blends designed to enhance vitality and mood. Damiana should be used in moderation. Overuse can lead to mild hallucinations or dizziness. It is important to source damiana from a reputable supplier to ensure its quality.

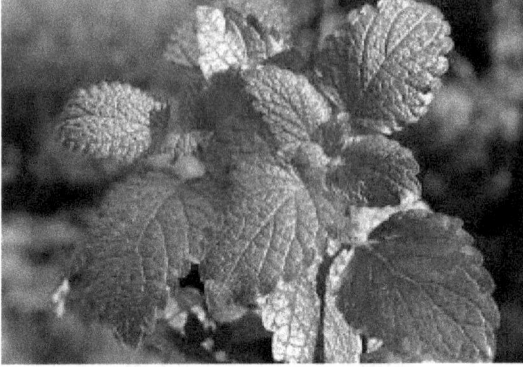

Peppermint (Mentha piperita)

Respiratory Relief

Peppermint is highly effective for clearing the respiratory tract, reducing congestion, and soothing the lungs. When smoked, it provides a cooling sensation that can relieve respiratory discomfort.

Digestive Support

Smoking peppermint can help alleviate symptoms of indigestion, nausea, and other digestive issues.

Mental Clarity

The invigorating effects of peppermint can enhance mental clarity, focus, and concentration.

Cultural and Historical Significance

Peppermint has been a part of African American herbal traditions, used both as a culinary herb and for its medicinal properties. It is often included in remedies for respiratory and digestive health. Peppermint is generally safe to smoke, but it should be used in moderation. Excessive use can lead to throat irritation.

Safe and Respectful Use of Smoking Herbs

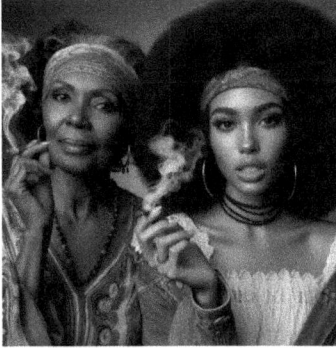

Smoking herbs can be a powerful way to connect with nature, support health, and tap into ancient traditions. However, it is important to approach this practice with respect and caution. Always source your herbs from reputable suppliers, ensure they are organic and free from pesticides, and use them in moderation. Smoking herbs is not without risks, and it's essential to be mindful of how your body responds.

Final Warnings and Instructions

Moderation: Start with small amounts and pay attention to how your body reacts. Each person's body is different, and what works for one person may not work for another. **Pregnancy and Health Conditions:** If you are pregnant, breastfeeding, or have pre-existing health conditions, consult with a healthcare provider before smoking any herbs. Some herbs can have strong effects on the body and may not be safe for everyone. **Environment:** Always smoke herbs in a well-ventilated area to avoid inhaling too much smoke. Consider using a pipe or rolling your herbs in organic papers to minimize the intake of harmful substances. **Mindfulness:** Smoking herbs should be done with intention and mindfulness. Approach it as a ritual that honors both your body and the plant's healing properties.

Herbs like mugwort, raspberry leaf, rose, lavender, and others offer a holistic way to support health through smoking, connecting us to ancient traditions and natural healing. By understanding their effects, cultural significance, and the importance of respectful use, we can incorporate these practices into our lives in a way that honors their origins and promotes overall well-being. Always approach the use of smoking herbs with caution, respect, and mindfulness, ensuring that you are enhancing your health and well-being in a safe and intentional manner.

Therapeutic Marijuana Smoking

Marijuana, derived from the Cannabis plant, has long been valued in herbal medicine for its therapeutic properties. When approached from a holistic and mindful perspective, marijuana smoking can offer significant health benefits. However, it is essential to balance these benefits with an understanding of potential risks and to incorporate supportive herbal practices.

Chronic Pain Management

Marijuana is highly effective for managing chronic pain conditions. The active compounds THC and CBD interact with the body's endocannabinoid system to reduce pain perception. Herbalists may enhance this effect by combining marijuana with other pain-relieving herbs like turmeric and ginger, known for their anti-inflammatory properties.

Marijuana smoking can offer significant therapeutic benefits. By integrating supportive herbs, adopting alternative consumption methods, and practicing mindful use, individuals can harness the healing properties of marijuana while maintaining overall health and well-being.

Anxiety and Stress Reduction

Certain strains of marijuana can help alleviate anxiety and stress. Indica strains, in particular, are known for their calming effects. Herbalists often recommend integrating marijuana with adaptogenic herbs such as ashwagandha and valerian root to further support stress management and promote relaxation. ***Mood Enhancement:*** Marijuana can elevate mood and promote a sense of well-being. Herbs like St. John's wort and lavender can be used alongside marijuana to enhance its mood-stabilizing effects.

Sleep Support

Insomnia Relief: Marijuana, particularly strains high in THC, can be effective in treating insomnia by promoting deeper and more restful sleep. Combining marijuana with sleep-supportive herbs such as chamomile and passionflower can create a more comprehensive approach to managing sleep disorders.

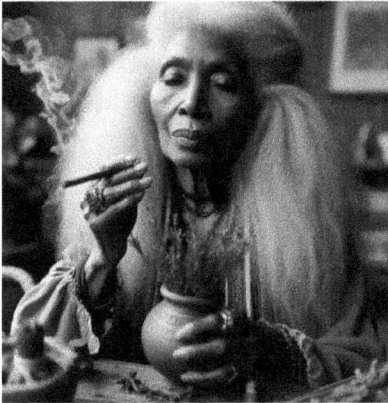

Appetite Stimulation and Nausea Reduction

Marijuana is well-known for its ability to stimulate appetite and reduce nausea, making it beneficial for individuals undergoing treatments like chemotherapy. Herbalists may suggest combining marijuana with digestive-supportive herbs like peppermint and ginger to enhance these effects and promote overall digestive health.

Respiratory Health Considerations

While marijuana smoking can provide therapeutic benefits, it also presents respiratory health considerations. Herbalists recommend several strategies to mitigate these risks.

Alternative Consumption Methods

Vaporization: Using a vaporizer to consume marijuana can significantly reduce the intake of harmful combustion by-products compared to traditional smoking. *Edibles and Tinctures:* Consuming marijuana as edibles or tinctures eliminates respiratory risks entirely, providing a safer alternative for those concerned about lung health.

Supportive Herbs for Respiratory Health

Mullein: Known for its ability to soothe irritated lung tissues and clear mucus, mullein can be a valuable herb for individuals who smoke marijuana. *Eucalyptus:* Inhaling eucalyptus oil vapors can help open airways and promote easier breathing, complementing the therapeutic effects of marijuana. *Thyme:* With its antiseptic properties, thyme can help clear respiratory infections and mucus.

119

Enhancing Therapeutic Effects with Herbal Blends

Combining marijuana with other medicinal herbs can create synergistic effects, enhancing its therapeutic benefits. Some recommended herbal blends.

Pain Relief Blend

Marijuana, Turmeric, and Ginger: This combination leverages the anti-inflammatory properties of turmeric and ginger to complement marijuana's pain-relieving effects.

Stress and Anxiety Relief Blend

Marijuana, Ashwagandha, and Valerian Root: This blend combines the calming effects of marijuana with the adaptogenic properties of ashwagandha and the relaxing qualities of valerian root.

Sleep Support Blend

Marijuana, Chamomile, and Passionflower: This combination promotes deep and restful sleep, addressing insomnia and sleep disorders effectively.

Harm Reduction and Mindful Use

To maximize the therapeutic benefits of marijuana while minimizing potential risks, herbalists advocate for mindful use and harm reduction strategies.

Limiting Frequency and Quantity

Using marijuana in moderation can help reduce the risk of dependency and adverse effects. ***Strain Selection***: Choosing strains with balanced THC-to-CBD ratios can help manage side effects such as anxiety and paranoia.

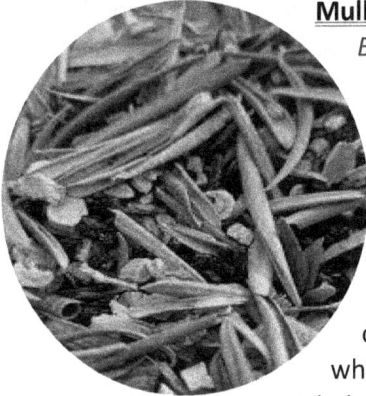

Mullein Leaf

Benefits Soothes the respiratory tract, reduces inflammation *Treatment* Known for its ability to reduce inflammation and soothe irritation in the respiratory tract, helping to relieve cough and congestion.

Thyme

Benefits Antimicrobial properties, helps clear mucus *Treatment* Contains thymol, which acts as a natural expectorant and antimicrobial agent, making it effective in clearing mucus and fighting respiratory infections.

Peppermint

Benefits Contains menthol, which opens airways and eases breathing *Treatment* Menthol in peppermint acts as a natural decongestant, relaxing the muscles of the respiratory tract and facilitating easier breathing.

Eucalyptus

Benefits Acts as a decongestant, reduces inflammation *Treatment* Eucalyptus oil helps open up the airways, reduces inflammation, and has antimicrobial properties that can help clear respiratory infections.

Ginger

Benefits Anti-inflammatory, helps reduce throat and airway irritation *Treatment* Ginger's anti-inflammatory properties help soothe irritated airways and reduce coughing and bronchial spasms.

Licorice Root

Benefits Soothes mucous membranes, has anti-inflammatory properties *Treatment* Contains glycyrrhizin, which soothes and protects mucous membranes and reduces inflammation in the respiratory tract.

Turmeric

Benefits Anti-inflammatory, may reduce airway inflammation *Treatment* Curcumin in turmeric has powerful anti-inflammatory effects that can help reduce inflammation and swelling in the airways.

Echinacea

Benefits Boosts immune system, may help prevent respiratory infections *Treatment* echinacea can help prevent and shorten the duration of respiratory infections. Known for its immune-boosting properties,

Garlic

Benefits Antimicrobial and anti-inflammatory, supports immune function *Treatment* Garlic has strong antimicrobial properties and can help fight respiratory infections while reducing inflammation.

Elderberry

Benefits Antiviral properties, helps reduce symptoms of colds and flu *Treatment* Contains antioxidants and vitamins that boost the immune system and help reduce the severity and duration of respiratory infections like colds and flu.

Osha Root

Benefits Helps clear mucus, supports respiratory function *Treatment* Known as a lung tonic, it helps clear mucus from the lungs and supports overall respiratory health.

Schisandra

Benefits Supports respiratory health, acts as an adaptogen *Treatment* Helps protect the lungs from oxidative stress and enhances respiratory function by supporting overall lung health.

Yarrow

Benefits Antimicrobial and anti-inflammatory properties *Treatment* Helps reduce fever, clears mucus, and has astringent properties that can aid in treating respiratory infections.

Black Seed Oil

Benefits Anti-inflammatory and immune-boosting properties *Treatment* Contains thymoquinone, which has potent anti-inflammatory and antioxidant effects that can support respiratory health and reduce asthma symptoms.

Plantain

Benefits Soothes mucous membranes, has antimicrobial properties *Treatment* Acts as a demulcent and expectorant, helping to soothe and protect the respiratory tract while clearing mucus.

Gaia-Grown Nettle
Benefits Supports respiratory health, anti-inflammatory properties *Treatment* Nettle is rich in nutrients and acts as an anti-inflammatory agent, helping to alleviate symptoms of allergies and other respiratory conditions.

Oil of Oregano
Benefits Strong antimicrobial and antiviral properties *Treatment* Contains carvacrol and thymol, which have strong antimicrobial properties that can help fight respiratory infections and reduce inflammation.

Mullein Flower
Benefits Helps with coughs, bronchitis, and other lung issues *Treatment* Similar to mullein leaf, it soothes the respiratory tract and helps reduce inflammation, making it effective in treating coughs and bronchitis.

Elecampane Root
Benefits Expectorant and antimicrobial properties *Treatment* Helps clear mucus from the lungs and has antimicrobial properties that can help treat respiratory infections.

Marshmallow Root & Leaf
Benefits Soothes mucous membranes, acts as a demulcent *Treatment* Contains mucilage, which coats and soothes the mucous membranes, reducing irritation and inflammation in the respiratory tract.

Common Mallow
Benefits Soothes and protects the mucous membranes, reduces inflammation *Treatment* Acts as a demulcent, providing a soothing film over mucous membranes, which helps relieve irritation and inflammation in the respiratory tract.

White Horehound
Benefits Stimulant action on mucus production, antimicrobial properties, works on both upper and lower respiratory systems *Treatment* Stimulates the production of mucus, helping the body expel it, and contains antimicrobial properties that support respiratory health.

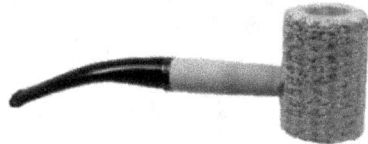

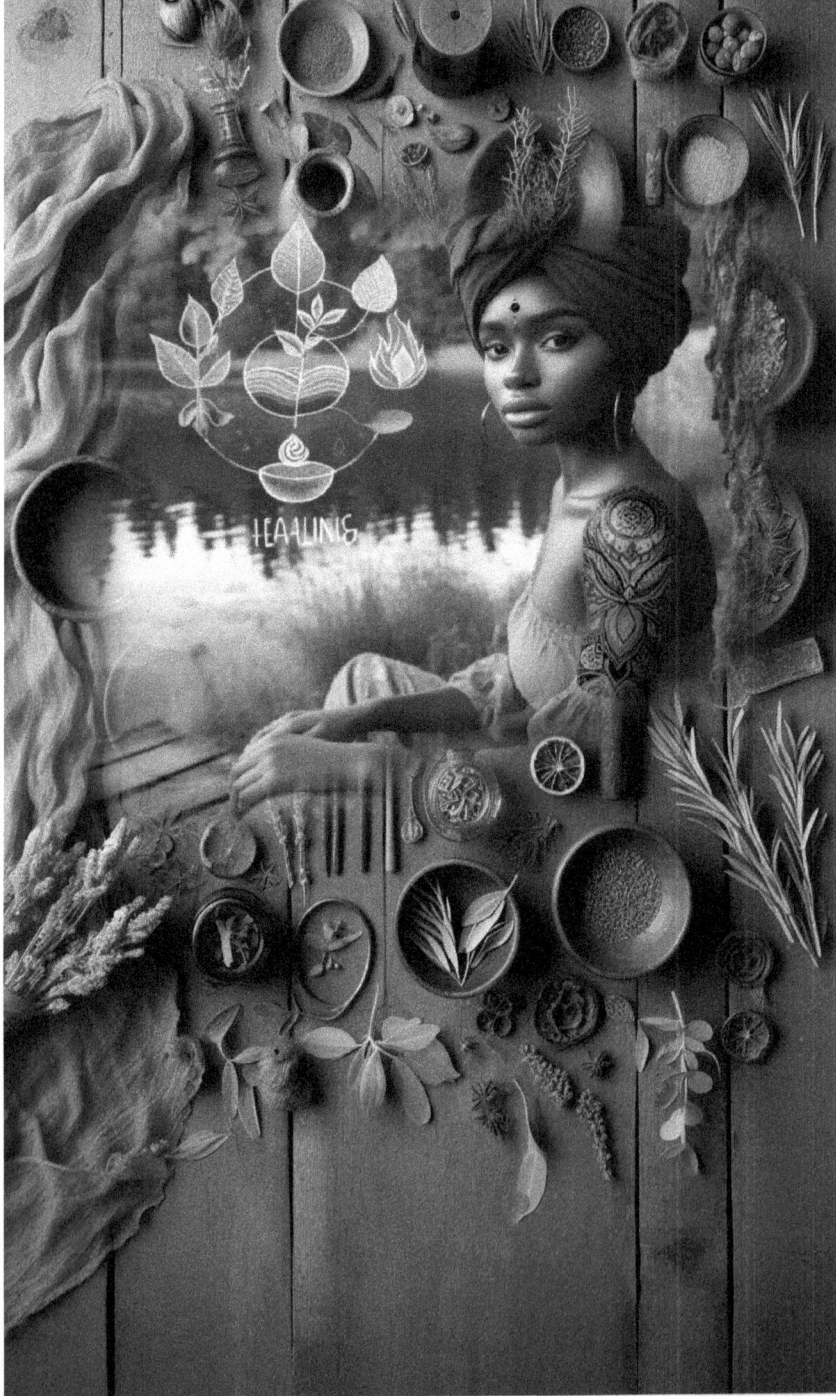

Chapter 6
Journey Into the Elements for Healing

Ether the Fifth Element

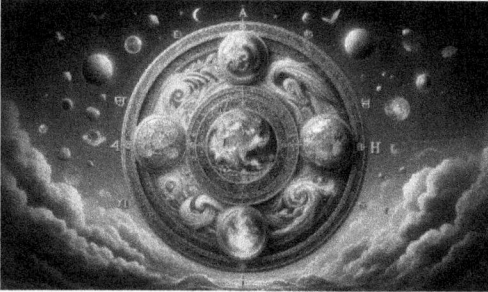

The ether, often referred to as the "fifth element" or "quintessence," has roots in ancient philosophies and sciences. In various cultures, the ether was believed to be the subtle, invisible force that filled the universe, existing beyond the physical elements of earth, water, fire, and air. Before the 1920s, the concept of ether was prevalent in both Eastern and Western thought, seen as the medium through which light and energy traveled, and as the substance that connected all living beings to the cosmos.

In ancient healing traditions, particularly those from Africa and other non-Western cultures, the ether was associated with the unseen aspects of health and wellness—the spiritual and energetic dimensions that modern medicine often overlooks. For African American health and well-being, reconnecting with the concept of ether can be profoundly empowering. It encourages a holistic approach to health, one that goes beyond the physical symptoms to address the spiritual and energetic imbalances that may underlie illness.

Ether, as an ancient concept, reminds us that health is not just about the body but also about the mind, spirit, and the energy that flows within and around us. Practices such as meditation, deep breathing, and spending time in nature can help us tap into this etheric energy, promoting a sense of balance and well-being that is essential for healing. By embracing a more holistic understanding of health—one that includes the subtle energies that connect us to the universe—we can cultivate a more complete and profound sense of wellness.

The Fifth Element for our Bodies

Acknowledging and harnessing the concept of ether can serve as a powerful means of reconnecting with ancestral wisdom that has been passed down through generations. This wisdom, rooted in traditional African healing practices, often emphasized the importance of the spiritual and energetic aspects of health. By recognizing the significance of ether, African Americans can tap into this legacy, integrating ancient practices into modern health routines.

One way to harness this energy is by incorporating rituals and practices that honor the connection between the physical and spiritual realms. For example, meditation, prayer, and energy-based therapies like Reiki can be used to align the body's energies, promote healing, and maintain balance. Additionally, engaging with nature, such as spending time near water or under the open sky, can help in accessing the etheric energy that surrounds us, providing a sense of grounding and spiritual rejuvenation.

Incorporating these practices into modern health routines allows African Americans to reclaim a holistic approach to wellness that respects both the body and the spirit. This can lead to more personalized and culturally resonant health practices that address not just physical symptoms but also the deeper, often overlooked, aspects of well-being. By integrating this ancient wisdom with contemporary health practices, African Americans can create a more comprehensive and empowering approach to health that honors their cultural heritage and promotes overall wellness

Air: The Vital Role of Clean, Fresh Air

Air Clean, fresh air is essential for respiratory health and overall well-being. Breathing exercises and spending time in nature can increase oxygen intake and improve mental clarity. Practice deep breathing exercises, spend time outdoors in clean air environments, and use air purifiers at home.

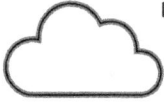

Air is a fundamental element essential for life and well-being. Clean, fresh air supports respiratory health, enhances mental clarity, and contributes to overall vitality. Our respiratory system relies on the intake of oxygen from the air to fuel cellular functions and maintain bodily processes. Ensuring access to clean air and integrating practices that improve air quality can have significant benefits for physical and mental health.

Respiratory Health

Clean air is crucial for maintaining healthy respiratory function. Pollutants, allergens, and other airborne contaminants can negatively impact the lungs and respiratory system, leading to conditions such as asthma, bronchitis, and chronic obstructive pulmonary disease (COPD). Fresh, unpolluted air supports optimal lung function, reduces the risk of respiratory infections, and improves overall respiratory health. Regular exposure to clean air helps the lungs expel toxins more efficiently and maintain their ability to perform essential functions.

Mental Clarity

Adequate oxygen intake is essential for cognitive function and mental clarity. Fresh air enhances the delivery of oxygen to the brain, which can improve concentration, memory, and cognitive performance. Spending time in nature and breathing in clean air has been shown to reduce mental fatigue, alleviate stress, and enhance mood. The restorative effects of natural environments contribute to improved mental well-being and a heightened sense of clarity and focus.

Benefits of Deep Breathing Exercises

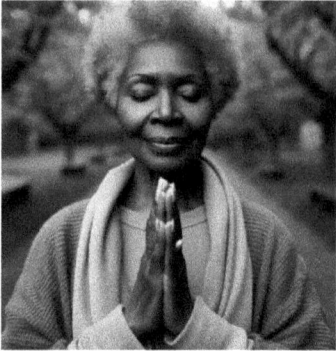

Deep breathing exercises are a practical way to increase oxygen intake and promote relaxation. These exercises help to expand the lungs, improve oxygenation of the blood, and reduce stress. By engaging in deep, controlled breathing, you can enhance your body's ability to utilize oxygen more effectively and support overall respiratory health. Deep breathing also activates the parasympathetic nervous system, which can promote a state of calm and relaxation.

How to Incorporate Clean Air Practices

Practice Deep Breathing Exercises

Incorporate deep breathing exercises into your daily routine to enhance oxygen intake and support respiratory health. Try practices such as diaphragmatic breathing, where you breathe deeply into the diaphragm rather than shallow breaths into the chest. Perform these exercises for a few minutes several times a day, especially during moments of stress or mental fatigue. Techniques like the 4-7-8 method or box breathing can also help improve focus and relaxation.

Spend Time Outdoors

Make time to spend outdoors in clean, natural environments. Activities such as walking in parks, hiking in nature reserves, or simply sitting outside in fresh air can provide significant benefits for respiratory and mental health. Aim to spend at least 30 minutes a day in nature to experience the restorative effects of fresh air. If you live in an area with poor air quality, consider visiting nearby natural spaces that are less affected by pollution.

Use Air Purifiers

Air purifiers can help maintain a clean indoor environment by filtering out pollutants, allergens, and particulate matter. Invest in high-quality air purifiers with HEPA filters to reduce indoor air pollution and improve air quality in your home. Regularly clean or replace filters as recommended to ensure the effective operation of your air purifier. Additionally, maintain good ventilation by opening windows or using exhaust fans to promote air circulation and reduce indoor pollutants.

Create Air Quality Zones

Designate specific areas in your home or workplace as air quality zones. Use air purifiers and Houseplants such as spider plants, peace lilies, and snake plants can naturally improve indoor air quality by absorbing pollutants and releasing oxygen. Ensure that these zones are well-ventilated and free from excessive dust and smoke. Houseplants that help filter and clean the air in these areas.

Monitor Air Quality

Stay informed about local air quality levels, especially if you live in areas prone to air pollution. Use air quality monitoring apps or websites to track pollution levels and take appropriate actions to minimize exposure. On days with high pollution levels, limit outdoor activities or use protective measures such as masks if necessary.

Fire (Heat/Thermotherapy): The Power of Heat

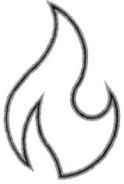

Fire (Heat/Thermotherapy) Heat can relieve muscle tension, improve circulation, and promote relaxation. It can also aid in detoxification through sweating. Use saunas, hot baths, or heating pads. Practice safe sun exposure for vitamin D synthesis.

Heat therapy, also known as thermotherapy, is a powerful tool for promoting health and well-being through the application of heat. The use of heat can offer a wide range of benefits, from relieving muscle tension and improving circulation to aiding in detoxification and enhancing relaxation. By understanding and utilizing heat effectively, you can support your body's healing processes and improve your overall quality of life.

Tension Relief of Muscle

One of the primary benefits of heat therapy is its ability to relieve muscle tension and reduce pain. Applying heat to sore or stiff muscles helps to increase blood flow to the affected area, which can alleviate discomfort and facilitate faster healing. Heat therapy works by relaxing the muscles, reducing spasms, and improving flexibility. This can be particularly beneficial for individuals experiencing muscle strain, chronic pain conditions, or tension from stress.

Improved Circulation

Heat therapy enhances circulation by dilating blood vessels and increasing blood flow. This improved circulation helps to deliver oxygen and nutrients to tissues, while also removing waste products. Enhanced blood flow can contribute to faster recovery from injuries and support overall cardiovascular health. The increased warmth also helps to soothe aching joints and promote the healing of damaged tissues.

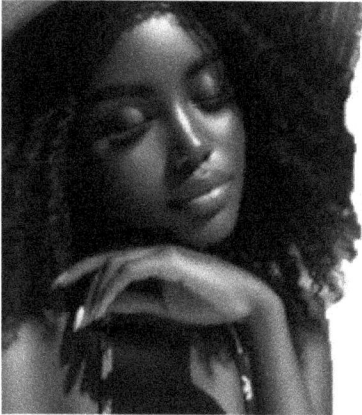

Promotion of Relaxation

The soothing effect of heat can have a profound impact on relaxation and stress reduction. Warm baths, saunas, and hot packs create a comforting environment that can help calm the nervous system and promote a sense of well-being. This relaxation response can be particularly beneficial for individuals dealing with high levels of stress, anxiety, or insomnia. By incorporating heat therapy into your routine, you can create a calming experience that supports both physical and mental relaxation.

Detoxification Through Sweating

Heat exposure can aid in the body's natural detoxification processes through sweating. Saunas and steam rooms induce sweating, which helps to flush out toxins and impurities from the body. This process of sweating not only supports detoxification but also contributes to improved skin health and a general sense of rejuvenation. Regular use of saunas or steam baths can enhance the body's ability to eliminate waste products and promote overall health.

Sun Exposure for Vitamin D Synthesis

In addition to direct applications of heat, safe sun exposure is another way to benefit from the power of fire. Sunlight is a natural source of ultraviolet (UV) rays, which are essential for the synthesis of vitamin D in the skin. Vitamin D plays a crucial role in bone health, immune function, and overall well-being. It is important to practice safe sun exposure by using sunscreen, wearing protective clothing, and avoiding excessive sun exposure to minimize the risk of skin damage while reaping the benefits of vitamin D.

How to Practice Heat Therapy

Saunas

Using a sauna is a popular method of heat therapy that can promote relaxation and support detoxification. Saunas use dry or moist heat to induce sweating and provide a range of health benefits. Aim to use the sauna for 15-20 minutes per session, allowing your body to acclimate to the heat. Stay hydrated before, during, and after your sauna session to support the detoxification process and prevent dehydration.

Hot Baths

Taking a warm bath can be a simple yet effective way to relieve muscle tension and promote relaxation. Add Epsom salts or essential oils to the bathwater to enhance its therapeutic effects. Soak in the bath for 15-30 minutes to enjoy the calming and soothing benefits of heat.

Heating Pads

Heating pads provide localized heat to specific areas of the body, such as the back, neck, or shoulders. Use a heating pad for 15-20 minutes at a time, ensuring that it is not too hot to avoid burns. Heating pads can be particularly useful for managing chronic pain or muscle soreness.

Safe Sun Exposure

To benefit from vitamin D synthesis, aim for moderate sun exposure. Spend 10-30 minutes in the sun, depending on your skin type and location, while protecting your skin with sunscreen. Avoid peak sun hours and use protective clothing if necessary.

Electricity: Balancing the Body's Electric Field

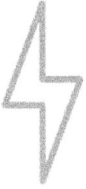

Electricity The body's natural electric field can be balanced by grounding, which may reduce inflammation, improve sleep, and enhance overall health. Use grounding mats or sheets, walk barefoot on natural surfaces, and avoid excessive exposure to artificial electromagnetic fields.

Electricity, in the form of the body's natural electric field, plays a crucial role in maintaining physiological balance and overall health. The concept of grounding, or earthing, involves aligning the body's electrical state with the Earth's natural electric field. This practice has been associated with various health benefits, including reduced inflammation, improved sleep, and enhanced well-being. Understanding how to harness the benefits of grounding and manage exposure to artificial electromagnetic fields can support a healthier lifestyle.

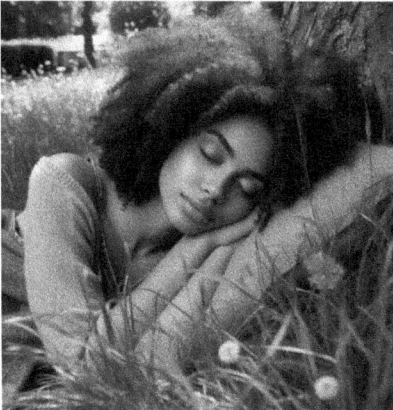

Balancing the Body's Electric Field

The human body generates its own electric field, which is essential for various bodily functions, including nerve signaling, muscle contraction, and cellular processes. Grounding helps to balance this electric field by connecting the body to the Earth's natural electric charge. This connection allows for the transfer of electrons from the Earth to the body, which can neutralize free radicals and reduce oxidative stress. This process is thought to alleviate inflammation, improve immune function, and support overall health.

133

Reducing Inflammation

Inflammation is a common underlying factor in many chronic diseases and conditions. Grounding has been shown to reduce inflammation by neutralizing free radicals and improving the body's electrical balance. By maintaining a proper electric field through grounding, the body can better manage inflammatory responses and promote healing. This can be particularly beneficial for individuals with chronic inflammatory conditions or those recovering from injuries.

Improving Sleep

Quality sleep is vital for overall health and well-being. Grounding can enhance sleep quality by promoting a more balanced electric field, which may help regulate circadian rhythms and improve sleep patterns. Studies suggest that grounding can lead to faster sleep onset, longer sleep duration, and reduced wakefulness during the night. This is achieved by aligning the body's electrical state with the Earth's natural rhythms, which can support more restful and restorative sleep.

Enhancing Overall Health

Beyond specific benefits such as reducing inflammation and improving sleep, grounding can contribute to overall health and well-being. By maintaining a balanced electric field, the body can better manage stress, improve energy levels, and support general health. Grounding practices can also foster a sense of connection with nature, which can enhance mental and emotional well-being.

How to Incorporate Grounding Practices

Grounding Mats and Sheets

Grounding mats and sheets are designed to connect the body with the Earth's electric field while indoors. These products are made from conductive materials that allow the transfer of electrons from the Earth to the body. To use a grounding mat, place it on a bed or floor and ensure that it is connected to a grounding point (such as a grounded outlet). Sleep on the mat or use it while sitting or working for at least a few hours a day to experience the benefits.

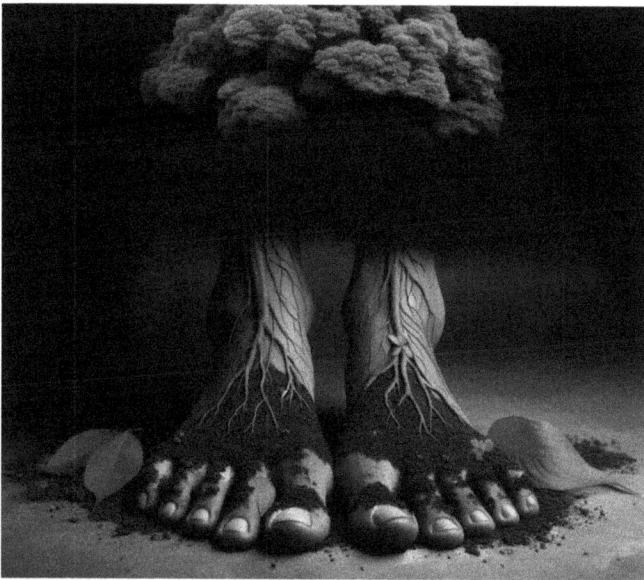

Walking Barefoot on Natural Surfaces

One of the simplest and most natural ways to ground is by walking barefoot on natural surfaces such as grass, soil, or sand. Aim to spend 20-30 minutes a day walking barefoot in a natural environment. This practice allows direct contact with the Earth's surface and promotes the transfer of electrons to the body. If walking barefoot outside is not feasible, consider creating a small indoor area with natural materials like sand or gravel for grounding purposes.

Avoiding Excessive Exposure to Artificial

Electromagnetic Fields

Artificial electromagnetic fields (EMFs) are emitted by various electronic devices, such as smartphones, computers, and Wi-Fi routers. Excessive exposure to EMFs can disrupt the body's natural electric field and contribute to various health issues. To minimize exposure, practice measures such as reducing screen time, using speakerphone or headphones during phone calls, and keeping electronic devices at a distance while sleeping.

Creating Grounding Spaces

Set up dedicated grounding areas in your home or workplace where you can spend time in direct contact with natural materials. This could include using grounding mats, sitting on natural surfaces, or incorporating elements of nature into your living space. Regularly spending time in these spaces can help maintain a balanced electric field and support overall health.

Water: The Essence of Life and Health

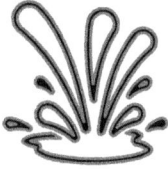

Water Water is crucial for hydration, detoxification, and overall bodily functions. It can also have a calming and healing effect when used in baths or hydrotherapy. Drink at least 8 glasses of water a day, take regular baths, and consider hydrotherapy treatments like hot tubs or spa sessions.

Water is a fundamental component of life, playing a critical role in virtually every bodily function. Its importance extends far beyond merely quenching thirst; water is essential for hydration, detoxification, and the overall maintenance of bodily functions. Proper hydration ensures that our cells, tissues, and organs operate efficiently. Each day, our bodies lose water through various processes such as breathing, sweating, and digestion, making it vital to replenish this loss to maintain optimal health.

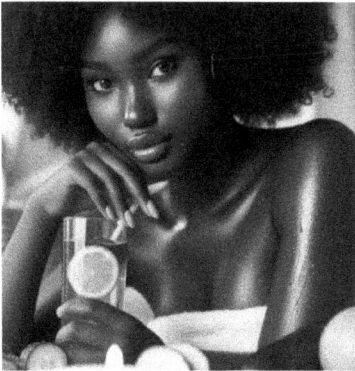

Hydration

One of the primary benefits of water is its role in hydration. Every cell in the human body relies on water to function correctly. Adequate hydration helps to regulate body temperature, lubricate joints, and support metabolic processes. It also aids in the transportation of nutrients and oxygen to cells, and in the removal of waste products from the body. Dehydration, even in its mild forms, can impair physical performance, cognitive function, and mood. Severe dehydration can lead to serious health complications, emphasizing the importance of regular water intake.

Detoxification

Water is a natural detoxifier, facilitating the elimination of toxins from the body. The kidneys, liver, and other organs depend on water to filter and expel waste products. Drinking sufficient water helps to maintain the health and efficiency of these organs. It supports kidney function by preventing kidney stones and urinary tract infections, which can result from concentrated urine. Additionally, water assists in bowel regularity and prevents constipation, further aiding in the body's detoxification processes.

Calming and Healing Effects

Beyond its physiological functions, water also has calming and healing properties, particularly when used in baths or hydrotherapy. Immersing the body in water can provide a sense of relaxation and stress relief. Warm baths can soothe sore muscles, alleviate tension, and promote a sense of well-being. Hydrotherapy, which involves the use of water in various forms (such as hot tubs, whirlpools, and steam baths), is a therapeutic approach that harnesses the healing properties of water to treat conditions such as arthritis, muscle pain, and stress-related ailments. The buoyancy of water also reduces the strain on joints and muscles, making it an excellent medium for physical therapy and rehabilitation.

Incorporating Water into Your Daily Routine

Drinking 8 Glasses a Day

To maintain proper hydration, it is recommended to drink at least eight 8-ounce glasses of water daily, commonly referred to as the "8x8 rule." This guideline ensures that the body receives an adequate supply of water to support its various functions. However, individual water needs can vary based on factors such as age, gender, weight, climate, and physical activity levels. It's essential to listen to your body's signals and drink water whenever you feel thirsty. For those who engage in intense physical activities or live in hot climates, the need for water may be higher.

Regular Baths

Taking regular baths can be a simple yet effective way to harness the therapeutic benefits of water. A warm bath can help to relax the body and mind, relieve muscle tension, and promote a restful night's sleep. Adding Epsom salts or essential oils to the bath can enhance its therapeutic effects, providing additional benefits such as reducing inflammation and improving skin health.

Hydrotherapy Treatments

Hydrotherapy treatments, such as hot tubs, spa sessions, and contrast baths, can offer profound health benefits. Hot tubs and whirlpools can soothe sore muscles and joints, enhance circulation, and promote relaxation. Contrast baths, which involve alternating between hot and cold water, can stimulate blood flow and reduce inflammation. Spa sessions that include steam rooms or saunas can aid in detoxification through sweating, improve respiratory function, and provide a deep sense of relaxation.

The Power of the Earth/Soil/Clay/Ground

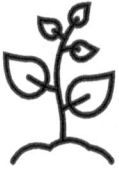

Earth/Soil/Clay/Ground Contact with soil or clay can provide minerals, promote relaxation, and reduce inflammation. Grounding connects the body to the Earth's electrons, promoting balance. Walk barefoot on grass, use clay masks for skin health, and engage in gardening or soil-based activities.

Engaging with the Earth through soil, clay, and natural ground offers profound benefits for physical and mental well-being. The practice of grounding, or earthing, involves direct physical contact with the Earth's surface, such as walking barefoot on grass or using clay. These practices harness the Earth's natural energy to support health and promote balance.

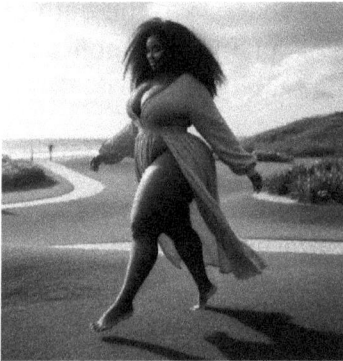

Contact with Soil and Clay

Direct interaction with soil and clay can provide a range of health benefits. The Earth is rich in minerals that are essential for bodily functions, including magnesium, potassium, and calcium. When we come into contact with soil, these minerals can be absorbed through the skin, supporting various physiological processes. Clay, in particular, has been used for centuries in traditional medicine for its therapeutic properties. It can help draw out toxins from the skin, reduce inflammation, and improve overall skin health.

Grounding and Electron Transfer

Grounding involves connecting the body directly with the Earth's surface to allow the transfer of electrons. This practice is believed to reduce inflammation, improve sleep, and enhance overall well-being by balancing the body's electrical charge. The Earth's electrons have antioxidant properties that can neutralize free radicals and reduce oxidative stress, contributing to reduced inflammation and improved health. Grounding can also promote a sense of calm and relaxation by reducing stress and improving mood.

Promoting Relaxation

Spending time in natural environments, such as walking barefoot on grass or engaging in gardening, can have a calming effect on the mind and body. The act of connecting with nature helps to reduce stress, anxiety, and mental fatigue. Natural settings provide a sensory experience that engages sight, sound, and touch, which can enhance relaxation and mental clarity. The simplicity of being in nature, away from the hustle and bustle of daily life, allows for a restorative and grounding experience.

Engaging in Gardening and Soil-Based Activities

Gardening and soil-based activities offer both physical and mental health benefits. Physical engagement with soil through gardening provides moderate exercise, which can improve cardiovascular health, strengthen muscles, and enhance flexibility. Additionally, interacting with soil exposes individuals to beneficial microbes that can support immune function and contribute to overall health. Gardening also provides a sense of accomplishment and satisfaction, further enhancing mental well-being.

How to Incorporate Earth-Based Practices

Walking Barefoot

To practice grounding, find a natural surface such as grass, sand, or soil. Spend 20-30 minutes walking barefoot, allowing your body to make direct contact with the Earth. This practice can be particularly beneficial in natural settings such as parks or gardens. If walking barefoot outside is not possible, consider using grounding mats or sheets designed to simulate the effects of direct contact with the Earth's surface.

Using Clay Masks

Clay masks can be used to improve skin health and detoxify the skin. Apply a thin layer of natural clay (such as bentonite or green clay) to the face or other areas of the body, and leave it on for 10-15 minutes before rinsing off. Clay masks help to draw out impurities, reduce inflammation, and improve skin texture. Use clay masks once a week for optimal results.

Gardening and Soil-Based Activities

Engage in gardening or other soil-based activities to reap the benefits of physical exercise and connection with the Earth. Whether tending to a vegetable garden, planting flowers, or simply digging in the soil, these activities provide a sense of connection to nature and promote physical and mental health. Aim to spend time in the garden regularly to maintain the benefits.

Grounding Practices

In addition to walking barefoot, consider other grounding practices such as sitting or lying on natural surfaces, such as grass or soil. Integrate grounding into your daily routine by spending time outdoors, engaging in nature walks, or participating in outdoor activities.

How To Practice Grounding

Walk barefoot on grass, sand, or soil for at least 30 minutes a day to experience grounding benefits. Use grounding mats, sheets, or patches that connect to the Earth's electrical field. Engage in gardening activities with direct contact with soil to benefit from grounding and exposure to beneficial microbes. Swim in natural bodies of water like oceans, lakes, or rivers to experience grounding through water.

Elemental Healing Practices

Air

Health Benefits Respiratory health, mental clarity *How To Practice* Deep breathing exercises, outdoor activities, air purifiers

Water

Health Benefits Hydration, detoxification, relaxation *How To Practice* Drink water, baths, hydrotherapy

Fire

Health Benefits Muscle relaxation, improved circulation, detoxification *How To Practice* Saunas, hot baths, heating pads, safe sun exposure

Earth

Health Benefits Mineral absorption, relaxation, inflammation reduction *How To Practice* Walking barefoot, clay masks, gardening

Electricity

Health Benefits Inflammation reduction, sleep improvement, overall balance *How To Practice* Grounding mats/sheets, barefoot walking, minimizing EMF exposure.

Instructions for Grounding

Choose a natural surface such as grass, sand, or soil. Avoid concrete or asphalt. Take off your shoes and socks to allow direct contact with the Earth. Walk, stand, or sit with your bare feet in contact with the ground for at least 30 minutes. Incorporate grounding into your daily routine to maximize health benefits. Use grounding time for meditation, deep breathing, or simply enjoying nature to enhance the experience.

The Importance of Copper

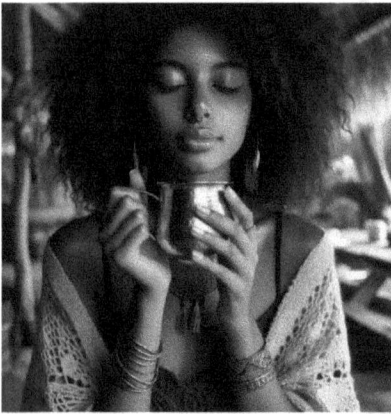

Copper is an essential mineral that supports a wide range of bodily functions, from red blood cell formation to brain health. Maintaining adequate copper levels is vital for overall well-being. By consuming a balanced diet rich in copper-containing foods, they can ensure they receive the necessary amount of this crucial mineral and enjoy its numerous health benefits.

Functions of Copper in the Body

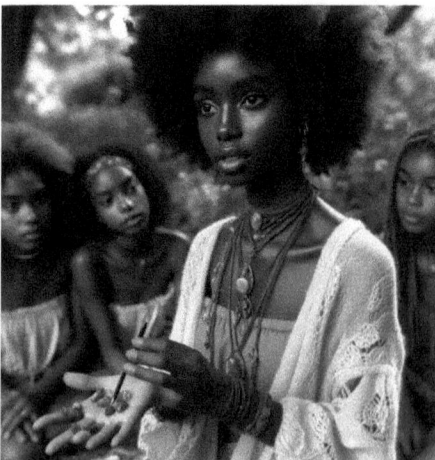

Copper is crucial for several physiological processes :**Red Blood Cell Formation** Copper helps in the production and maintenance of red blood cells. **Iron Absorption** It aids in the absorption and utilization of iron, preventing anemia.

Connective Tissue Health Copper is involved in the formation of collagen and elastin, essential for skin, bone, and joint health. *Brain Function* It supports neurodevelopment and cognitive function by aiding in the formation of neurotransmitters. *Antioxidant Defense* Copper is a component of superoxide dismutase, an antioxidant enzyme that protects cells from damage.

Copper Deficiency Symptoms

Copper deficiency, though rare, can lead to several health issues. Symptoms include: *Anemia* Due to impaired iron absorption and utilization. *Weak Immune System* Increased susceptibility to infections. *Bone and Joint Problems* Osteoporosis and joint pain due to poor collagen formation. *Neurological Issues* Problems such as numbness, tingling, and cognitive difficulties. *Skin Depigmentation* Loss of skin pigmentation and the development of gray hair.

Sources of Copper

Copper is found in a variety of foods, including: *Shellfish* Such as oysters, crabs, and lobster. *Nuts and Seeds* Including almonds, sunflower seeds, and sesame seeds. *Whole Grains* Such as quinoa, brown rice, and oats. *Dark Chocolate* A tasty source of copper. *Organ Meats* Such as liver.

Benefits of Adequate Copper Intake

Ensuring sufficient copper intake can provide several health benefits for Black women: *Enhanced Energy Levels* Improved red blood cell production boosts overall energy. *Better Skin and Hair Health* Supports collagen production and prevents premature graying. *Stronger Immune System* Helps in maintaining a robust immune response. *Improved Brain Function* Supports cognitive health and prevents neurodegenerative conditions. *Bone and Joint Health* Promotes healthy connective tissue, reducing the risk of osteoporosis and arthritis.

The Importance of Magnesium

Magnesium is an essential mineral that plays a crucial role in numerous bodily functions. Maintaining adequate magnesium levels is particularly important due to its significant impact on overall health, including gut health.

Functions of Magnesium in the Body

Magnesium play a role in over 300 biochemical reactions in the body. Key functions include: *Muscle and Nerve Function* Magnesium helps regulate muscle contractions and nerve signals. *Energy Production* It is essential for the production of adenosine triphosphate (ATP), the body's main energy source. *Bone Health Magnesium* contributes to bone formation and influences the activities of osteoblasts and osteoclasts. *Blood Sugar Control* It plays a role in glucose metabolism and insulin regulation. Heart Health Magnesium helps maintain a steady heartbeat and supports overall cardiovascular health.

Magnesium Deficiency Symptoms

Magnesium deficiency, also known as hypomagnesemia, can manifest in various ways. Common symptoms include: *Muscle Cramps and Spasms* Frequent muscle cramps, especially in the legs, can be a sign of low magnesium levels. *Fatigue and Weakness* A deficiency can lead to general fatigue and muscle weakness. *Irritability and Anxiety* Low magnesium levels can affect mood and increase feelings of irritability and anxiety. *Irregular Heartbeat* Magnesium deficiency can cause arrhythmias or irregular heartbeats. *Poor Bone Health* Long-term deficiency can contribute to osteoporosis and weakened bones.

Risks of Magnesium Overdose

While magnesium is essential, excessive intake can be harmful. Symptoms of magnesium overdose include: *Diarrhea* High doses of magnesium, particularly from supplements, can cause diarrhea. *Nausea and Vomiting* Overconsumption may lead to gastrointestinal distress. *Low Blood Pressure* Excessive magnesium can cause a significant drop in blood pressure. *Heart Problems* Severe overdose can lead to heart issues, including irregular heartbeat and cardiac arrest.

Benefits of Topical Magnesium

Topical magnesium, often applied as magnesium oil, offers several benefits: *Muscle Relaxation* It helps relieve muscle tension and cramps. *Improved Sleep* Magnesium oil can promote relaxation and improve sleep quality. *Skin Health* Topical application can enhance skin hydration and reduce inflammation. *Pain Relief* It can alleviate joint pain and muscle soreness.

Gut Health and Magnesium

Magnesium plays a vital role in maintaining gut health: *Digestive Function* It supports regular bowel movements and prevents constipation. *Microbiome Balance* Adequate magnesium levels contribute to a healthy gut microbiome. *Inflammation Reduction* Magnesium helps reduce gut inflammation and supports the integrity of the gut lining.

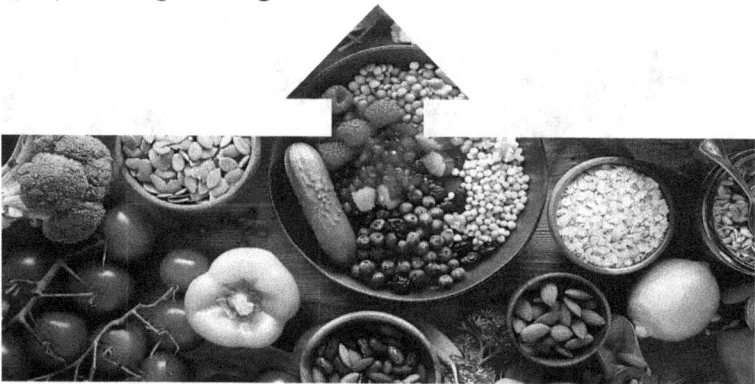

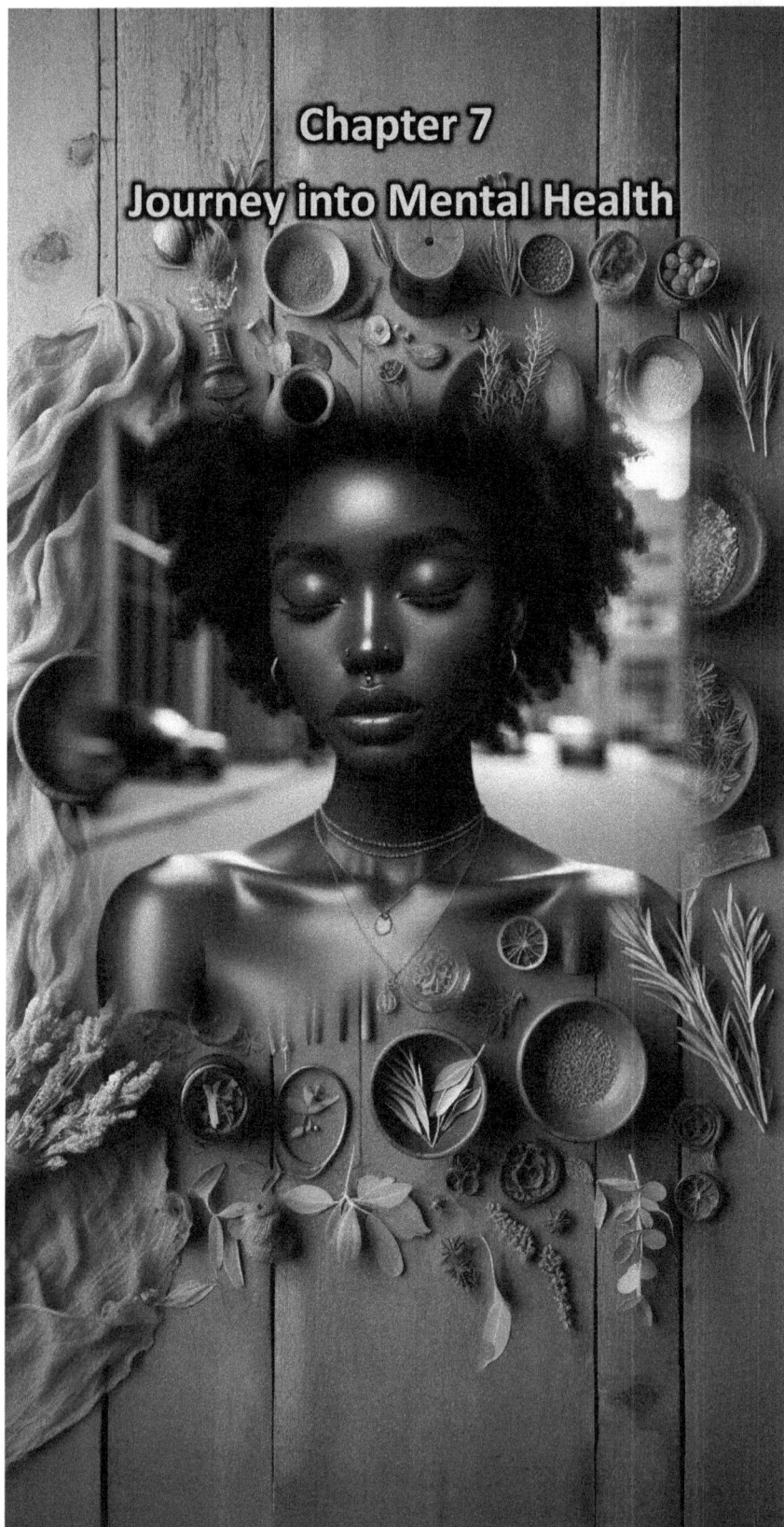

Chapter 7
Journey into Mental Health

Black women often face unique stressors that can impact their mental health, stemming from societal pressures, discrimination, and cultural expectations. These stressors can lead to several common mental health challenges. Many Black women manage high levels of stress due to daily responsibilities and the effects of systemic racism. This stress can lead to anxiety, a condition characterized by excessive worry, restlessness, and physical symptoms such as increased heart rate and sweating. Addressing stress and anxiety often requires a combination of lifestyle changes and therapeutic interventions. Herbal remedies like ashwagandha, which helps reduce stress, and CBD oil, known for its calming effects, can be beneficial.

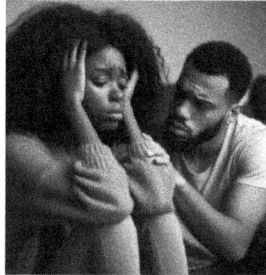

CHANNEL YOUR INNER POWER!   **YOU ARE NOT CRAZY!**

Depression is another significant concern, marked by persistent feelings of sadness, hopelessness, and a loss of interest in activities. Hormonal imbalances and chemical changes in the brain can contribute to depression. It's crucial to recognize the signs of depression early and seek help. Holistic approaches like regular exercise, mindfulness meditation, and natural supplements such as St. John's Wort can help alleviate symptoms. Professional therapy is also a critical component of effective treatment.

Societal standards can heavily influence body image, leading many Black women to struggle with self-acceptance. Embracing body positivity involves rejecting unrealistic beauty standards and appreciating one's body for its uniqueness. Engaging in self-love practices and seeking supportive communities can foster a healthier body image. Herbal remedies like chamomile tea can help reduce anxiety associated with body image issues.

Attention Deficit Hyperactivity Disorder (ADHD)

ADHD is a condition that affects focus, self-control, and other important skills. There are different types of ADHD, including inattentive, hyperactive-impulsive, and combined types. Symptoms include difficulty concentrating, hyperactivity, and impulsiveness. ADHD can be managed through a combination of behavioral strategies, therapy, and natural supplements like omega-3 fatty acids and ginkgo biloba, which may support brain health and improve symptoms.

Maintaining mental health requires a holistic approach that integrates various strategies to promote overall well-being. Prioritizing self-care is essential. This includes setting aside time for rest, engaging in hobbies, and participating in activities that bring joy. Simple practices such as taking a relaxing bath, reading a book, or spending time in nature can significantly improve mental health. Seeking professional help from therapists, particularly those who are culturally competent, can provide valuable support. Therapy offers a safe space to explore emotions, develop coping strategies, and address underlying issues.

Building a strong support network of family and friends is crucial. Community support can provide emotional strength, practical assistance, and a sense of belonging. Connecting with others who share similar experiences can be particularly empowering. Online platforms can offer support and connection with others facing similar challenges. These communities provide a space for sharing experiences, advice, and encouragement. Community groups and non-profits focused on mental health can offer resources, support, and advocacy. These organizations often provide workshops, counseling services, and support groups. Confidential hotlines can offer immediate support for those in crisis. Having access to these helplines can be a critical resource for anyone feeling overwhelmed or in need of urgent help.

If you are feeling suicidal, it is vital to reach out for help. Text, write a letter, or email someone to express your feelings. Remember that you are enough, and your feelings are valid. You have touched many lives, whether you personally know it or not. There were no mistakes made when you were created; your journey may be challenging, but it is purposeful. Reaching out can provide the support you need during difficult times.

Dear Melanin Gurlll,

I know you're going through a really tough time right now, and I want you to know that you're not alone. Sometimes, life can feel overwhelming, and the pain you're experiencing can seem unbearable. But I believe in you, and I want you to stay with us because your life is incredibly valuable.

Your life has a purpose, and you are meant to be here. The world needs you, with all your beautiful imperfections and unique qualities. There is so much more for you to experience, so many more sunsets to watch, laughter to share, and dreams to chase.

You are stronger than you think, and you have the power to overcome this. Hold on to hope, even if it feels faint right now. Trust that things can and will get better, because they truly can. And always remember, you are loved, you are important, and you matter.

Please stay. The world is a better place with you in it.

~ October Reign

Engaging in a mental health workbook exercise designed to promote healing could include journaling about your feelings, setting goals for self-care, and reflecting on positive affirmations. Such exercises can help in processing emotions and developing a proactive approach to mental wellness. Grounding practices, such as walking barefoot on grass, can connect you to the earth and provide a sense of calm and stability. Spending time in sunlight is another natural way to improve mood and overall well-being. These practices can help reduce stress and enhance mental clarity. Racism can significantly impact mental health, contributing to feelings of stress, anxiety, and depression. It is essential to acknowledge these experiences and seek supportive environments that validate and empower you. Encouraging messages and affirmations remind you of your strength, resilience, and worth. Embrace your journey, knowing that you are powerful and deserving of love and respect.

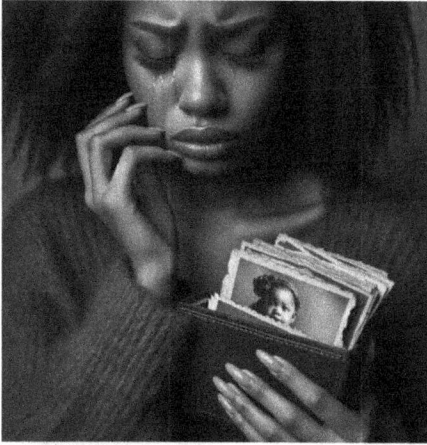

Understanding Grief and Broken Heart

Grief and a broken heart can profoundly impact anyone, but Black women often face unique challenges. This section aims to provide comprehensive insights into understanding, processing, and overcoming these intense emotions. We will explore the symptoms, physical and mental effects, and healing strategies, including herbal and holistic remedies.

Grief is a natural response to loss. It is the emotional suffering experienced when something or someone significant is taken away. Grief can result from various losses, including the death of a loved one, the end of a relationship, or the loss of a job. A broken heart, often stemming from romantic relationships, is a form of intense emotional pain or suffering following a deep disappointment or loss. It can be as devastating as grief and sometimes overlap with it.

Emotional symptoms of grief and a broken heart include profound sadness, anger, guilt, anxiety, and depression. Physical symptoms can include fatigue, insomnia, appetite changes, and unexplained aches and pains. Grief can cause a range of physical reactions due to the stress it places on the body. The brain releases stress hormones like cortisol, which can weaken the immune system, increase blood pressure, and lead to other health issues. Also known as Takotsubo cardiomyopathy, broken heart syndrome is a temporary heart condition triggered by extreme emotional stress. Symptoms mimic those of a heart attack, including chest pain and shortness of breath, but it typically does not cause permanent damage.

Severe grief and broken heart syndrome can lead to serious health issues such as heart disease, high blood pressure, and weakened immune responses. In extreme cases, the stress and physiological strain can be fatal, particularly in those with preexisting health conditions. To heal, it is important to acknowledge your pain, seek support, prioritize self-care, and consider professional help. Herbal remedies like chamomile, St. John's Wort, and valerian root can also aid in managing symptoms. Holistic approaches such as meditation, yoga, and acupuncture can promote emotional stability and mental health.

Lion's Mane mushroom (Hericium erinaceus) has been studied for various potential health benefits, including its effects on brain health. While there is some research suggesting that Lion's Mane may have neuroprotective properties and could potentially support cognitive function and mood, there isn't direct scientific evidence specifically linking it to grief relief. Compounds in Lion's Mane, such as hericenones and erinacines, have been shown in animal studies to stimulate nerve growth factor (NGF) production, which is crucial for the growth, maintenance, and survival of neurons. Some studies suggest that Lion's Mane extract may improve cognitive function, including memory and learning ability, possibly due to its effects on nerve growth and brain plasticity. While not directly studied for grief, Lion's Mane has shown potential in reducing symptoms of anxiety and depression in some animal studies. Improved cognitive function and reduced anxiety could indirectly help with emotional resilience. Chronic inflammation is associated with various mental health conditions. Lion's Mane has anti-inflammatory properties that could potentially contribute to overall brain health and emotional stability.

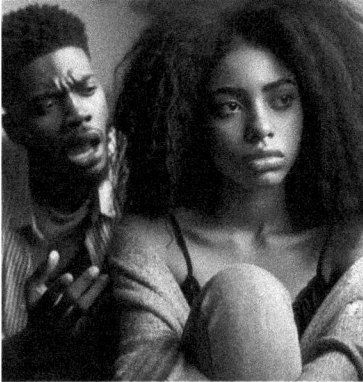

Understanding Different Forms of Abuse

Domestic Abuse

Domestic abuse is a pervasive issue that affects individuals across all demographics, including race, age, and socioeconomic status. Escaping from an abusive situation is challenging, but it is crucial for physical and emotional well-being. This section provides comprehensive tips and resources to help individuals, particularly Black women, navigate the difficult process of leaving an abusive relationship and finding safety and support.

Domestic abuse can take many forms, including physical, emotional, psychological, sexual, and financial abuse. Each type of abuse can have severe and long-lasting effects on the victim's health and well-being. Recognizing the signs of abuse is the first step toward seeking help. The impact of domestic abuse extends beyond physical injuries. It can lead to severe psychological trauma, including depression, anxiety, PTSD, and a diminished sense of self-worth. Understanding the broad impact of abuse highlights the importance of seeking help and escaping the situation.

Physical Abuse

Physical abuse involves the deliberate use of force that causes bodily harm or injury to another person. This can include hitting, punching, slapping, kicking, or any other form of physical violence. Signs of physical abuse may include visible injuries such as bruises, cuts, or broken bones, as well as behavioral changes like withdrawal or fearfulness. Physical abuse is never justified and is not a demonstration of love. In many cases, it tends to escalate over time and rarely improves without intervention.

Mental or Psychological Abuse

Mental or psychological abuse is characterized by behaviors aimed at exerting control and manipulation over another person's thoughts, feelings, and actions. This can include tactics such as gaslighting, constant criticism, belittling, threats, or intimidation. Victims of mental abuse may experience feelings of confusion, self-doubt, and worthlessness. They may also blame themselves for the abuse, believing they deserve mistreatment. Mental abuse is not a sign of love or care, and it can have severe and long-lasting effects on a person's mental well-being.

Financial Abuse

Financial abuse occurs when someone exploits or controls another person's financial resources without their consent. This can involve stealing money, withholding financial assets, or coercing someone into signing financial documents. Victims of financial abuse may feel powerless and dependent on the abuser for their financial security. They may also experience shame or embarrassment about their financial situation. Financial abuse is a form of power and control, and it can severely impact a person's ability to live independently and make choices for themselves.

Emotional Abuse

Emotional abuse involves behaviors that undermine an individual's self-esteem, emotional well-being, and sense of identity. This can include verbal insults, threats, manipulation, gaslighting, or isolation from friends and family. Victims of emotional abuse may feel trapped in the relationship, experiencing fear or anxiety about the abuser's reactions. They may also blame themselves for the abuse, believing they are responsible for the abuser's behavior. Emotional abuse is not a display of love or affection, and it can have profound effects on a person's mental health and self-worth.

Sexual Abuse

Sexual abuse involves any unwanted sexual activity or behavior, including rape, molestation, or forced sexual acts. It can have severe physical and psychological effects, leaving the victim feeling violated, ashamed, and traumatized. Recognizing the signs of sexual abuse and seeking help from trusted individuals or professional resources is crucial for healing and recovery. Reporting the abuse to authorities and accessing support services can provide protection and necessary care.

Overcoming Drug Abuse

Overcoming drug abuse is a complex process that requires a multifaceted approach. Recognizing the problem and seeking help is the first critical step. Support from healthcare professionals, therapy, and support groups can aid in recovery. Holistic remedies, such as mindfulness practices, exercise, and proper nutrition, can complement traditional treatments and promote overall well-being. Embracing a supportive community and setting achievable goals can empower individuals to overcome addiction and rebuild their lives.

EVERYONE DESERVES SAFETY AND SERENITY!
Recognizing Manipulation Tactics and Overcoming Fear

Abusers often use manipulation tactics to maintain control over their victims. These tactics may include gaslighting, where the abuser denies or distorts reality to make the victim doubt their perceptions or sanity. Victims may also experience feelings of self-blame, believing they are somehow responsible for the abuse or that they deserve mistreatment. Additionally, abusers may use threats, intimidation, or embarrassment to maintain power and control over their victims. Overcoming fear and seeking help can be challenging, but it's essential to remember that abuse is not love, and it rarely gets better without intervention.

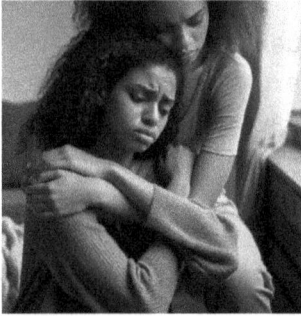

You cannot change or fix a person who does not want to change themselves. It's important to prioritize your safety and well-being and seek support from trusted friends, family members, or professionals. If verbal communication is difficult, consider expressing your feelings through writing, texting, or emailing someone you trust.

Remember that you deserve to be treated with respect, dignity, and kindness, and there are people who can help you break free from the cycle of abuse. Abuse in any form is unacceptable and can have devastating consequences for victims. It's essential to recognize the signs of abuse and take steps to protect yourself and seek help. Remember that abuse is not love, and you deserve to live a life free from fear, intimidation, and control. If you are experiencing abuse, know that you are not alone, and there are resources and support systems available to help you. You deserve to be treated with kindness, respect, and dignity, and there are people who can help you on your journey to healing and recovery.

Escaping Domestic Abuse

Safety Planning Creating a safety plan is essential for anyone considering leaving an abusive relationship. A well-thought-out plan can help minimize risks and increase the chances of a successful escape. **Identifying a Safe Place** Know where you can go in an emergency, such as a friend's house, a family member's home, or a domestic violence shelter. **Packing an Emergency Bag** Prepare a bag with essential items, including identification, important documents, money, keys, medication, and basic personal items. Keep this bag in a safe, accessible place. **Memorizing Important Numbers** Memorize the phone numbers of trusted friends, family members, and local shelters. **Create a Code Word** Establish a code word with trusted individuals to signal when you need help.

Financial Preparation

Financial independence is often a significant barrier to leaving an abusive relationship. Preparing financially can help reduce this barrier. **Save Money:** Save small amounts of money whenever possible and keep it in a safe place. **Open a Separate Bank Account:** If possible, open a separate bank account in your name. **Gather Financial Documents:** Collect important financial documents, such as bank statements, credit cards, and insurance policies.

Support Networks

Building a strong support network is crucial for escaping and recovering from domestic abuse. **Friends and Family:** Reach out to trusted friends and family members who can provide emotional support and practical assistance. **Support Groups:** Join support groups for survivors of domestic abuse to connect with others who have had similar experiences and gain strength from shared stories. **Professional Counseling:** Seek counseling or therapy to help process the trauma and rebuild self-esteem.

DON'T FEEL GUILTY PUT YOURSELF 1ST

Legal Resources

Understanding your legal rights and accessing legal resources can be pivotal in escaping an abusive situation. **Protective Orders** Apply for a protective order (restraining order) to legally prevent the abuser from contacting or approaching you. *Legal Aid*: Utilize legal aid services that offer free or low-cost legal assistance for domestic abuse survivors. *Child Custody and Divorce:* If applicable, seek legal advice on child custody and divorce to protect your rights and your children's well-being.

Utilizing Community Resources

Shelters and Safe Houses Domestic violence shelters and safe houses provide immediate safety and support for those escaping abuse. **Finding a Shelter:** Use national hotlines, such as the National Domestic Violence Hotline (1-800-799-7233), to locate nearby shelters. **Services Provided:** Shelters often provide food, clothing, counseling, legal advocacy, and assistance with finding long-term housing. **Hotlines and Crisis Centers** Hotlines and crisis centers offer immediate assistance, emotional support, and resources for those in danger.

National Domestic Violence Hotline
Provides confidential support and resources 24/7
(1-800-799-7233).
Local Crisis Centers
Many communities have local crisis centers that offer emergency assistance and referrals to additional services.

Building a New Life

Leaving an abusive relationship is a significant step, but the journey to recovery continues as you build a new life. **Secure Housing:** Find stable, long-term housing through shelters, housing programs, or rental assistance services. **Employment:** Seek employment or vocational training to achieve financial independence. **Health Care:** Address any physical and mental health needs by seeking medical care and counseling.

MOVE FORWARD DON'T LOOK BACK

Healing and Self-Care

Healing from the trauma of domestic abuse takes time and self-care. **Therapy and Counseling:** Continue therapy or counseling to work through emotional trauma and build resilience. **Support Networks:** Maintain connections with support networks, including friends, family, and support groups. **Self-Care Practices:** Engage in self-care practices that promote well-being, such as exercise, meditation, journaling, and hobbies. Escaping domestic abuse is a challenging but necessary step towards reclaiming your life and well-being. By preparing a safety plan, seeking support, utilizing community resources, and focusing on healing, survivors can overcome the trauma of abuse and build a brighter, safer future.

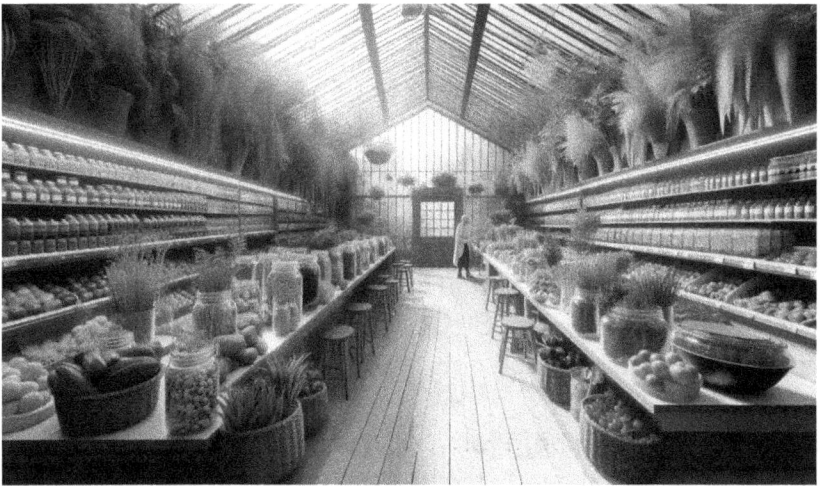

Ashwagandha Reduces stress and anxiety- Improves cognitive function- Supports mood stability
Adaptogen with calming effects; supports adrenal function.

Bacopa Monnieri Enhances memory and cognitive function- Reduces anxiety- Supports focus and attention; Adaptogen; traditionally used in Ayurvedic medicine for cognitive enhancement.

Brahmi (Gotu Kola) Improves cognitive function- Enhances memory and concentration- Supports calmness and mental clarity Adaptogenic herb; traditionally used in Ayurvedic medicine for brain health.

Caffeine (from Coffee) Improves alertness and concentration- Enhances cognitive function temporarily Stimulant, can improve focus but may cause jitteriness in some individuals.

Chamomile Calming and anti-anxiety properties- Promotes relaxation and sleep Gentle sedative; commonly consumed as tea.
Ginkgo Biloba Enhances cognitive function- Improves memory and concentration- Supports circulation to the brain Antioxidant properties; improves blood flow to the brain.

Green Tea (L-theanine) Promotes relaxation and reduces stress- Improves attention and focus_Contains caffeine; L-theanine promotes relaxation without drowsiness.

Lavender Calming and relaxing effects- Reduces anxiety and stress- Supports focus and attention Aromatic herb; often used in aromatherapy and teas.

Lemon Balm Calming and relaxing effects- Reduces anxiety and stress- Supports cognitive function and focus Mild sedative properties; often used in combination with other herbs for anxiety.

Magnesium Calms the nervous system- Reduces anxiety and promotes relaxation Mineral essential for nerve function; often deficient in modern diets.

Omega – 3 Fatty Acids Supports brain health and cognitive function- Reduces inflammation- May improve focus and attention Found in fish oil and flaxseed oil; essential for brain function.

Passionflower Reduces anxiety and insomnia- Calming effect on the nervous system Mild sedative; can be used to promote sleep.
Rhodiola Rosea Enhances mood- Reduces fatigue and stress- Improves cognitive function Adaptogen that increases resistance to stress.

St. John Wort Improves mood and emotional balance- Reduces symptoms of mild to moderate depression Increases serotonin levels; interacts with certain medications.

Tumeric Curcumin Anti-inflammatory effects- Supports brain health and cognitive function- Potential for improving focus and attention Contains curcumin, which has neuroprotective properties.

Valerian Root Reduces anxiety and insomnia- Calms the nervous system Mild sedative; often used in combination with other herbs for anxiety and sleep.

Understanding and Overcoming Fatigue

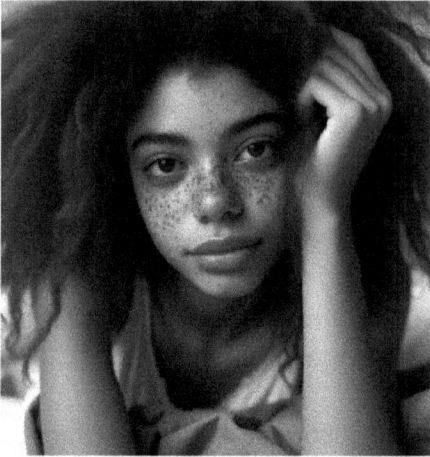

Feeling tired all the time is a common complaint among many individuals, but it can be particularly prevalent and concerning among Black people and Black women. Fatigue can stem from a variety of causes, ranging from lifestyle factors to underlying health conditions. Understanding these causes and exploring natural, holistic, and alkaline-based, animal-free remedies can help in managing and overcoming fatigue.

Recognizing and Addressing Vitamin B12 Deficiency

Vitamin B12 deficiency is a condition that can significantly impact your overall health and well-being. It's important to recognize the symptoms and understand the importance of this crucial vitamin for maintaining various bodily functions.

Symptoms of Vitamin B12 Deficiency

If you consistently feel sleepy or low on energy, experience confusion or neurological issues, or have difficulty remembering things, you might be suffering from a vitamin B12 deficiency. Additional symptoms include: **Muscle Weakness**: Unexplained weakness in your muscles. **Mouth Sores**: Sores that appear in your mouth without any clear cause. **Paresthesia**: Pins and needles sensations that start in your fingertips and toes and can spread to other parts of your extremities. These symptoms occur because vitamin B12 plays a vital role in maintaining nerve health and connectivity. It is essential for DNA formation and the production of red blood cells.

Causes and Importance of Vitamin B12

Vitamin B12 is found in animal-based proteins. However, many people, especially those following vegetarian or vegan diets, may not get enough vitamin B12 from their food. Even individuals who consume animal products can have low vitamin B12 levels due to absorption issues. Vitamin B12 is important for: **Nerve Health:** It helps in maintaining the myelin sheath, which protects nerve fibers and ensures proper signal transmission. **DNA Formation:** This vitamin is crucial for the synthesis of DNA, which is vital for cell production and function. **Red Blood Cell Formation:** Adequate levels of vitamin B12 are necessary for the production of healthy red blood cells, which carry oxygen throughout the body.

Addressing Vitamin B12 Deficiency

If you suspect you have a vitamin B12 deficiency, it's essential to consult a healthcare professional for proper diagnosis and treatment. Here are some steps you can take to address and prevent vitamin B12 deficiency: **Dietary Changes**: Include B12-rich foods in your diet, such as fortified cereals, nutritional yeast, and plant-based milk alternatives. If you consume animal products, ensure you're eating sufficient amounts of meat, fish, dairy, and eggs. **Supplements**: Vitamin B12 supplements can be an effective way to boost your levels, especially for those who follow a vegan or vegetarian diet. **Regular Check-ups**: Routine blood tests can help monitor your vitamin B12 levels and ensure they remain within a healthy range.

Constant Fatigue Common Causes

Fatigue can be a persistent issue affecting many individuals, particularly Black people and Black women. Understanding the various causes of constant tiredness and exploring natural, holistic, and alkaline-based, animal-free remedies can help in managing and overcoming this condition. Common causes of constant fatigue include iron deficiency anemia, which is a condition where the body lacks enough healthy red blood cells to carry adequate oxygen to tissues. Symptoms of iron deficiency anemia include fatigue, weakness, pale skin, shortness of breath, and dizziness. Hypothyroidism, an underactive thyroid gland that doesn't produce enough thyroid hormones, also leads to fatigue, weight gain, cold intolerance, dry skin, and hair loss.

Chronic stress

Chronic stress is another significant cause of fatigue, as prolonged stress can lead to hormonal imbalances that affect energy levels. This results in constant tiredness, difficulty sleeping, irritability, and headaches. Poor sleep quality, resulting from conditions like insomnia, sleep apnea, or other sleep disorders, can cause daytime fatigue, trouble concentrating, irritability, and waking up tired. Dehydration, due to not consuming enough water, leads to decreased blood volume, affecting energy and concentration, and presenting symptoms such as fatigue, dizziness, dry mouth, and dark urine.

Nutritional deficiencies

Lacking essential nutrients like magnesium, potassium, or omega-3 fatty acids, also contribute to fatigue. This can cause tiredness, muscle cramps, cognitive issues, and a weakened immune system. Depression, a mental health condition, significantly impacts energy levels and overall motivation, with symptoms including persistent sadness, fatigue, loss of interest in activities, and changes in appetite.

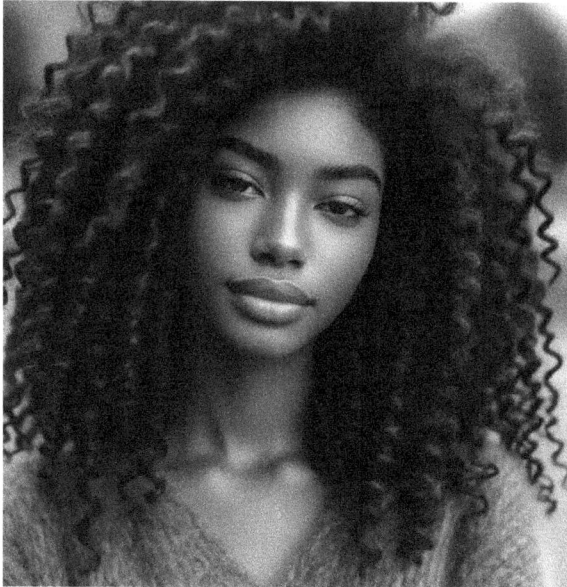

Adrenal fatigue

Adrenal fatigue is a theory suggesting that chronic stress leads to overworked adrenal glands, resulting in inadequate hormone production. Symptoms include body aches, fatigue, nervousness, sleep disturbances, and digestive problems. Diabetes, a condition where the body either doesn't produce enough insulin or can't use it effectively, leads to high blood sugar levels and symptoms like fatigue, frequent urination, excessive thirst, and unexplained weight loss.

Chronic Fatigue Syndrome (CFS)

CFS is a complex disorder characterized by extreme fatigue that can't be explained by any underlying medical condition. Symptoms of CFS include severe tiredness, memory problems, muscle pain, and headaches.

Addressing these causes through natural remedies and lifestyle changes can significantly improve energy levels. Alkaline foods such as spinach, lentils, and pumpkin seeds can help manage iron deficiency anemia, while sea vegetables and adaptogenic herbs like ashwagandha support hypothyroidism. Chronic stress can be alleviated with practices like meditation and yoga, and herbs like holy basil and Rhodiola rosea. Improving sleep quality might involve using valerian root, chamomile tea, and maintaining good sleep hygiene. To combat dehydration, incorporating coconut water, watermelon, and herbal teas is beneficial.

For nutritional deficiencies, a balanced diet with a variety of fruits, vegetables, nuts, and seeds is essential. Depression can be managed with St. John's Wort, saffron, and regular physical exercise, while adrenal fatigue can be addressed with adaptogens like holy basil and a balanced diet. Managing diabetes involves consuming low glycemic index foods, cinnamon, and regular physical activity. Chronic Fatigue Syndrome might benefit from ginseng, CoQ10, and omega-3 fatty acids.

When consulting a healthcare professional about persistent fatigue, it's crucial to ask questions about the underlying causes and request specific tests. Inquire whether the fatigue could be related to nutritional deficiencies, thyroid function, or adrenal fatigue. Request tests such as a Complete Blood Count (CBC), thyroid function tests, iron studies, vitamin and mineral level assessments, blood glucose tests, sleep studies, and mental health screenings.

Iron Deficiency Anemia Alkaline foods like spinach, lentils, and pumpkin seeds; herbal teas like nettle and dandelion root.

Hypothyroidism Sea vegetables (kelp, nori), Brazil nuts (selenium), adaptogenic herbs like ashwagandha.

Chronic Stress Meditation, yoga, ashwagandha, holy basil, Rhodiola rosea, magnesium-rich foods like dark leafy greens.

Poor Sleep Quality Valerian root, chamomile tea, lavender oil, melatonin-rich foods like cherries, sleep hygiene practices.

Dehydration Coconut water, watermelon, cucumber, and herbal teas; aim for at least 8 glasses of water daily.

Nutritional Deficiencies Balanced diet with a variety of fruits, vegetables, nuts, and seeds; consider a multivitamin if necessary.

Depression St. John's Wort, saffron, omega-3 fatty acids from flaxseed and chia seeds, regular physical exercise.

Adrenal Fatigue Adaptogens like holy basil, Rhodiola, and licorice root; balanced diet, regular sleep patterns.

Diabetes Low glycemic index foods, cinnamon, fenugreek, regular physical activity, avoiding processed sugars.

Chronic Fatigue Syndrome Ginseng, CoQ10, omega-3 fatty acids, regular gentle exercise like walking or tai chi, adequate rest.

?QUESTIONS TO ASK HEALTHCARE PROVIDERS?

What could be the underlying cause of my fatigue?
Could my fatigue be related to a nutritional deficiency?
Are there any lifestyle changes or natural remedies that could help?
Should I be tested for thyroid function or adrenal fatigue?
Could my fatigue be related to a sleep disorder?

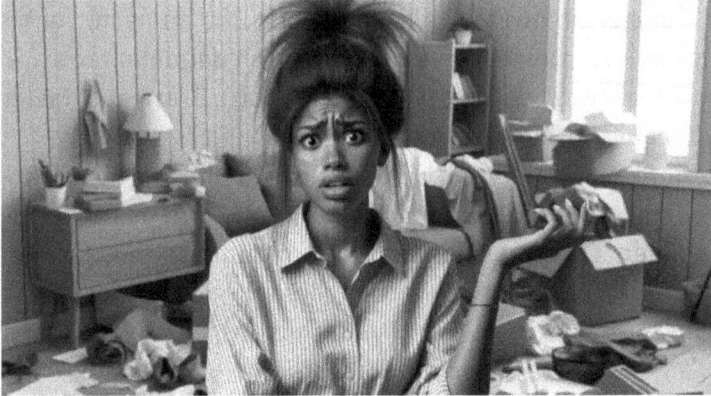

Complete Blood Count (CBC): To check for anemia and overall health.
Thyroid Function Tests: To assess thyroid hormone levels.
Iron Studies: To check for iron deficiency.
Vitamin and Mineral Levels: To assess levels of key nutrients like vitamin D, magnesium, and potassium.
Blood Glucose Test: To check for diabetes.
Sleep Study: To evaluate sleep disorders such as sleep apnea.
Mental Health Screening: To assess for depression or anxiety. Fatigue can be debilitating, affecting daily life and overall well-being.

Understanding Executive Dysfunction

Executive dysfunction is a term used to describe challenges with cognitive processes like planning, organizing, focusing, and completing tasks. In Black women, experiences with executive dysfunction may be shaped by unique factors, including genetic predisposition, environmental stressors, and systemic barriers to healthcare. Conditions that often involve executive dysfunction include ADHD, bipolar disorder, obsessive-compulsive disorder (OCD), anxiety disorders, borderline personality disorder (BPD), and depression. Understanding executive dysfunction holistically can reveal natural healing pathways and empower Black women to take charge of their mental health with the support of both traditional and alternative approaches.

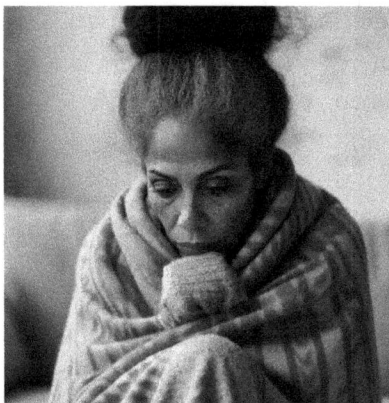

Bipolar Disorder

Bipolar disorder is characterized by shifts between manic and depressive phases, where motivation, energy, and focus can vary drastically. **Manic phase** Often, there is an intense surge of energy and motivation, yet this can lack focus, leading to impulsivity. Depressive phase This phase typically involves low energy, reduced motivation, and struggles with completing even basic tasks.

Obsessive-Compulsive Disorder (OCD)

OCD involves recurrent, intrusive thoughts (obsessions) and repetitive behaviors (compulsions). **Decision paralysis** The constant fear of making the "wrong" choice can paralyze decision-making, resulting in task avoidance and procrastination. **Anxiety Disorders** High levels of anxiety affect focus and task initiation, often making it difficult for individuals to start or complete tasks. **Coping mechanisms** Procrastination can act as a way to avoid situations that trigger anxiety, leading to a cycle of avoidance.

Borderline Personality Disorder (BPD)

BPD often involves emotional dysregulation, leading to inconsistent performance on tasks. **Emotional influence** Extreme emotional shifts can affect motivation and concentration, making it challenging to maintain productivity. **Depression** can deeply impact motivation and energy levels, often making task completion a monumental effort. **Energy depletion** Individuals with depression may lack the energy to perform basic tasks, often finding even simple decisions overwhelming.

A Perspective on Executive Dysfunction

An herbalist's approach to executive dysfunction would center on addressing both the mental and physical aspects through natural remedies, detoxification, and dietary adjustments. Practitioners in natural healing believe in cleansing the body to remove toxins that disrupt mental clarity and affect the nervous system. They may recommend herbs that support brain function, nervous system health, and hormonal balance.

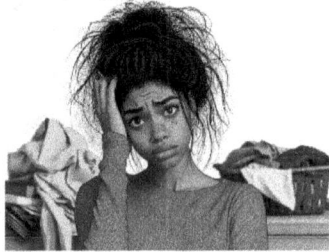

Detoxification as a Foundation

Detoxification removes accumulated toxins in the body, believed to contribute to mental fog, irritability, and lack of focus. Detox protocols may include: **Juicing:** Fresh juices of fruits and vegetables to cleanse the liver and improve mental clarity. **Herbal teas:** Dandelion and burdock root teas help support liver detox, aiding in clearing mental fog.

Emotional Balancing through Adaptogens

Adaptogenic herbs help the body resist stress and stabilize mood. Ashwagandha: Known to reduce anxiety and enhance focus. Rhodiola: Improves cognitive function and mitigates fatigue associated with executive dysfunction.

An Approach to Healing Executive Dysfunction

A healthy alkaline diet could restore the body to its natural state, thereby reducing symptoms associated with various ailments. A plant-based diet rich in natural herbs and minerals to address deficiencies that might contribute to mental health conditions, including those with symptoms of executive dysfunction.

Alkaline Diet: Eating an alkaline, plant-based diet rich in leafy greens, fruits, and vegetables helps restore pH balance in the body, which is believed to reduce inflammation and improve mental clarity. **Natural Mineral Intake:** The importance of minerals like magnesium and iron to support brain and nerve function. **Sea Moss:** Rich in minerals, sea moss is a key to aid in overall body nourishment, including mental health.

Suggested Herbs

Sarsaparilla Root: Known for its high iron content, this herb supports blood health and, by extension, mental function. **Bladderwrack:** Often used alongside sea moss, bladderwrack provides a wealth of nutrients that support cognitive function and reduce fatigue. **Ginkgo Biloba:** Improves blood flow to the brain and has been noted to enhance memory and focus.

? QUESTIONS TO ASK YOUR DOCTOR ?

What specific tests could help diagnose my executive dysfunction symptoms? Request cognitive assessments, mental health screenings, and blood work to evaluate nutrient deficiencies.

Could nutrient deficiencies or thyroid imbalances be contributing to my symptoms? Certain deficiencies, like those in Vitamin B12, iron, and magnesium, can impact cognitive function and mental health.

What treatment options are available that address executive dysfunction specifically? Inquire about therapy, lifestyle changes, and medication options designed to target executive dysfunction and associated symptoms.

Can we explore herbal supplements that might support focus and mental clarity? Discuss any herbs of interest, ensuring there are no contraindications with other medications.

How might changes in diet and exercise help manage my symptoms? Lifestyle modifications, including diet and physical activity, can play a significant role in managing symptoms.

Herbs for Supporting Mental Clarity and Executive Function

Ginkgo Biloba Increases blood flow to the brain, enhances memory **Suggested Use** Capsule or tea

Ashwagandha Reduces anxiety and supports mood balance **Suggested Use** Capsule or powder in smoothies

Rhodiola Reduces mental fatigue, enhances focus **Suggested Use** Capsule or tea

Lion's Mane Promotes nerve regeneration, improves cognitive health **Suggested Use** Capsule or as a mushroom extract

Gotu Kola Improves concentration and mental clarity **Suggested Use** Tea or capsule

Holy Basil (Tulsi) Reduces stress and enhances mental focus **Suggested Use** Tea or capsule

Bacopa Monnieri Boosts memory and cognitive function **Suggested Use** Capsule or tea

Sarsaparilla Root Provides high iron content, believed to support focus **Suggested Use** Capsule or tea

Bladderwrack Rich in minerals, supports cognitive function **Suggested Use** Capsule or as a powder with sea moss

Executive dysfunction, especially as experienced by Black women, often intersects with multiple aspects of mental and physical health. Taking a holistic approach—integrating both conventional and natural healing methods—can empower individuals to manage symptoms effectively. Whether through herbal remedies, nutrient-dense diets, or proactive healthcare conversations, Black women can reclaim control over their mental clarity and productivity by addressing executive dysfunction in a balanced, individualized manner.

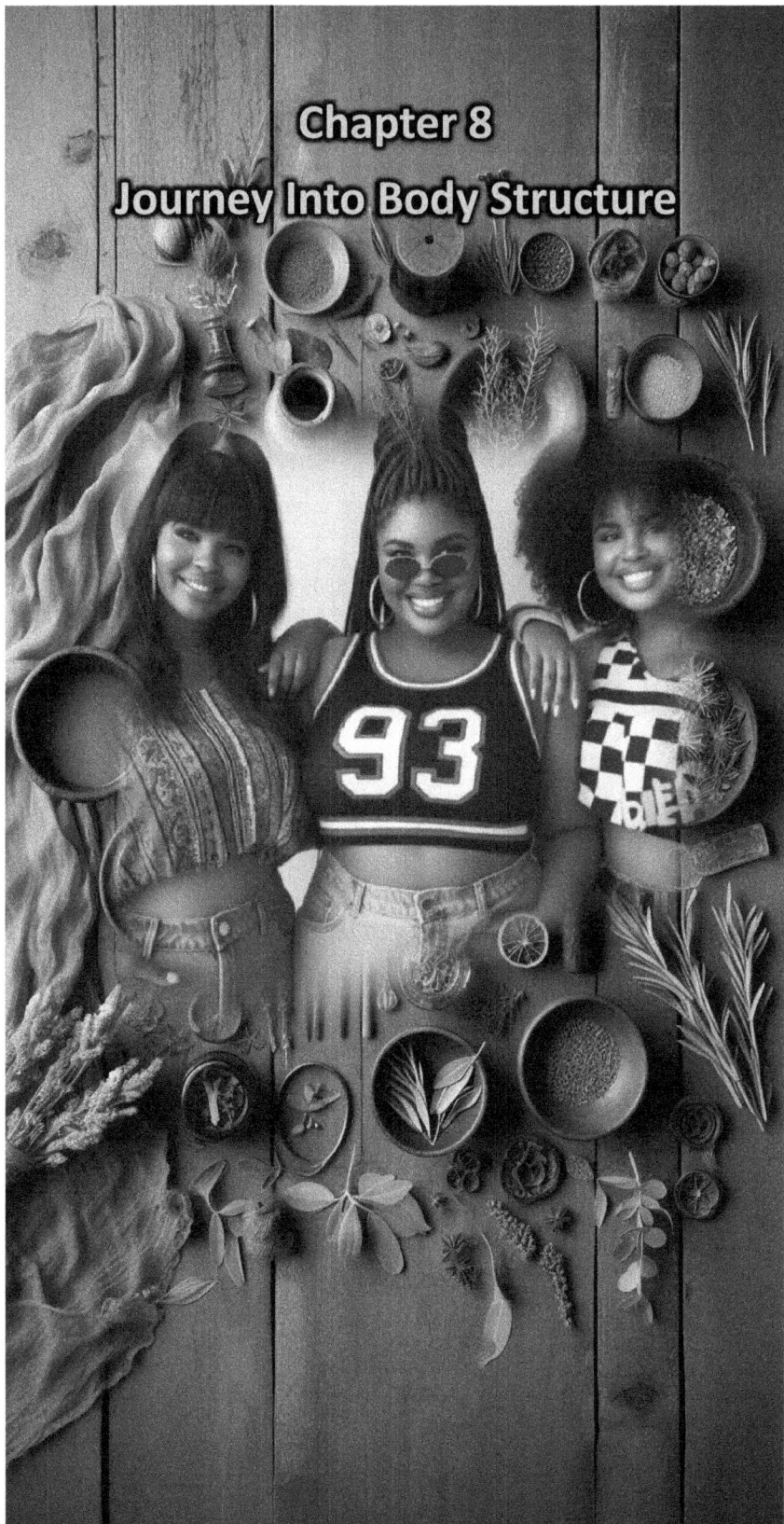

Chapter 8
Journey Into Body Structure

The Skeletal System
BONES JOINTS TEETH

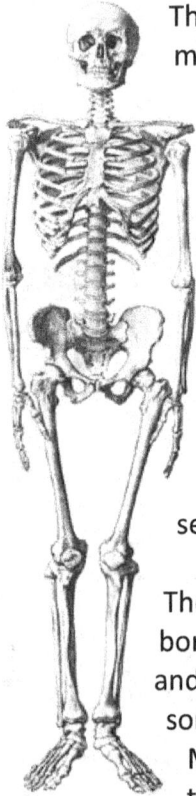

The skeletal system, also known as the musculoskeletal system, is the body's foundational support structure, comprising bones, joints, and other integral tissues. It plays a vital role in providing structure, protection, and movement, as well as housing essential minerals and producing blood cells. For Black women, understanding the skeletal system from a holistic and natural perspective can enhance overall health and well-being. Bones are living organs composed of cells, protein fibers, and minerals. They provide the structural framework for the body, protect vital internal organs, and serve as reservoirs for calcium, iron, and fat.

The adult human skeleton consists of 206 named bones, including those in the skull, spine, ribs, arms, and legs. In children, the skeleton has more bones, some of which fuse together as they grow. Maintaining bone health is particularly crucial due to the higher bone density often observed in this population, which can influence dietary and exercise needs. Ensuring adequate intake of nutrients such as calcium and vitamin D, alongside regular physical activity, supports strong and healthy bones.

Holistic Approaches to Bone Health

Calcium-Rich Foods: Incorporate plant-based calcium sources such as dark leafy greens (kale, collards), almonds, and fortified plant milks into the diet. *Vitamin D:* Since higher melanin levels can reduce vitamin D synthesis from sunlight, it is important to ensure adequate sun exposure and consider plant-based vitamin D supplements. *Weight-Bearing Exercises:* Engage in regular weight-bearing activities like walking, jogging, and resistance training to strengthen bones and improve overall musculoskeletal health. *Joints: Enabling Movement* Joints are the connections between two bones, allowing for movement and flexibility. They vary in their range of motion, from immovable joints like sutures in the skull to highly mobile joints such as those in the shoulders and hips. Proper joint health is essential for maintaining mobility and preventing conditions such as arthritis.

Holistic Approaches to Joint Health

Anti-Inflammatory Diet: Consuming an anti-inflammatory diet rich in omega-3 fatty acids (found in flaxseeds, chia seeds, and walnuts), antioxidants, and spices like turmeric and ginger can help reduce joint inflammation. *Hydration:* Maintaining adequate hydration is essential for joint lubrication and overall joint health. *Regular Exercise:* Low-impact exercises such as yoga, swimming, and tai chi can improve joint flexibility and strength without putting excessive strain on the joints. *Other Tissues: Supporting Structure and Function* The skeletal system also includes other crucial tissues such as cartilage, tendons, ligaments, muscles, nerves, and blood vessels. These components work together to support the body, facilitate movement, protect internal organs, and produce blood cells.

Holistic Approaches to Supporting Tissues

Collagen-Boosting Foods: Consuming foods that support collagen production, such as berries, citrus fruits, and garlic, can strengthen connective tissues. *Herbal Remedies:* Using herbs like comfrey and nettle can support tissue repair and reduce inflammation. *Massage and Physical Therapy:* Regular massage and physical therapy can help maintain tissue health, improve circulation, and reduce pain.

Collagen-Boosting Smoothie

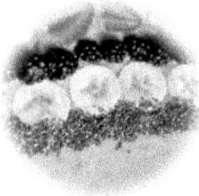

Ingredients: 1 cup mixed berries, 1 banana, 1 tablespoon chia seeds, 1 tablespoon flaxseed meal, 1 cup coconut water **Instructions:** Blend all ingredients until smooth. Drink daily to boost collagen production and support the health of connective tissues.

Anti-Inflammatory Joint Tea

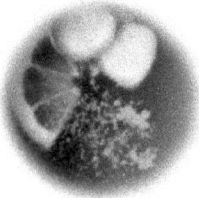

Ingredients: 1 teaspoon turmeric powder, 1/2 teaspoon ginger powder, 1 teaspoon lemon juice, 1 teaspoon honey, 2 cups hot water **Instructions:** Mix turmeric and ginger powder in hot water. Add lemon juice and honey to taste. Drink twice daily to reduce joint inflammation and support overall joint health.

Natural Anti-Inflammatory Cream for Joint Health

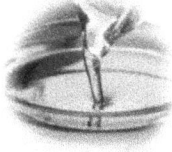

Ingredients: 1/2 cup coconut oil, 1/4 cup shea butter, 10 drops eucalyptus oil, 10 drops peppermint oil. Instructions: Melt coconut oil and shea butter, add essential oils, and let cool. Apply to joints to reduce inflammation and pain.

Herbal Bone Strengthening Tea

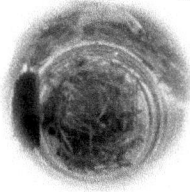

Ingredients: 1 tsp horsetail, 1 tsp nettle leaf, 1 tsp oat straw, 2 cups water. **Instructions:** Boil water and add herbs. Simmer for 10 minutes, strain, and drink twice daily to support bone density and joint health

Bone Strengthening Elixir

Ingredients: 1 cup almond milk, 1 tablespoon chia seeds, 1 tablespoon tahini, 1 teaspoon blackstrap molasses, 1/2 teaspoon cinnamon **Instructions:** Blend all ingredients until smooth. Drink daily to support bone health with a rich source of calcium and other essential nutrients

Understanding Osteoporosis

African American women are at risk for osteoporosis, a metabolic bone disease that causes low bone mass and makes bones fragile. Although Black women tend to have higher bone mineral density (BMD) than women of other ethnic backgrounds throughout life, they are more likely to die after a hip fracture, and their risk of hip fracture doubles every seven years as they age. Despite their higher bone density, osteoporosis remains underrecognized and undertreated in Black women. Therefore, it is essential for Black women to focus on bone health to prevent osteoporosis and fractures.

Bone Health Despite Higher Bone Density

While Black women generally have higher bone density compared to women of other ethnic backgrounds, it is essential not to develop a false sense of security. Without proper care, bones can still weaken over time. Therefore, maintaining a nutrient-rich diet, engaging in regular physical activity, and making healthy lifestyle choices are vital practices for mitigating the risk of bone-related problems. In summary, African American women must remain vigilant about their bone health despite their generally higher bone density. By focusing on adequate nutrition, regular exercise, and healthy lifestyle choices, they can prevent osteoporosis and maintain strong, healthy bones throughout their lives.

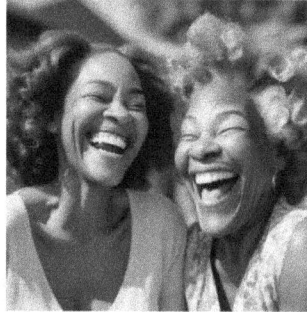

Importance of Calcium and Vitamin D

Calcium: This mineral is vital for maintaining strong bones. Black women can consume calcium-rich plant-based foods like dark leafy greens (e.g., kale, collard greens), sea vegetables (e.g., sea moss), and fortified plant milks.

Calcium-Rich Plant-Based Foods

Dark Leafy Kale Collard Greens, Spinach, Bok Choy, Mustard Greens Turnip Greens

Sea Vegetables Sea Moss, Wakame, Nori, Dulse, Kombu

Fortified Plant Milks Almond Milk, Soy Milk, Oat Milk, Rice Milk, Coconut Milk, Hemp Milk

Calcium-Rich Foods Tofu(calcium-set),Tempeh, Almonds, Chia Seeds, Figs, Oranges, White Beans, Sesame Seeds (including tahini)

Vitamin D--Rich Plant-Based Foods

Dark Leafy Greens Spinach, Kale, Collard, Greens

Sea Vegetables Sea Moss, Nori, Dulse

Fortified Plant Milks Almond Milk, Soy Milk, Oat Milk, Rice Milk, Coconut Milk, Hemp Milk

Other Sources Mushrooms (exposed to sunlight), Fortified Cereals, Fortified Orange Juice

Vitamin D: This vitamin helps the body absorb calcium. Black women may need to ensure adequate sun exposure or take plant-based supplements, as darker skin can reduce vitamin D synthesis. Foods like mushrooms exposed to sunlight can also be beneficial.

Gout and Uric Acid Reduction

Gout, a form of inflammatory arthritis caused by elevated levels of uric acid in the blood, disproportionately affects African Americans, especially men. Gout can lead to sudden, painful flare-ups, usually in the big toe, ankle, or knee. Dietary choices and chronic health conditions such as hypertension and metabolic syndrome are more prevalent with African American and can increase the risk of gout. There also may be a genetic predisposition that affects the body's ability to process uric acid efficiently.

Being overweight or obese, inactive lifestyle and insulin resistance can contribute to metabolic syndrome which is related to risk factors such as waist size, triglycerides, HDL cholesterol, blood pressure and fasting blood sugar.

Dietary Changes to Reduce Uric Acid

To manage gout effectively, it's crucial to reduce high-purine foods, as they increase uric acid levels. Avoid red meats like beef, lamb, pork, and venison, as well as organ meats such as liver and kidneys. High-purine seafood like anchovies, sardines, and scallops should also be limited. Instead, opt for plant-based proteins and whole grains. Other foods to skip include game meats, turkey, meat gravies, and yeast products. Beverages like beer, grain liquors, and sugary sodas also contribute to higher uric acid, so it's best to avoid them. Increasing hydration with water helps flush out uric acid, while incorporating alkaline foods like leafy greens and cucumbers can help balance the body's pH and reduce acidity.

Purines: chemicals found in some foods and beverages that the body uses to produce uric acid. High levels of uric acid in the blood causes gout.

Reduce Uric Acid!

Natural approaches using dietary changes, natural remedies, and lifestyle adjustments can effectively manage gout, reducing flare-ups without heavy reliance on medications. Consuming cherries or tart cherry juice helps lower uric acid levels due to their strong anti-inflammatory properties. Nettle tea acts as a natural anti-inflammatory and diuretic, aiding in uric acid reduction. Spices like turmeric and ginger are excellent for easing pain and inflammation.

Regular exercise, stress management, and ensuring adequate levels of vitamin D and magnesium are also important, as these nutrients support joint and bone health, which can be particularly beneficial for African Americans who may be prone to deficiencies that exacerbate gout symptoms.

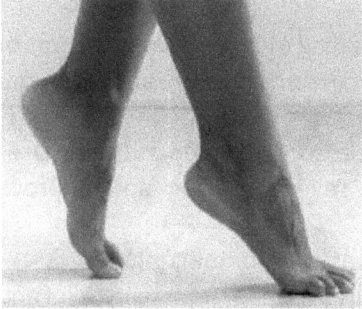

Why Do So Many Black Women's Feet Hurt?

Foot pain in Black women is a common issue due to various factors such as genetics, lifestyle, and footwear choices. Conditions like plantar fasciitis, flat feet, bunions, and even wearing high heels frequently can contribute to chronic foot pain. Genetics also play a role, as inherited foot structures and biomechanics can contribute to pain and discomfort. Conditions like flat feet or high arches are often hereditary and can predispose individuals to various types of foot pain. *Arnica* and *peppermint oil* can be used topically to relieve pain and inflammation. *Epsom salt* baths can also soothe sore feet.

Managing Foot Pain

Proper Footwear: Choose supportive shoes that provide adequate arch support and cushioning. Avoid high heels and tight shoes that can exacerbate pain. *Foot Exercises*: Regularly perform stretching and strengthening exercises for the feet and calves. *Orthotics:* Custom orthotics can provide support and alleviate pain caused by flat feet or other structural issues. *Rest and Ice*: Resting the feet and applying ice can reduce inflammation and pain.

Arnica (Arnica montana)

Anti-inflammatory - **Benefits** Reduces inflammation and swelling **Uses** Used topically in creams, ointments, or gels to treat bruises, sprains, strains, and muscle soreness.

Pain Relief - **Benefits** Relieves pain associated with bruises, injuries, and arthritis **Uses** Applied externally to alleviate sore muscles, joint pain, and post-surgical discomfort.

Bruise Treatment - **Benefits** Speeds up healing of bruises **Uses** Creams or gels applied to affected areas to reduce discoloration and promote recovery.

Muscle Soreness - **Benefits** Eases muscle soreness and stiffness **Uses** Used in liniments or massage oils to relieve tension and improve circulation in sore muscles.

Joint Pain - **Benefits** Alleviates pain from arthritis or joint injuries **Uses** Topical applications or diluted tinctures used for joint pain relief and improved mobility.

Wound Healing - **Benefits** Promotes healing of minor wounds and cuts **Uses** Applied topically to clean wounds and promote faster recovery without causing irritation.

Swelling Reduction - **Benefits** Helps reduce swelling from injuries or surgeries **Uses** Used as compresses or in topical preparations to minimize edema and inflammation.

Skin Care - **Benefits** Soothes skin irritations and sunburns **Uses** Creams or - salves applied to calm irritated skin and accelerate healing.

Hair Care - **Benefits** Strengthens hair follicles and promotes hair growth **Uses** Added to shampoos or hair rinses to improve scalp health and stimulate hair growth.

Insect Bites - **Benefits** Relieves itching and inflammation caused by insect bites **Uses** Applied topically to soothe bites and reduce swelling.

Scalp Health - **Benefits** Treats dandruff and improves scalp condition **Uses** Arnica-infused hair products used to reduce flakiness, itching, and maintain scalp health.

Note: *Arnica should only be used externally on unbroken skin due to its potential toxicity if ingested. Avoid using Arnica on open wounds or mucous membranes.*

Muscular System
SKELETAL MUSCLES SMOOTH MUSCLE TISSUES

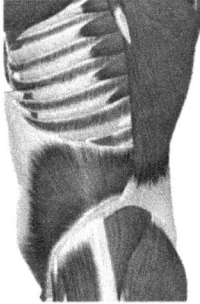

The muscular system, a complex network composed of more than 600 muscles, plays a pivotal role in bodily movement, posture maintenance, and blood circulation. Understanding this system from a holistic and natural perspective is essential for optimizing health and overall well-being. The muscular system includes three main types of muscle tissue: skeletal, cardiac, and smooth muscles.

Skeletal muscles are attached to bones by tendons and ligaments and are the only muscles under voluntary control. When these muscles contract, they pull attachment points closer together, facilitating bone movement. These muscles are also known as striated muscles due to their distinctive red and white line patterns. Skeletal muscles serve multiple functions, such as supporting body weight, protecting internal organs, and regulating body temperature. For instance, when the body is cold, skeletal muscles contract and relax to generate heat, thereby restoring normal body temperature. This thermogenic function is crucial for maintaining homeostasis.

Cardiac muscle, found in the heart's middle layers, operates involuntarily. This muscle type is unique to the heart and is responsible for pumping blood throughout the body. The rhythmic contractions of cardiac muscle ensure a continuous supply of oxygen and nutrients to tissues while removing waste products. The health of the cardiac muscle is vital for overall cardiovascular health, which can be supported through a balanced diet, regular physical activity, and stress management techniques.

Smooth muscles, also involuntary, line the insides of various organs, including the intestines, stomach, and blood vessels. These muscles also appear in the walls of airways and the urinary tract.

Smooth muscles work automatically, contracting in a coordinated sequence to form waves of contractions known as peristalsis. Peristalsis moves food through the digestive system and urine through the urinary tract, playing a critical role in the body's waste elimination processes.

Skeletal Muscles
Voluntary movement, posture, heat production
Plant-based protein diet, strength training, yoga

Cardiac Muscle
Involuntary pumping of blood through the heart
Balanced diet, cardiovascular exercise, stress management

Smooth Muscles
Involuntary movement of food and waste through organs
Anti-inflammatory diet, hydration, regular physical activity

Approaches to Muscular Health

Maintaining muscle health involves a comprehensive approach that includes diet, exercise, and natural remedies. A nutrient-rich diet with a focus on plant-based proteins can provide the necessary building blocks for muscle maintenance and repair. Foods such as beans, lentils, quinoa, and tofu are excellent sources of protein. Additionally, incorporating anti-inflammatory foods like turmeric, ginger, and green leafy vegetables can help reduce muscle soreness and inflammation.

Regular physical activity is essential for maintaining muscle strength and flexibility. Engaging in a mix of aerobic exercises, strength training, and flexibility exercises such as yoga can promote overall muscular health. It is crucial to choose activities that are enjoyable and sustainable, ensuring long-term adherence to an active lifestyle.

Understanding Obesity

Obesity is a significant health issue that affects many people, but it is particularly prevalent among Black women. It is defined as having a Body Mass Index (BMI) of 30 or higher. Several factors contribute to the higher rates of obesity in Black women, including genetic predispositions, socioeconomic challenges, cultural dietary preferences, and limited access to healthy foods and recreational facilities. Understanding these factors is crucial in addressing the issue effectively.

Your Body is Beautiful

Impact on the Body

Knees and Joints Carrying excess weight puts substantial strain on the joints, particularly the knees. The knees bear the brunt of the body's weight, and every extra pound adds about four pounds of pressure on these joints. This increased pressure can lead to the development of osteoarthritis, a condition characterized by the deterioration of cartilage that cushions the ends of the bones. Osteoarthritis can cause pain, stiffness, and decreased mobility, significantly impacting the quality of life. Spinal Cord and Back Obesity also affects the spinal cord and back. Excess weight can alter the natural curve of the spine, leading to lower back pain and other spinal issues. The additional weight can cause herniated discs and spinal stenosis, which are conditions that compress the nerves in the spine, causing pain, numbness, and sometimes, disability.

Maintaining a healthy weight is essential to reduce the risk of these painful and debilitating conditions. Heart Health The heart is another critical organ affected by obesity. Excess body weight increases the risk of developing cardiovascular diseases, such as hypertension (high blood pressure), coronary artery disease, and heart failure. Obesity is associated with increased levels of bad cholesterol (LDL) and triglycerides, and decreased levels of good cholesterol (HDL). This imbalance can lead to the buildup of plaque in the arteries, narrowing them and making it harder for blood to flow. Over time, this can result in heart attacks or strokes.

Other Health Concerns

Diabetes Obesity is a major risk factor for Type 2 diabetes, a condition where the body becomes resistant to insulin or does not produce enough insulin to maintain normal blood glucose levels. Black women have higher rates of Type 2 diabetes, which can lead to complications such as kidney disease, vision problems, and nerve damage. Weight management through diet and exercise can help prevent and manage diabetes. Respiratory Issues Carrying excess weight can also affect respiratory function. Fat deposits around the chest and abdomen can restrict lung capacity and make it harder to breathe. This can lead to conditions like sleep apnea, where breathing stops and starts repeatedly during sleep, leading to poor sleep quality and increased risk of cardiovascular problems.

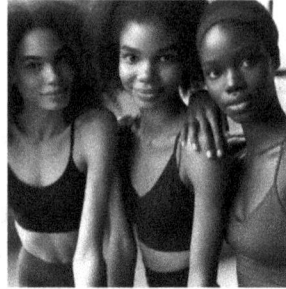

Mental Health Obesity can also have significant psychological impacts. Black women experiencing obesity may face societal stigma and discrimination, leading to issues such as low self-esteem, depression, and anxiety. The mental health burden associated with obesity can further complicate efforts to lose weight and maintain a healthy lifestyle.

Black women often have higher muscle mass, which is beneficial for overall strength and metabolic health. Muscle mass helps in burning calories, maintaining a healthy weight, and reducing the risk of chronic diseases.

Muscle Mass and Physical Fitness

Regular Exercise: Engaging in strength training exercises like body-weight exercises (push-ups, squats, lunges), resistance band workouts, and yoga helps maintain and build muscle mass. **Metabolic Health**: Maintaining muscle mass is crucial for metabolic health. It helps in managing blood sugar levels, blood pressure, and cholesterol levels.

Metabolic Health

Maintaining muscle mass is crucial for metabolic health, playing a significant role in managing various bodily functions. Muscle tissue helps regulate blood sugar levels by enhancing insulin sensitivity, allowing the body to use glucose more effectively. This process is essential in preventing and managing type 2 diabetes. Muscle mass also contributes to maintaining healthy blood pressure and cholesterol levels by supporting cardiovascular health and improving lipid metabolism. To support muscle maintenance and overall metabolic health, regular strength training exercises are recommended alongside a balanced diet rich in protein. Incorporating herbal remedies can further enhance metabolic health.

For instance, consuming fenugreek seeds can help improve blood sugar control, while hawthorn berries can support heart health and blood pressure regulation. Additionally, incorporating turmeric into the diet can aid in reducing inflammation and improving cholesterol levels. These natural approaches, combined with a healthy lifestyle, can significantly enhance metabolic health and reduce the risk of chronic diseases.

Understanding and maintaining muscle mass is crucial for overall health and vitality. Muscle mass refers to the amount of muscle tissue in the body, which plays a significant role in metabolism, strength, and mobility. Due to factors like higher bone density and muscle mass compared to other populations, Black women have unique dietary, and exercise needs to preserve their muscular strength and function. Engaging in regular strength training exercises, such as weightlifting, resistance band exercises, and bodyweight exercises, is essential to stimulate muscle growth and prevent muscle loss over time.

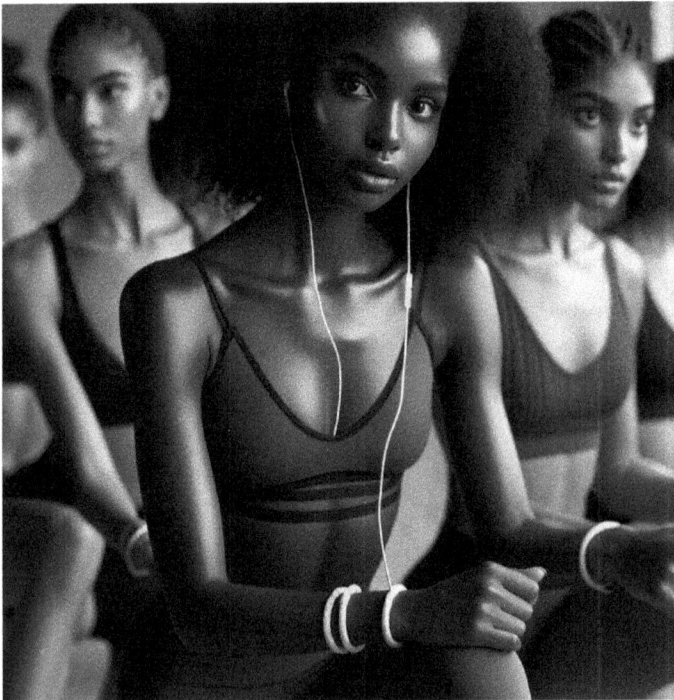

Additionally, consuming an adequate amount of protein from plant-based sources such as legumes, tofu, tempeh, and nuts can support muscle repair and growth. By prioritizing strength training and incorporating plant-based protein sources into their diets, Black women can effectively maintain muscle mass, supporting their overall health and well-being.

Exercise Recommendations

Regular physical activity is essential for maintaining overall health and well-being. Engaging in cardiovascular exercises, such as walking, running, and dancing, can significantly improve cardiovascular health by strengthening the heart and lungs. Strength training, which involves building muscle strength through the use of weights or resistance bands, is crucial for maintaining muscle mass and supporting metabolic health. Additionally, incorporating flexibility exercises, like yoga or stretching routines, into your fitness regimen helps enhance mobility, reduce the risk of injury, and promote relaxation.

Importance of Physical Activity

Physical activity offers numerous benefits that contribute to a healthier lifestyle. It plays a pivotal role in weight management by helping to maintain a healthy weight through the burning of calories and increasing metabolism. Engaging in regular exercise also strengthens bones, thereby preventing conditions such as osteoporosis, which is particularly important as one ages. Moreover, physical activity has significant mental health benefits, including the reduction of stress levels and the improvement of mood. By promoting the release of endorphins, exercise can help alleviate symptoms of depression and anxiety, fostering a more positive mental state. Overall, incorporating regular physical activity into daily routines is vital for both physical and mental health.

Warm-up and Cool-down

To prevent injuries, it is crucial to begin each cardio workout with a 5-10 minute warm-up and conclude with a cool-down. This prepares your muscles and cardiovascular system for exercise and helps in recovery post-workout.

Hydration

Staying hydrated is essential before, during, and after your workout. Proper hydration supports optimal physical performance and aids in recovery.

Consistency

For effective cardio fitness, aim for at least 150 minutes of moderate-intensity or 75 minutes of high-intensity cardio exercise each week. Consistency in your exercise routine is key to achieving and maintaining fitness goals.

Mix It Up

Vary your workouts to target different muscle groups and to keep your exercise routine engaging. Incorporating different types of cardio activities helps prevent boredom and ensures a comprehensive fitness regimen.

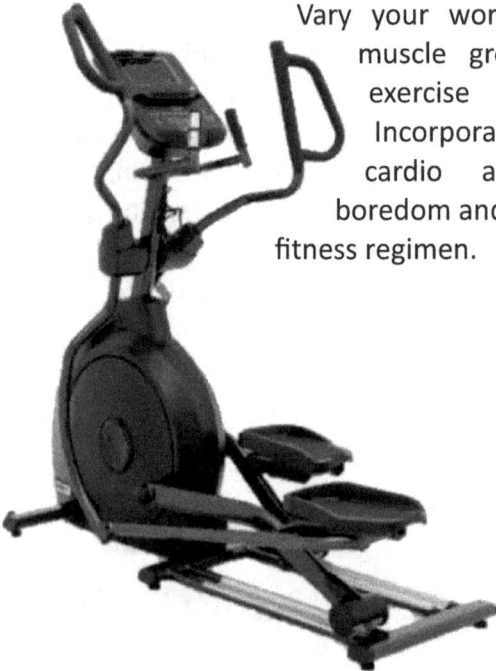

Endocrine System
GLANDS THAT SECRETE HORMONES INTO THE BLOOD

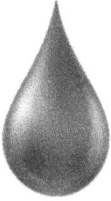

The endocrine system is an intricate network of glands and organs that produce and secrete hormones into the bloodstream, functioning as the body's chemical messengers to regulate numerous physiological processes. This system plays a critical role in maintaining homeostasis and influencing almost every cell, organ, and function of the body. Understanding the endocrine system from a holistic and natural standpoint can provide valuable insights into managing and optimizing hormonal health.

Hormones are natural substances that carry information and instructions from one set of cells to another. They are essential in regulating growth and development, metabolism, reproduction, sexual function, sleep, hunger, mood, energy levels, and the body's response to injury and stress. Glands, which are distributed throughout the body, including the hypothalamus, pituitary gland, pancreas, ovaries, and adrenal glands, are responsible for producing these hormones. Receptors in various organs and tissues recognize and respond to these hormones, ensuring that the body's functions are precisely regulated.

The hypothalamus, located in the brain, plays a pivotal role in controlling the endocrine system by sending signals to the pituitary gland, often referred to as the master gland. The pituitary gland, in turn, releases hormones that influence other glands throughout the body. For instance, the pancreas produces insulin, a hormone that signals muscle cells to rapidly absorb glucose, thus regulating blood sugar levels. The ovaries produce estrogen, which is crucial for uterine growth and the development of female secondary sex characteristics.

Approaches to Endocrine Health

Maintaining endocrine health requires an approach that includes diet, lifestyle changes, and natural remedies. A nutrient-dense diet rich in whole foods can support hormonal balance. Incorporating foods such as flaxseeds, which are high in phytoestrogens, can help modulate estrogen levels. Additionally, foods rich in omega-3 fatty acids, such as chia seeds and walnuts, can support hormone production and reduce inflammation.

Regular physical activity is also essential for maintaining endocrine health. Exercise helps regulate hormones such as insulin and cortisol, enhancing overall metabolic health. For Black women, engaging in activities that reduce stress, such as yoga and meditation, can be particularly beneficial as chronic stress can lead to hormonal imbalances.

Hypothalamus *Hormone Produced* Various releasing hormones *Function* Controls pituitary gland *Health Tips* Stress management, meditation

Pituitary Gland *Hormone Produced* Growth hormone, others *Function* Regulates other glands *Health Tips* Regular exercise, balanced diet

Pancreas *Hormone Produced* Insulin *Function* Regulates blood sugar levels *Health Tips* Low-glycemic diet, regular meals

Ovaries Hormone *Hormone Produced* Estrogen, progesterone *Function* Regulates menstrual cycle, fertility *Health Tips* Phytoestrogen-rich foods, hormonal balancing herbs

Adrenal Glands Hormone *Hormone Produced* Cortisol, adrenaline *Function* Stress response, metabolism *Health Tips* Adaptogens like ashwagandha, adequate sleep

The endocrine system, which regulates hormones responsible for controlling various bodily functions, plays a crucial role in maintaining overall health. When the endocrine system malfunctions, it can trigger a range of disorders that disrupt the body's normal processes, leading to widespread symptoms affecting multiple organs and systems. Endocrine disorders are primarily caused by an imbalance in hormone levels—either an excess or deficiency of particular hormones. This imbalance can lead to several health issues.

Thyroid Disorders

The thyroid gland, which regulates metabolism, can become overactive (hyperthyroidism) or underactive (hypothyroidism). Hyperthyroidism causes symptoms like rapid heart rate, weight loss, anxiety, and heat intolerance. Hypothyroidism, on the other hand, leads to fatigue, weight gain, depression, and cold sensitivity. Both conditions affect the body's energy balance and overall metabolic health.

Diabetes

One of the most well-known endocrine disorders, diabetes results from the pancreas failing to produce sufficient insulin (type 1 diabetes) or the body becoming resistant to insulin's effects (type 2 diabetes). This disrupts glucose regulation, leading to elevated blood sugar levels. If untreated, diabetes can cause complications such as nerve damage, cardiovascular disease, kidney failure, and vision loss.

Adrenal Disorders

The adrenal glands produce cortisol, a hormone that helps the body respond to stress. Disorders like Cushing's syndrome (excess cortisol production) can lead to symptoms such as rapid weight gain, high blood pressure, and weakened bones. Addison's disease, a result of insufficient cortisol, causes fatigue, low blood pressure, and weight loss. These conditions significantly affect the body's ability to manage stress and maintain energy balance.

Polycystic Ovary Syndrome (PCOS)

PCOS is a common endocrine disorder among women of reproductive age, caused by an imbalance in sex hormones like estrogen and androgens. Symptoms include irregular periods, infertility, excessive hair growth, and acne. PCOS is often linked to insulin resistance, which increases the risk of type 2 diabetes and metabolic syndrome.

Growth Disorders

The pituitary gland, known as the "master gland," regulates growth hormone. Overproduction of growth hormone can cause acromegaly in adults (enlargement of bones and tissues) or gigantism in children. A deficiency in growth hormone, however, can result in stunted growth and delayed development.

Reproductive Health Issues

Imbalances in estrogen, progesterone, and testosterone can affect reproductive health. For women, conditions like estrogen dominance can lead to fibroids, heavy menstruation, and fertility issues. In men, low testosterone levels may result in reduced muscle mass, fatigue, and sexual dysfunction. These hormone imbalances can affect overall health, including mood, energy, and sexual health.

Mood and Mental Health Disorders

Hormones play a critical role in regulating mood. Imbalances in cortisol, thyroid hormones, and sex hormones can contribute to anxiety, depression, and other mood disorders. For example, women experiencing hormonal fluctuations during menopause or menstrual cycles may experience mood swings or anxiety. Thyroid imbalances are also linked to depression or heightened anxiety.

Bone Health Issues

Hormonal imbalances, especially in sex hormones like estrogen and testosterone, can lead to osteoporosis, a condition where bones become weak and brittle. Low estrogen levels, often seen in postmenopausal women, accelerate bone loss, increasing the risk of fractures. The impact of an improperly functioning endocrine system is widespread, as hormones control almost every bodily process. When these systems are out of balance, symptoms often overlap, affecting energy levels, metabolism, growth, mood, reproductive health, and the body's ability to manage stress. Managing endocrine health holistically through lifestyle changes, diet, and stress management can help restore balance and prevent more severe health complications.

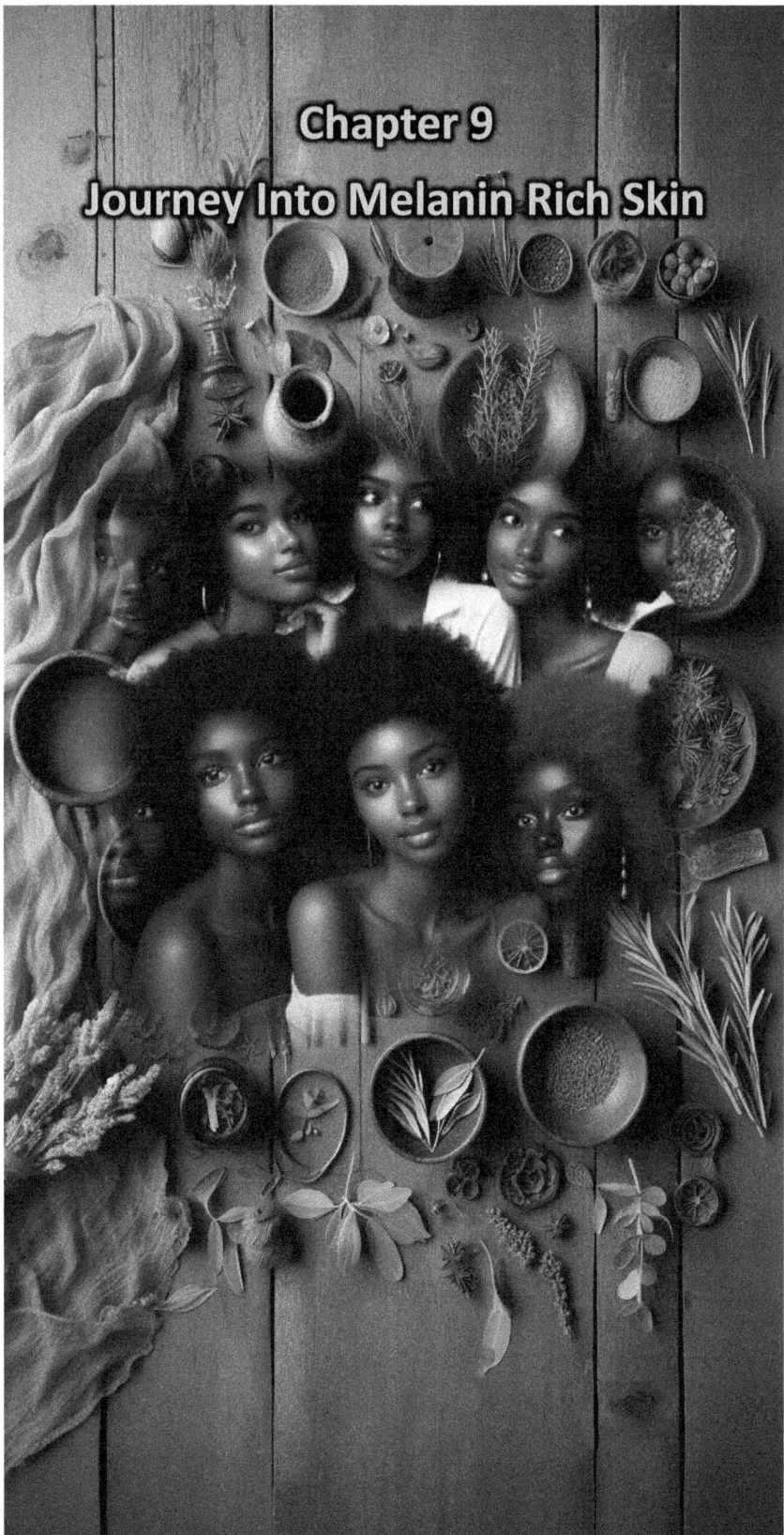

Chapter 9
Journey Into Melanin Rich Skin

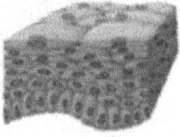

The Integumentary System

SKIN HAIR   NAILS

The integumentary system is the body's outermost layer of organs, which includes the skin, hair, and nails. These structures, composed of similar types of cells, work together to protect the body from injury, germs, and water evaporation. They also assist other body systems, such as the immune and respiratory systems, in maintaining overall health. For Black women, understanding and caring for the integumentary system through a holistic and natural lens can enhance health and well-being.

The skin is the largest and heaviest organ in the body, consisting of three layers: the epidermis, dermis, and subcutaneous tissue. The epidermis serves as the outer protective layer, the dermis provides structural support and contains nerves that detect sensations, and the subcutaneous layer insulates the body and stores fat. The skin plays a crucial role in protecting the body from infections and germs and has the remarkable ability to regenerate itself approximately every 27 days. Maintaining skin health is particularly important due to the unique properties of melanin-rich skin, which provides additional protection against UV radiation but can also be prone to specific conditions such as hyperpigmentation and keloids.

Natural Remedies for Skin Health

Hydration and Moisturization: Drinking adequate water and using natural moisturizers like shea butter and coconut oil can keep the skin hydrated and supple. **Exfoliation:** Natural exfoliants like sugar scrubs and oatmeal can help remove dead skin cells and promote healthy skin regeneration. **Diet:** A diet rich in antioxidants, vitamins A, C, and E, and omega-3 fatty acids supports skin health and reduces inflammation. **Hair:** Protection and Sensory Function Hair, made of keratin, is a protein that also forms the cells of the skin and nails. Hair helps keep the body warm, protects the eyes from water and dirt, and contains nerve endings that detect touch, pressure, and temperature. For Black women, hair care involves not only aesthetic considerations but also addressing specific issues such as dryness, breakage, and scalp health.

Natural Remedies for Hair Health

Nutrient-Rich Diet: Incorporating foods rich in vitamins and minerals, such as lean meats, fish, eggs, legumes, dark leafy greens, and nuts, can promote hair strength and growth. *Hydration:* Adequate water intake supports hair hydration and reduces breakage. *Natural Oils:* Applying oils like argan oil, jojoba oil, and castor oil can nourish the scalp and hair, promoting shine and reducing dryness. *Nails:* Protection and Functionality Nails, also composed of keratin, protect the ends of the fingers and toes. They consist of several segments, including the nail plate, nail bed, cuticle, nail folds, lunula, and matrix. Healthy nails are essential for performing daily tasks and protecting the delicate skin at the tips of the fingers and toes.

Natural Remedies for Nail Health

Diet: Consuming a balanced diet rich in biotin, zinc, and iron supports nail strength and growth. Foods like eggs, nuts, and whole grains are excellent sources of these nutrients. *Moisturization*: Regularly moisturizing the nails and cuticles with natural oils like almond oil and coconut oil can prevent dryness and brittleness. *Avoiding Harsh Chemicals*: Limiting exposure to harsh chemicals found in some nail polishes and removers can help maintain nail health. *Glands:* Essential for Homeostasis The integumentary system also includes various glands, such as sweat glands and sebaceous glands, which release materials like water, salt, or oil from under the skin to the surface. These glands play a vital role in regulating body temperature, maintaining skin hydration, and protecting the skin from infections.

Natural Remedies for Gland Health

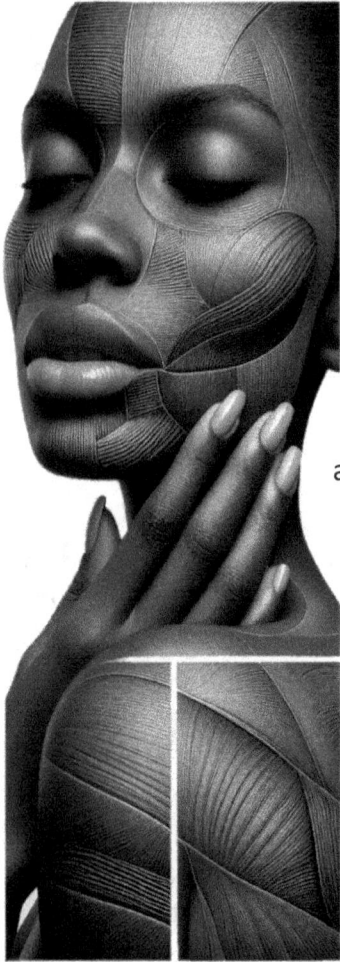

Herbal Teas: Consuming herbal teas like chamomile and green tea can support the detoxification processes and promote glandular health. *Balanced Diet:* A diet rich in fruits, vegetables, and whole grains supports the function of glands by providing essential nutrients and antioxidants. *Proper Hygiene:* Maintaining good hygiene practices, such as regular washing and using natural, gentle cleansers, can help prevent infections and support gland health.

Maintaining the health of melanin-rich skin requires understanding its unique properties and needs. By following proper skin care practices, using natural remedies, and protecting against UV damage, Black women can achieve and maintain healthy, radiant skin. Empowering oneself with this knowledge not only enhances physical health but also boosts confidence and well-being. Remember, your skin is a reflection of your inner health and deserves the best care possible. Embrace your natural beauty and take pride in your unique skin.

Melanin Rich Skin Health

The skin of Black women contains more melanin, which provides some protection against UV radiation but also requires specific care to prevent conditions like hyperpigmentation and keloids.

Moisturization

Regular use of emollients to prevent dryness and ashy skin. Regular moisturization is essential for maintaining the health and appearance of melanin-rich skin. Emollients, such as shea butter, cocoa butter, and coconut oil, help prevent dryness and ashy skin by replenishing the skin's natural moisture barrier. By forming a protective layer on the skin's surface, these emollients lock in moisture, keeping the skin hydrated and supple. Consistent use of moisturizers, especially immediately after bathing when the skin is still damp, helps prevent moisture loss and promotes soft, smooth skin.

Sun Protection

Use of broad-spectrum sunscreen to prevent sun damage and hyperpigmentation. Sun protection is paramount for preserving the health and beauty of melanin-rich skin. Broad-spectrum sunscreen with SPF 30 or higher should be applied daily to shield the skin from harmful UV radiation. Sunscreen helps prevent sunburn, premature aging, and hyperpigmentation by blocking both UVA and UVB rays. Ingredients like zinc oxide and titanium dioxide provide effective and gentle protection without causing irritation or clogging pores. Incorporating sunscreen into the daily skincare routine, regardless of weather conditions, is essential for maintaining skin health and preventing sun-related damage.

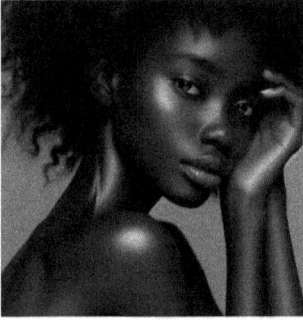

Gentle Exfoliation

Avoiding harsh scrubs to reduce the risk of skin irritation and scarring. Exfoliation is a crucial step in any skincare routine, but for melanin-rich skin, it's essential to use gentle exfoliants to avoid irritation and scarring. Harsh scrubs and abrasive exfoliating agents can cause micro-tears in the skin, leading to inflammation and post-inflammatory hyperpigmentation. Gently remove dead skin cells without disrupting the skin's barrier function. Exfoliation should be performed no more than 1-2 times per week to prevent over-exfoliation and maintain skin health.

Skin Layer

Epidermis *Description* Outermost layer of the skin.- Composed of multiple sub-layers including the stratum corneum, stratum granulosum, stratum spinosum, and stratum basale. *Function* Provides a waterproof barrier.- Protects against UV radiation.- Regulates body temperature.- Houses melanocytes (produce melanin) and Langerhans cells.

Dermis *Description* Thicker layer beneath the epidermis.- Contains blood vessels, hair follicles, and sweat glands.- Composed of connective tissue (collagen and elastin fibers). *Function* Provides structural support and elasticity.- Contains nerve endings for sensation.- Supplies nutrients to the epidermis.

Hypodermis (Subcutis) *Description* Deepest layer of the skin.- Composed of fat cells (adipocytes) and connective tissue.- Attaches the skin to underlying muscle and bone.- Contains blood vessels and nerves. *Function* Insulates the body.- Cushions and protects organs.- Stores energy as fat.- Provides passage for blood vessels and nerves to reach the skin layers.

Common Skin Concerns for Black Women
Hyperpigmentation

Darker patches on the skin caused by excess melanin production, often triggered by inflammation, acne, or sun exposure. Hyperpigmentation refers to the darkening of patches on the skin caused by an overproduction of melanin. This condition often occurs as a result of various factors such as inflammation, acne, or prolonged sun exposure. When the skin experiences these triggers, melanocytes— the cells responsible for melanin production— become hyperactive, leading to localized areas of increased pigmentation. These dark patches can be challenging to manage and may persist if not addressed properly, impacting the overall complexion and skin tone.

Keloids

Overgrowth of scar tissue that forms at the site of a skin injury, more common in melanin-rich skin. Keloids are abnormal growths of scar tissue that form at the site of a skin injury or trauma. They occur when the body produces excessive collagen during the healing process, resulting in raised, thickened scars that extend beyond the boundaries of the original wound. Keloids are more common in individuals with melanin-rich skin and can develop after various types of skin injuries, including surgical incisions, burns, piercings, or even minor cuts and scratches. While keloids are not harmful, they can be cosmetically bothersome and may cause discomfort or itching.

Dryness and Ash

Due to lower levels of ceramides, the skin's natural moisture barrier can be compromised, leading to dryness and an ashy appearance. Dryness and ashy skin are common concerns for individuals with melanin-rich skin due to lower levels of ceramides—a type of lipid that helps maintain the skin's natural moisture barrier. When the skin lacks sufficient ceramides, its ability to retain moisture is compromised, leading to dry, rough, and flaky skin. This can result in an ashy appearance, especially in areas prone to friction or environmental exposure. Proper hydration and moisturization are essential for addressing dryness and restoring the skin's moisture balance, helping to alleviate discomfort and improve overall skin health and appearance.

Key Skin Care Recommendations

Moisturization Prevents dryness and ashy skin, maintaining the skin's natural barrier. *How to Moisturize:* Use emollients like shea butter, cocoa butter, or coconut oil. Apply immediately after bathing to lock in moisture. **Sun Protection** Despite natural protection from melanin, UV radiation can still cause damage and lead to hyperpigmentation. *How to Protect:* Use a broad-spectrum sunscreen with SPF 30 or higher. Look for sunscreens with ingredients like zinc oxide or titanium dioxide. **Gentle Exfoliation** Removes dead skin cells and promotes cell turnover without causing irritation. *How to Exfoliate:* Use gentle exfoliants like lactic acid or fruit enzymes. Avoid harsh scrubs that can damage the skin and increase the risk of scarring. Dry skin, or xerosis, can be caused by a variety of factors, including genetics, health conditions, habits, and nutrient deficiencies. Understanding these causes can help in effectively managing and treating dry skin.

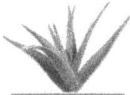

Aloe Vera	**Properties:** Anti-inflammatory and moisturizing. **Usage:** Apply gel directly to the skin to soothe irritation and provide hydration.
Turmeric	**Properties:** Anti-inflammatory and brightening. **Usage:** Use in masks or as a paste with honey to reduce hyperpigmentation and improve skin tone.
Shea Butter	**Properties:** Rich in fatty acids and vitamins A and E. **Usage:** Use as a daily moisturizer to maintain skin hydration and elasticity.
Tea Tree Oil	**Properties:** Antimicrobial and anti-inflammatory. **Usage:** Dilute with a carrier oil and apply to acne-prone areas to reduce breakouts and prevent scarring.

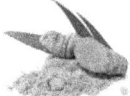

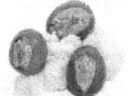

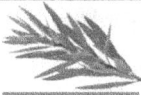

Understanding Dry Skin: Causes and Management

Symptoms and Impact: Dry skin is quite common and can affect individuals of all ages. Symptoms include redness, flakiness, and itchiness, which can be uncomfortable. If left untreated, dry skin can lead to complications such as infections or permanent skin changes.

Management and Treatment Most cases of dry skin can be managed with self-care measures, including: **Hydration:** Drink plenty of water to keep the skin hydrated. *Moisturizers*: Use moisturizers regularly to maintain skin moisture. *Avoiding Irritants:* Avoid hot showers, fragranced products, and excessive washing. *Diet:* Ensure adequate intake of vitamins and minerals. In severe cases, where dry skin is inflamed, painful, has open sores, or disrupts daily activities, it is advisable to see a primary care provider or dermatologist.

Preventative Measures Hydration: Regular intake of water. *Balanced Diet:* Consuming a diet rich in vitamins and minerals. *Proper Skincare*: Using gentle, fragrance-free products and avoiding excessive washing.

Dry Skin Causes	Description
Genetics	Genetic predisposition can make some individuals more prone to dry skin.
Health Conditions	Various health conditions can cause dry skin as a symptom. These include: - Allergies: Reactions can lead to dry skin. - Eczema: Causes inflamed, itchy, cracked, and rough skin. - Diabetes: High blood sugar levels can lead to dry skin. - Kidney Disease: Can result in dry, itchy skin. - Thyroid Disease: Reduced sweat production can cause dryness. - Chemotherapy: Cancer treatments can result in dry skin.
Habits	Certain habits can contribute to skin dryness: - Taking hot showers - Wearing fragrance - Excessive hand washing - Drinking too much alcohol and not enough water - Incorrect use of skincare products
Nutrient Deficiencies	Deficiencies in vitamins and minerals such as vitamin D, vitamin A, niacin, zinc, iron, or vitamin E can cause dry skin.
Smoking	Smoking can accelerate skin aging and contribute to dryness.

Understanding Melanin

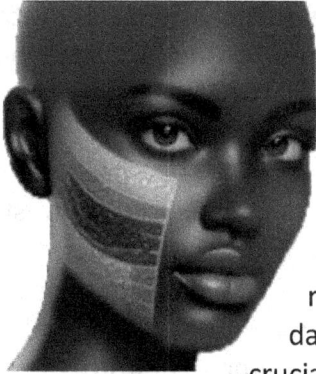

Melanin is a pigment produced by cells called melanocytes located in the epidermis, the outermost layer of the skin. It plays several critical roles.

Radiation

Melanin absorbs and dissipates UV radiation, reducing the risk of DNA damage and skin cancer. Melanin plays a crucial role in protecting the skin from the harmful effects of ultraviolet (UV) radiation. When the skin is exposed to UV rays, melanin absorbs and dissipates this radiation, effectively reducing the risk of DNA damage. This protective function lowers the likelihood of developing skin cancer and other UV-induced skin conditions. In essence, melanin acts as a natural sunscreen, shielding the skin from potential harm.

Antioxidant Properties

Melanin helps neutralize free radicals, reducing oxidative stress on the skin. Melanin also possesses significant antioxidant properties. Antioxidants are vital in combating free radicals, which are unstable molecules that can cause cellular damage and contribute to aging and various diseases. By neutralizing these free radicals, melanin reduces oxidative stress on the skin. This protective mechanism helps maintain the skin's overall health and resilience, preventing premature aging and other oxidative stress-related conditions.

Skin Color

The amount and type of melanin determine skin color, with eumelanin contributing to darker skin tones. The amount and type of melanin present in the skin are the primary determinants of an individual's skin color. There are two main types of melanin: eumelanin and pheomelanin. Eumelanin is responsible for darker skin tones, providing a rich, deep pigmentation. In contrast, pheomelanin contributes to lighter skin tones with reddish or yellowish hues. The higher concentration of eumelanin in the skin of Black women not only gives it its characteristic color but also enhances its protective functions against environmental stressors.

Facts About Melanin

Types of Melanin

There are two main types—eumelanin (black or brown) and pheomelanin (red or yellow). Melanin comes in two primary forms—eumelanin and pheomelanin. Eumelanin contributes to Black or brown skin tones, while pheomelanin is responsible for red or yellow hues. The relative amounts of these two types of melanin determine an individual's skin color, with higher levels of eumelanin resulting in darker skin tones.

Production

Melanin production is stimulated by UV exposure and certain hormones. Melanin production is regulated by various factors, including genetics, UV exposure, and hormonal influences. When the skin is exposed to UV radiation, melanocytes—the cells responsible for melanin production—are stimulated to produce more melanin. Additionally, certain hormones, such as melanocyte-stimulating hormone (MSH), can also influence melanin synthesis.

Health Benefits

Besides UV protection, melanin-rich skin tends to age slower and is less prone to wrinkles. Melanin-rich skin offers several health benefits beyond UV protection. Studies suggest that melanin acts as a natural defense mechanism against UV-induced damage, reducing the risk of skin cancer and other sun-related conditions. Moreover, melanin-rich skin tends to age slower and is less susceptible to premature aging signs like wrinkles and fine lines. This inherent protection against photoaging is attributed to melanin's ability to absorb and scatter UV radiation, minimizing its harmful effects on the skin cells.

Studies and Information on Melanin

UV Protection

Studies have shown that melanin can absorb up to 50-75% of UV radiation, offering significant protection compared to lighter skin tones. Research indicates that melanin provides substantial protection against the harmful effects of ultraviolet (UV) radiation. Studies have shown that melanin can absorb and scatter up to 50-75% of UV rays, depending on its concentration and distribution within the skin. This inherent UV protection is significantly higher compared to lighter skin tones, making melanin-rich skin less susceptible to sunburn, DNA damage, and the development of skin cancer. However, it's essential to note that while melanin offers significant UV protection, it is not foolproof, and individuals with darker skin tones still need to practice sun safety measures to minimize sun damage.

Antioxidant Benefits

Melanin's ability to neutralize free radicals helps protect against environmental damage and aging. Melanin possesses potent antioxidant properties that play a crucial role in maintaining skin health and combating oxidative stress. As an antioxidant, melanin helps neutralize free radicals—unstable molecules that can damage cells and contribute to premature aging and various skin disorders. By scavenging these harmful free radicals, melanin helps protect the skin from environmental damage, including UV radiation, pollution, and other sources of oxidative stress. This antioxidant defense system contributes to overall skin resilience, helping to maintain its youthful appearance and vitality.

Skin Cancer Rates

Despite its protective benefits, melanin does not make Black skin immune to skin cancer, highlighting the importance of sun protection. While melanin provides significant protection against UV radiation, it does not make individuals with darker skin tones immune to skin cancer. Despite having a lower incidence of skin cancer compared to lighter-skinned populations, Black individuals can still develop skin cancers, including melanoma, squamous cell carcinoma, and basal cell carcinoma. Factors such as genetics, family history, and environmental exposures play a role in skin cancer risk. Therefore, it's crucial for individuals with melanin-rich skin to prioritize sun protection measures, including wearing sunscreen, seeking shade, and wearing protective clothing, to reduce their risk of skin cancer and maintain skin health.

Skin Health Facts

Aging: Melanin-rich skin shows signs of aging later than lighter skin tones but may still experience issues like hyperpigmentation. Melanin-rich skin tends to show signs of aging later than lighter skin tones due to its increased natural protection against UV radiation. However, this does not mean that melanin-rich skin is immune to aging-related concerns. While melanin offers inherent UV protection, it does not entirely prevent the development of aging signs such as fine lines, wrinkles, and loss of elasticity. Additionally, melanin-rich skin may be more prone to issues like hyperpigmentation, which can exacerbate the appearance of aging. Therefore, it's essential for individuals with melanin-rich skin to adopt preventive skincare practices early on to maintain skin health and minimize the visible signs of aging.

Response to Treatment

Black skin may respond differently to certain treatments, making it crucial to choose products and methods specifically formulated for melanin-rich skin. Black skin may respond differently to certain skincare treatments and products compared to lighter skin tones. Factors such as melanin content, skin thickness, and sensitivity influence how the skin reacts to various ingredients and formulations. For example, certain exfoliating agents or chemical peels may be too harsh for melanin-rich skin, leading to irritation, inflammation, or post-inflammatory hyperpigmentation. Therefore, it's crucial for individuals with melanin-rich skin to choose skincare products and treatments specifically formulated for their unique needs. This includes opting for gentle, non-irritating formulations that address common concerns without causing undue harm or exacerbating existing skin issues

The Benefits of Ginger and Lemon for Tighter Skin and Stretch Mark Reduction

Ginger and lemon, two common kitchen ingredients, have long been valued not only for their culinary uses but also for their powerful health and beauty benefits. In holistic healing and natural skincare, ginger and lemon have become popular for their skin-tightening properties and their ability to reduce the appearance of stretch marks. This section delves into the potent skin-enhancing benefits of ginger and lemon, how they work to rejuvenate the skin, and how to create a natural oil recipe to tighten the skin and diminish stretch marks.

The Skin-Tightening and Healing Properties of Ginger

Ginger is rich in bioactive compounds such as gingerol, which has anti-inflammatory and antioxidant properties. These properties make ginger an effective ingredient for improving skin elasticity, reducing inflammation, and promoting the healing of damaged skin.

Key Benefits of Ginger for the Skin

Stimulates Circulation: Ginger enhances blood flow, which improves skin tone and firmness by ensuring that skin cells receive more oxygen and nutrients. **Antioxidant Powerhouse:** Its antioxidants combat free radicals that damage skin cells, thereby slowing down the aging process and helping to prevent wrinkles and sagging skin. **Collagen Production:** Ginger boosts the production of collagen, the structural protein responsible for maintaining skin elasticity and firmness. Increased collagen production can tighten the skin and reduce the appearance of stretch marks. **Heals Scars and Hyperpigmentation:** Ginger helps reduce the appearance of scars, including stretch marks, by promoting skin regeneration and fading hyperpigmentation over time.

The Skin-Brightening and Firming Benefits of Lemon

Lemon, a citrus fruit known for its high vitamin C content, offers numerous skin benefits. Vitamin C is essential for collagen production, skin brightening, and overall skin health.

Key Benefits of Lemon for the Skin

Vitamin C Boost: Lemon is rich in vitamin C, which plays a critical role in boosting collagen production, tightening the skin, and reducing fine lines. **Natural Astringent:** Lemon acts as a natural astringent, helping to tighten and firm the skin. This astringent property also shrinks pores, giving the skin a smooth appearance. **Lightens Dark Spots and Stretch Marks:** The citric acid in lemon acts as a natural exfoliant, helping to fade dark spots, stretch marks, and hyperpigmentation over time. **Detoxifying Effect:** Lemon detoxifies the skin, purging impurities that may contribute to sagging or uneven skin tone. This helps create a brighter and more even complexion.

Combining Ginger and Lemon for Tighter Skin and Stretch Mark Reduction

When used together, ginger and lemon create a powerful, natural remedy for improving skin elasticity, tightening loose skin, and reducing the appearance of stretch marks. The combination of ginger's collagen-boosting and circulation-enhancing properties with lemon's astringent and skin-lightening benefits makes them an effective duo for skin rejuvenation.

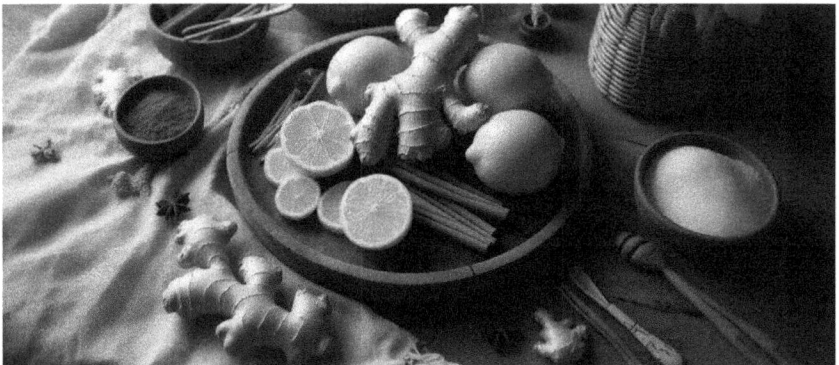

Why These Ingredients Work

Coconut Oil: Deeply moisturizes the skin, improves elasticity, and aids in the absorption of ginger and lemon. It also contains antioxidants that protect the skin from damage. *Jojoba Oil:* Mimics the skin's natural sebum and helps to balance moisture levels, while also promoting skin healing and regeneration. *Vitamin E Oil:* Promotes skin repair, reduces scarring, and protects the skin from free radical damage, making it a great addition for reducing stretch marks.

Additional Tips for Enhancing Results

Dry Brushing: Before applying the ginger-lemon oil, consider using a dry brush to exfoliate the skin. This will help remove dead skin cells and stimulate circulation, allowing the oil to penetrate more deeply.

Hydration: Drink plenty of water and eat foods rich in vitamins C and A to further support collagen production and skin health.

Consistency is Key: The natural process of reducing stretch marks and tightening skin takes time. Consistent use of the ginger-lemon oil, along with healthy lifestyle habits, will yield visible results over time.

Ginger and lemon offer a potent, natural solution for improving skin elasticity, tightening loose skin, and fading stretch marks. By regularly incorporating this ginger and lemon oil into your skincare routine, you can holistically support your skin's health and achieve a smoother, firmer appearance. Unlike chemical-laden commercial products, this natural remedy is free of harmful additives and works in harmony with your skin, allowing you to embrace the benefits of nature for your beauty and well-being.

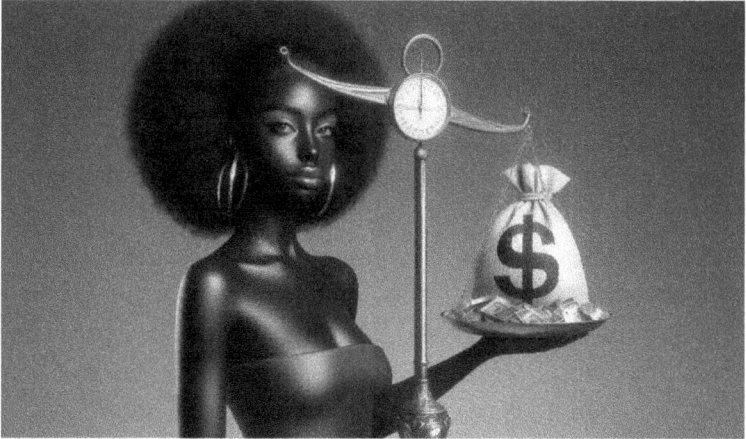

Protect Your Melanin

As stated in the section previously, melanin is a pigment found in the skin, hair, and eyes, contributing to the color of these tissues. While produced by all humans and animals, melanin is particularly abundant in Black and melanated skin. It plays a crucial role in protecting cells from ultraviolet (UV) radiation and maintaining cellular health, making it a vital asset to overall health and wellness.

Melanin Sourced for Commercial Usgage

Commercial melanin is typically extracted from non-human sources due to ethical concerns surrounding the extraction process. Squid ink is one of the primary non-human sources of melanin; it contains a type called eumelanin, which is also found in human hair and skin. This similarity makes squid ink a valuable resource for research and various industrial applications. However, reliance on squid ink poses sustainability challenges and risks disrupting marine ecosystems.

Laboratory and Synthetic Production

To address these sustainability and ethical issues, scientists have developed laboratory techniques for synthetic melanin production. Laboratory methods include: **Acid Precipitation and Base Dissolution:** These chemical processes help isolate melanin from natural sources. However, harsh acid treatments can damage melanin's structure, limiting its potential applications. **Cultivation of Melanocytes:** Some labs grow melanocytes (melanin-producing cells) in controlled environments to produce melanin sustainably, without requiring live animals or synthetic chemicals. These laboratory-based methods allow for a more sustainable approach to producing melanin while avoiding ethical concerns associated with live organisms.

Human Melanin Extraction

Melanin extraction from human skin is <u>not ethically viable</u>. It requires invasive procedures that would destroy skin cells essential to structure and function. This ethical challenge has led researchers to focus on alternative extraction and production methods, such as synthetic production, to meet the demand for melanin without compromising human or animal welfare.

Applications and Benefits of Melanin

Melanin's unique protective, antioxidative, and conductive properties make it valuable in various fields, from health and wellness to technology.

UV Protection In humans, melanin's primary function is to shield skin cells from UV radiation. By absorbing and dispersing UV rays, melanin reduces the risk of DNA damage, skin cancer, and premature aging. This protective function has led to its incorporation into skincare products and UV-blocking materials, including sunscreens, which aim to mimic melanin's natural protective barrier.

Medical and Pharmaceutical Research Melanin's protective properties make it promising for medical applications, particularly in radiation therapies. Its ability to shield cells from radiation has potential in cancer treatment, where it could protect healthy cells during radiation therapy. Additionally, melanin is explored as a stabilizing agent in drug delivery, helping to safeguard and transport therapeutic compounds within the body.

Electronic and Conductive Uses

Melanin's ability to conduct electricity under certain conditions has spurred interest in its use in electronic applications. As a biocompatible semiconductor, melanin has potential in: *Biodegradable Batteries:* A more sustainable battery alternative. *Biosensors and Implants:* Used in devices that interact directly with human tissue, melanin's compatibility with biological systems offers a safe, efficient material option.

Cosmetics and Pigments Thanks to its natural pigmentation, melanin is commonly used in cosmetics. Products such as hair dyes and skin-tone-matching foundations rely on melanin for creating deeper, natural shades for darker skin tones, making it valuable in creating inclusive cosmetic products.

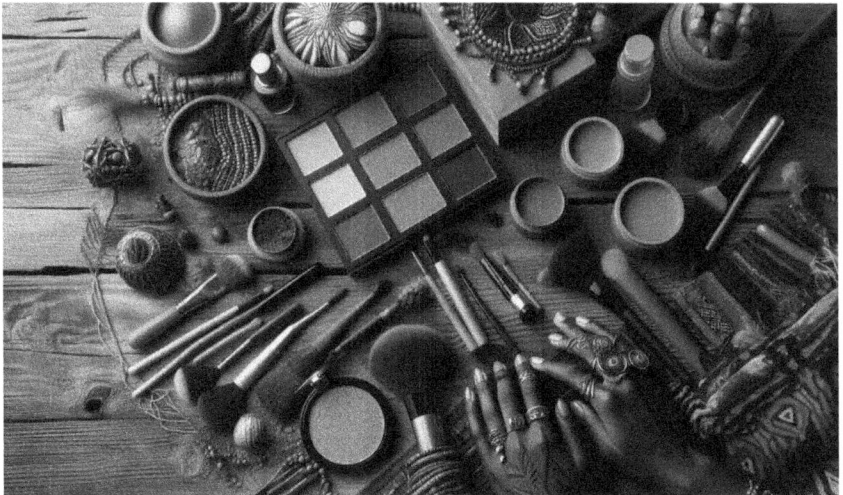

Anti-Oxidative and Anti-Inflammatory Properties Melanin's molecular structure gives it antioxidant capabilities, helping to neutralize free radicals and reduce cellular damage. This antioxidative effect, along with its anti-inflammatory potential, makes melanin an asset in therapeutic products aimed at reducing inflammation and combating oxidative stress, positioning it as a key component in anti-aging and restorative skincare products.

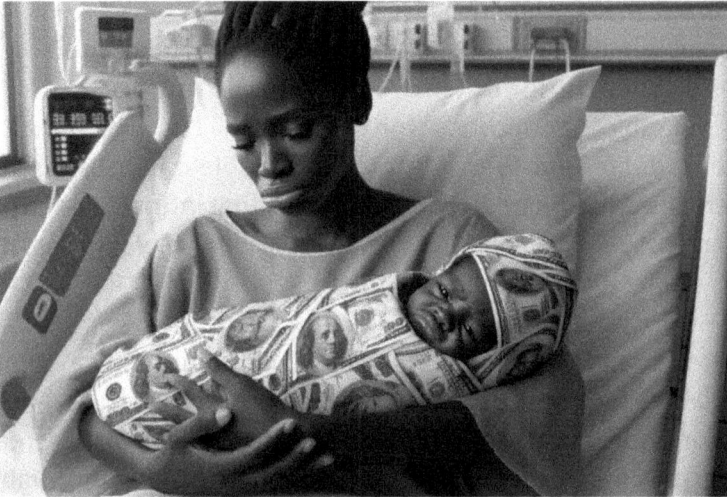

The Value of Melanin

Melanin's monetary value stems from its unique properties and high demand across various industries. As a natural UV protectant, antioxidant, and biocompatible semiconductor, melanin is sought after for applications in pharmaceuticals, cosmetics, and biocompatible electronics. These uses, combined with the challenging process of sustainable extraction and synthesis, have elevated melanin's market value, positioning it as a rare and valuable biological compound in both scientific and commercial sectors.

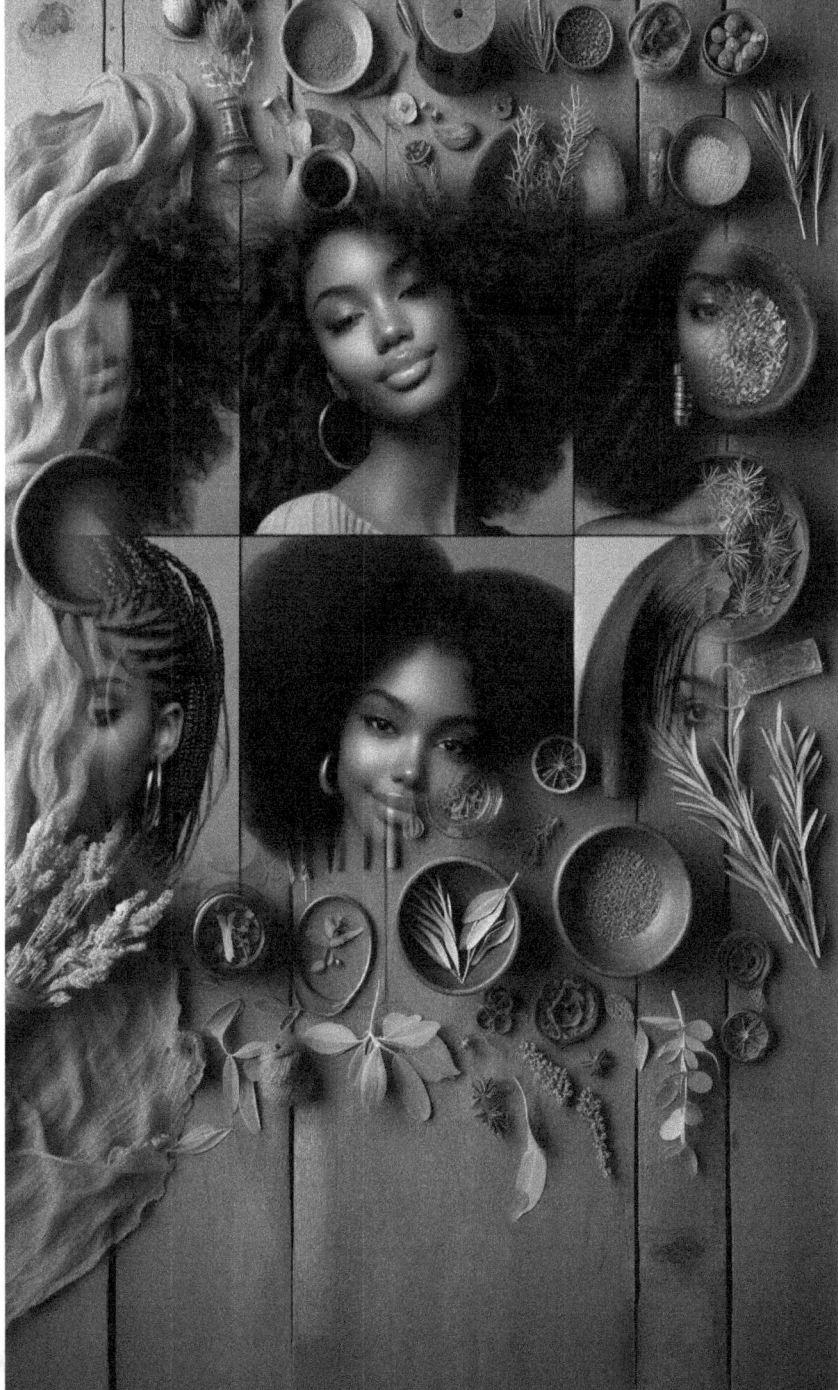

Chapter 10
Journey Into Hair and Scalp Health

The History of Black Hair and Cultural Appropriation

The history of Black women's hair is deeply intertwined with the painful experiences of slavery. During slavery, the cultural identity and dignity of enslaved Africans were systematically stripped away, with hair being a significant part of this dehumanization process. Enslaved women often had their heads shaved upon capture; a practice intended sever cultural ties. This act was profoundly humiliating and symbolized the erasure of their identity. The harsh conditions of slavery, including long hours of labor and inadequate nutrition, further damaged the health of their hair and scalp.

The Influence of Madam C.J. Walker

Madam C.J. Walker, born Sarah Breedlove, was a pioneering African American entrepreneur who made significant contributions to the history of Black hair. In the early 20th century, she developed a line of hair care products specifically for Black women, addressing their unique hair care needs. Walker's products and her promotion of scalp health and hair growth helped empower Black women to take pride in their hair. She also provided economic opportunities for Black women by creating jobs through her company. Walker's influence extended beyond hair care; she played a crucial role in the social and economic advancement of Black women in America.

Modern Workplace Discrimination

Despite progress, Black women continue to face discrimination based on their natural hair in professional settings. Many workplaces have historically enforced grooming policies that favor Eurocentric beauty standards, deeming natural hairstyles like afros, braids, locs, and twists as unprofessional. This bias often pressures Black women to alter their natural hair using chemical relaxers or heat styling to conform to these standards, leading to long-term damage and health risks.

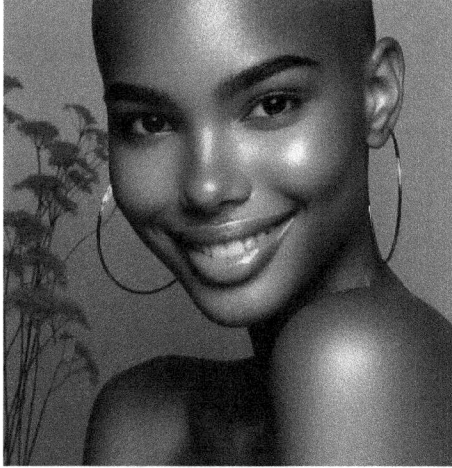

The CROWN Act

The CROWN (Creating a Respectful and Open World for Natural Hair) Act is a legislative effort to combat hair discrimination in workplaces and schools. First introduced in California in 2019, the CROWN Act prohibits discrimination based on hair texture and protective hairstyles associated with race.

Cultural Appropriation of Black Hairstyles

Black women's hair is a symbol of cultural identity and resilience. Understanding its unique needs and history is crucial for proper care and appreciation. Through protective styles, gentle handling, and nourishing products, Black women can maintain healthy, beautiful hair while honoring their heritage and individuality Black hairstyles such as braids, cornrows, and locs have often been appropriated by people outside the Black community, who adopt these styles without recognizing their cultural and historical importance. Appropriation is problematic and those who appropriate these styles are praised or seen as trendy, while Black women are penalized or discriminated against for wearing the same hairstyles. Be proud and always respect the history and honor the cultural journey.

Maintaining a healthy Scalp

Maintaining healthy hair and scalp for Black women involves a dedicated hair care routine that addresses common scalp issues such as dry scalp and dandruff, as well as other conditions like scalp psoriasis, scalp eczema, and contact dermatitis. A comprehensive routine includes proper cleansing, conditioning, moisturizing, and protective styling to ensure optimal hair and scalp health.

Common Scalp Conditions

Black women may experience a range of scalp conditions that require specific care: *Dry Scalp and Itchy Scalp:* These conditions are often due to lack of moisture, leading to itching and flaking. Using gentle, sulfate-free shampoos can help maintain the scalp's natural oils.

Dandruff: Characterized by white flakes on the scalp and hair, dandruff can be managed with anti-dandruff shampoos containing ingredients like zinc pyrithione or salicylic acid. **Scalp Psoriasis:** This is an autoimmune condition that causes red, scaly patches on the scalp. It may require medicated shampoos and topical treatments prescribed by a dermatologist. *Scalp* **Eczema:** Also known as seborrheic dermatitis, this condition causes inflamed, oily, and flaky skin.

Gentle cleansing and medicated treatments can help manage symptoms. **Contact Dermatitis:** This allergic reaction is caused by contact with certain hair products. Identifying and avoiding the allergen is crucial for treatment. **Lupus:** An autoimmune disease that can cause hair loss and scarring on the scalp. Treatment often involves medications prescribed by a doctor. **Scarring Alopecia:** This type of hair loss results from inflammation and destruction of hair follicles, leading to permanent hair loss. Early diagnosis and treatment are vital. *Favus:* A fungal infection leading to yellow crusts on the scalp, which requires antifungal medications.

Proper Scalp Cleansing

Proper scalp cleansing is essential to remove buildup of dirt, oils, and hair products. Black women should use a gentle, sulfate-free shampoo to cleanse their scalp without stripping away natural oils. Shampooing should be done regularly but not excessively to avoid over-drying. During cleansing, it's important to massage the scalp gently to improve blood circulation and ensure a thorough cleanliness.

Conditioning and Moisturizing

Conditioning is crucial for maintaining moisture and softness in Black hair. After shampooing, a good conditioner should be applied to the hair to replenish moisture. Deep conditioning treatments can be used weekly to provide extra hydration and strengthen the hair. Moisturizing the scalp with natural oils such as jojoba, coconut, or olive oil helps to prevent dryness and flakiness. These oils can be applied directly to the scalp and massaged in to promote healthy hair growth.

Protective Styling

Protective styling, such as braids, twists, and buns, can help minimize hair damage by reducing the need for constant styling and manipulation. These styles protect the ends of the hair and help retain length. However, it is important to avoid styles that are too tight, as they can cause traction alopecia, a condition where hair is lost due to excessive tension on the hair follicles.

Herbal Remedies

Herbal remedies can also be beneficial for scalp care. Aloe vera gel can soothe an itchy scalp, while a rinse made from rosemary or chamomile tea can help reduce dandruff. Regular use of these natural treatments can enhance scalp health and promote strong, healthy hair. Additionally, peppermint oil, when massaged into the scalp, can stimulate blood flow and promote hair growth.

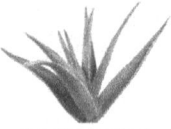
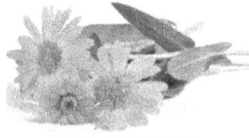
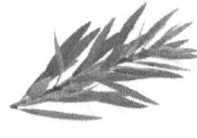

| ALOE VERA | CALENDULA | TEA TREE |

General Care Practices

Moisture Retention Deep conditioning, sealing with oils or butters, Prevents dryness and breakage , Aloe Vera and Shea Butter: Combination provides hydration and seals in moisture

Gentle Handling Minimizing heat and chemical treatments, using heat protectants, gentle detangling, Maintains hair health and prevents damage, Calendula: Soothes the scalp and reduces inflammation from styling. **Protective Styles** Braids, twists, updos, Protects hair from environmental damage and reduces manipulation, Tea Tree Oil: Keeps the scalp healthy and prevents dandruff while hair is in protective styles.

Different Hair Textures

Type 3 (Curly)

Type 3 hair ranges from loose curls (3A) to tight curls (3C). This hair type is characterized by a defined S-shape pattern. Type 3 hair can be prone to frizz and requires a balance of moisture and protein to maintain its shape and health. Regular deep conditioning and the use of leave-in conditioners can help retain moisture. Gentle detangling with a wide-tooth comb or fingers is recommended to prevent breakage.

3A: Loose, large curls that can benefit from lightweight leave-in conditioners and gels to enhance curl definition without weighing down the hair. **3B:** Tighter curls that need more moisture and can benefit from creams and custards to define curls and reduce frizz. **3C:** Tight, corkscrew curls that require heavier creams and butters to lock in moisture and define curls.

Type 4 (Coily)

Type 4 hair ranges from tightly coiled (4A) to Z-pattern coils (4C). This hair type is the most fragile and prone to shrinkage and dryness. Intensive moisture treatments, protective styling, and gentle handling are crucial for maintaining the health of Type 4 hair.

Moisturizing: Use sulfate-free shampoo and rich, creamy conditioners to retain moisture. **Styling**: Apply leave-in conditioners and curl creams to enhance and define curls. **Protection**: Sleep on a silk or satin pillowcase or use a satin bonnet to reduce friction and prevent breakage.

4A: Defined coils that benefit from moisture-rich creams and leave-ins. Regular deep conditioning and the use of light oils can help maintain hydration.

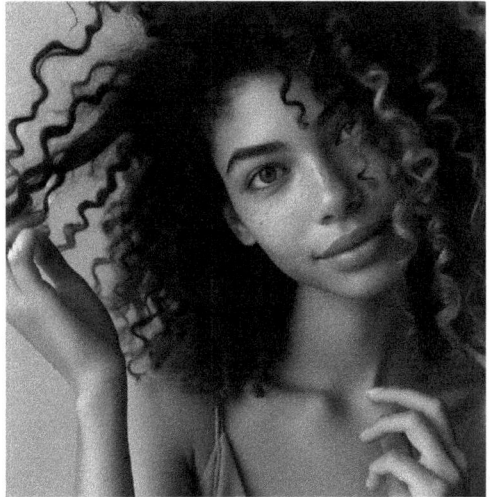

4B: Z-pattern coils that need intensive moisture treatments and heavy creams to combat dryness and shrinkage. Protective styles like twists and braids can help retain length.

4C: The most tightly coiled with a tendency for high shrinkage. This hair type requires frequent deep conditioning, heavy creams, and oils to lock in moisture. Low-manipulation styles and protective styling can help maintain hair health.

WHAT'S ON YOUR HAIR BINGO CARD?
BREAKAGE?

Skipping Trims **Damaging Protective Hairstyle** Improper Detangling **Dyeing Hair without Proper Aftercare**

LACK OF HAIR?

Tight Hairstyles **Washing Hair Routine (Hard Water)** Lack of Proper Moisturizer **Lack of Vitamin D/ Iron Deficiency**

GROWTH?

Improper Diet **Protective Hair Covering** Following Hair Growth Trends and Styles

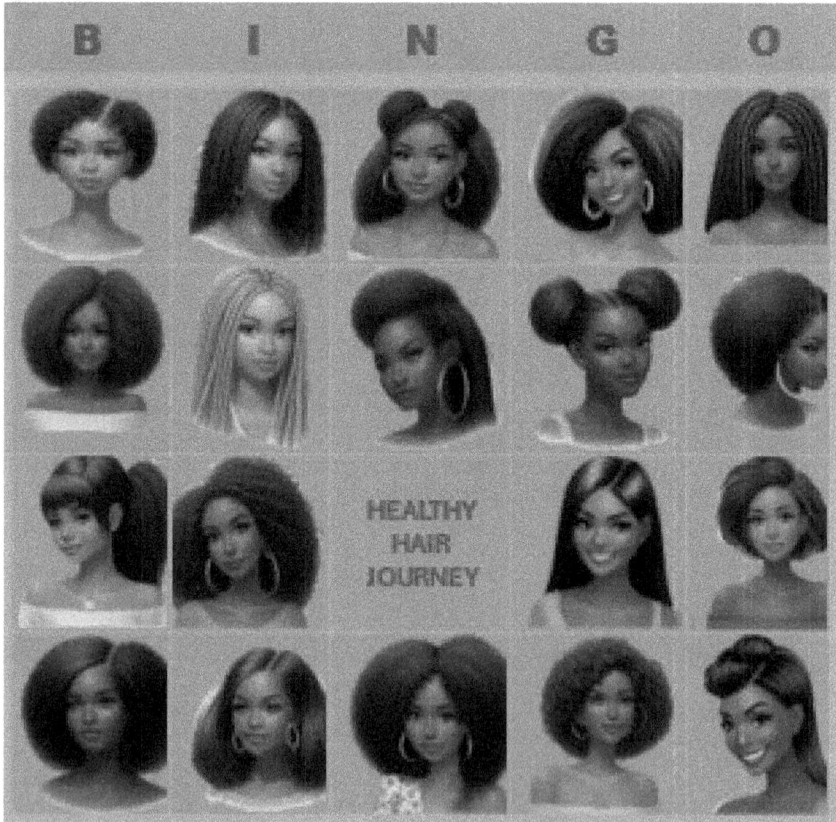

Type 4 (Coily)

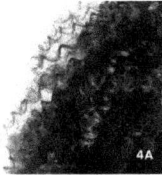

4A Dense, springy coils. Deep conditioning, heavier creams and oils for moisture retention. Shea Butter: Rich in vitamins, provides deep moisture and strengthens hair. Deep Conditioning

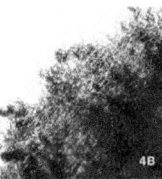

4B Z-pattern coils, less defined curl pattern. Intensive moisture, frequent protective styling to minimize breakage. Castor Oil: Promotes hair growth and retains moisture.

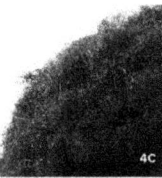

4C Tightest coils, prone to shrinkage. Maximum moisture retention, gentle detangling, and minimal manipulation. Aloe Vera and Jamaican Black Castor Oil: Combination provides hydration, strengthens roots, and locks in moisture.

Regular deep conditioning treatments with hydrating masks or hot oil treatments are essential. *Moisture and Seal:* Use the LOC (Liquid, Oil, Cream) method to lock in moisture. *Gentle Handling:* Detangle with fingers or a wide-tooth comb to minimize breakage and avoid styles that put too much tension on the hair.

Type 3 (Curly)

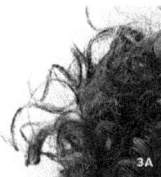

3A Loose, well-defined curls. Balance of moisture and protein. Aloe Vera: Provides hydration and soothes the scalp.

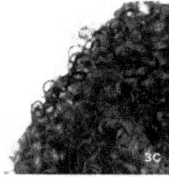

3B Tighter curls, more volume. Regular deep conditioning to maintain moisture. Hibiscus: Strengthens hair and prevents breakage.

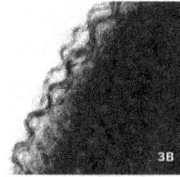

3C Tight corkscrew curls. Intensive moisture treatments and curl definition products. Marshmallow Root: Provides slip for easier detangling and hydration.

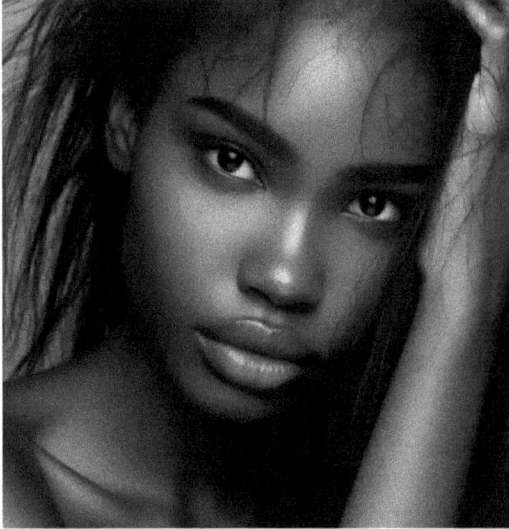

Hair Porosity

Low Porosity Hair with low porosity has tightly bound cuticles that repel moisture. This type of hair can feel resistant to water and products, often taking longer to dry. Care for low porosity hair includes using lightweight, water-based products that can penetrate the cuticle without weighing the hair down. Techniques such as using heat during conditioning (e.g., with a steamer or warm towel) can help open the cuticles and allow moisture to penetrate.

Low Porosity Hair Care Tips Clarify hair regularly to remove product buildup. Use warm water to help open the cuticles during washing and conditioning. Opt for lighter leave-in conditioners and avoid heavy butters and oils that can sit on top of the hair and cause buildup. *Warm Water* Rinses: Use warm water to help open the cuticles before applying conditioner. *Lightweight Products*: Opt for lightweight, water-based leave-in conditioners and avoid heavy butters that can weigh down the hair. *Steam Treatments*: Incorporate steam treatments to help moisture penetrate the hair shaft.

High Porosity High porosity hair has gaps and holes in the cuticles, making it more susceptible to moisture loss and damage. This hair type can absorb moisture quickly but also loses it just as fast. High porosity hair benefits from heavier products that can fill in the gaps and lock in moisture. Protein treatments can also help strengthen the cuticles and reduce porosity.

High Porosity Hair Care Tips Seal the hair with heavy creams and oils after moisturizing to lock in hydration. Use protein treatments periodically to strengthen the hair. Avoid excessive heat and chemical treatments that can further damage the cuticle layer. *Protein Treatments:* Regular protein treatments help to fill in gaps in the cuticle and strengthen the hair. *Heavy Moisturizers*: Use thicker creams and butters to seal in moisture. *Cold Water Rinses:* Finish with cold water rinses to help close the cuticles and retain moisture.

Low Porosity Lightweight, water-based products; heat to help products penetrate   Aloe Vera: Light moisturizer that penetrates easily when applied with heat. Tightly bound cuticles, repels moisture.

Medium Porosity Balanced care regimen with a mix of moisture and protein treatments Rosemary: Balances moisture and stimulates scalp circulation. Normal absorption and retention of moisture. **High Porosity** Heavier creams and oils; regular protein treatments to fill cuticle gaps Avocado Oil: Rich, nourishing oil that helps seal moisture and provides nutrients. Gaps in the cuticles, loses moisture quickly.

Hair Health and Blood Types

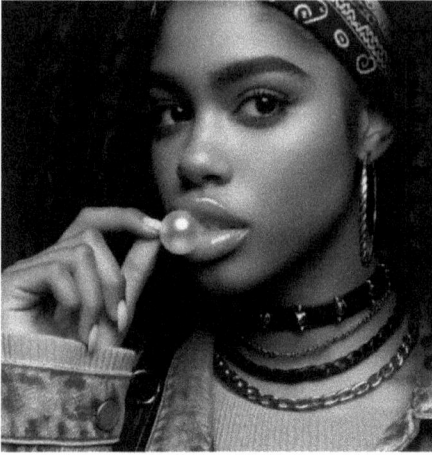

Understanding the nutritional needs based on blood type can offer a more tailored approach to maintaining hair health, ensuring that individuals receive the appropriate balance of nutrients necessary for strong, healthy hair growth. Herbal hair solutions include herbs like rosemary, nettle, and fenugreek promote hair growth and health. These herbs can be incorporated into oils, rinses, or hair masks to nourish the hair and scalp naturally.

Blood Type O

Individuals with Blood Type O might benefit from high-protein diets. Protein is essential for hair strength and growth, as hair is primarily made of keratin, a type of protein. Incorporating lean meats, fish, eggs, and legumes into the diet can help support healthy hair. Additionally, maintaining a balanced diet rich in iron, which supports circulation and oxygen delivery to hair follicles, is important for overall hair health.

Blood Type A

Those with Blood Type A might thrive on plant-based diets. Such diets are rich in vitamins and minerals that are essential for healthy hair, including vitamins A, C, and E, as well as iron and zinc. Consuming plenty of fruits, vegetables, whole grains, nuts, and seeds can provide the necessary nutrients for maintaining strong and healthy hair. Vitamin C helps with the absorption of iron from plant sources, and vitamin E promotes healthy scalp circulation.

Blood Type B

Individuals with Blood Type B are advised to have a balanced diet that includes a variety of both plants, calcium and vitamin D. While traditionally sourced from dairy, these nutrients can also be obtained from fortified plant-based milks, leafy greens, and sunlight exposure for vitamin D. A diet rich in green vegetables, eggs, and certain meats can help provide the necessary nutrients for hair health. Adequate intake of calcium and vitamin D is vital for hair growth and health.

Blood Type AB

Those with Blood Type AB can benefit from a diet that combines the recommendations for both Blood Type A and B. This means a diet that includes a variety of plant-based foods, as well as moderate amounts of fish, lean meats and calcium and vitamin D. While traditionally sourced from dairy, these nutrients can also be obtained from fortified plant-based milks, leafy greens, and sunlight exposure for vitamin D.. Such a diverse diet ensures a broad spectrum of vitamins, minerals, and proteins essential for healthy hair. Foods rich in omega-3 fatty acids, like fish and flaxseeds, are particularly beneficial for maintaining scalp health and preventing hair dryness and brittleness.

Hair Loss Causes and Natural Remedies

Understanding the causes of hair loss and using natural remedies can help maintain healthy hair. By incorporating a nutrient-rich diet, proper scalp care, and herbal treatments, it is possible to address hair loss and promote hair growth naturally.

Understanding Hair Loss

Hair loss can stem from various causes, including genetics, hormonal changes, medical conditions, and the frequent use of certain hairstyles and chemical treatments. These factors can lead to different types of hair loss, such as traction alopecia, androgenetic alopecia, and central centrifugal cicatricial alopecia (CCCA). *Traction Alopecia:* This type of hair loss occurs when there is constant tension on the hair shaft from tight hairstyles like braids, weaves, and ponytails. The tension damages the hair follicles, leading to hair loss, particularly around the hairline and edges.

Androgenetic Alopecia: Also known as female pattern baldness, this is a genetic condition that causes hair thinning, primarily at the crown and along the hairline. It is influenced by hormonal changes and can progress over time if left untreated. *Central Centrifugal Cicatricial Alopecia (CCCA):* CCCA is a type of scarring alopecia that starts at the crown of the head and spreads outward. It can result from inflammation and damage to the hair follicles, often exacerbated by certain hair care practices and products.

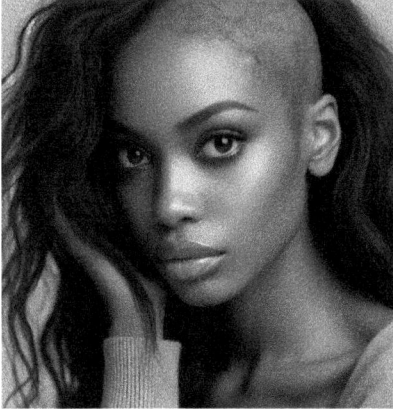

The Science Behind Hair Loss

Hair growth occurs in cycles: the anagen (growth) phase, catagen (transitional) phase, and telogen (resting) phase. Disruptions to this cycle can cause hair to fall out prematurely or not grow back at all. Factors such as hormonal imbalances, nutritional deficiencies, and scalp conditions can interfere with this cycle, leading to hair loss. *Hormonal Imbalances:* Changes in hormone levels, especially androgens, can shrink hair follicles and shorten the hair growth cycle, causing hair to become thinner and eventually fall out. *Nutritional Deficiencies:* Lack of essential nutrients like iron, vitamin D, and biotin can weaken hair follicles and impede hair growth. *Scalp Conditions:* Conditions such as seborrheic dermatitis and scalp infections can cause inflammation and damage to the hair follicles, resulting in hair loss.

Natural Remedies for Hair Loss

Natural remedies to treat hair loss emphasize the importance of a healthy diet, proper scalp care, and the use of herbal treatments. *Diet and Nutrition:* Consuming a balanced diet rich in essential nutrients supports hair health. Foods high in iron, zinc, vitamins A, C, D, and E, and omega-3 fatty acids can strengthen hair follicles and promote hair growth. Herbalists recommend including green leafy vegetables, nuts, seeds, and fatty fish in the diet. *Scalp Care:* Keeping the scalp clean and well-moisturized is crucial for healthy hair growth. Regularly washing the scalp with mild, natural shampoos and massaging with oils can improve blood circulation and strengthen hair follicles.

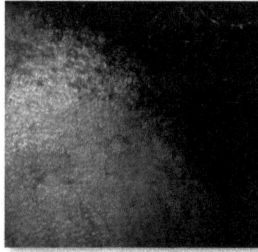

Traction Alopecia

Causes Tight hairstyles, excessive pulling
Mechanics Damage to hair follicles from tension **Herbal Remedies** Aloe vera, rosemary, peppermint oil **Natural Hair Oils** Castor oil, coconut oil **Will my hair grow back?** Yes, if treated early and properly **Is the hair loss permanent?** Not if treated early **Can I prevent it?** Avoid tight hairstyles **What treatments are effective?** Topical treatments, less tension **General Nutrients** Iron, Vitamin E, Omega-3 fatty acids **Specific Foods** Leafy greens, nuts, fish.

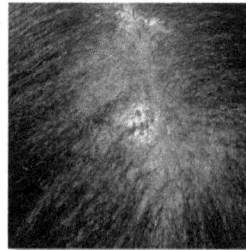

Central Centrifugal Cicatricial Alopecia (CCCA)

Causes Inflammatory conditions, genetics **Mechanics** Destruction of hair follicles due to inflammation **Herbal Remedies** Tea tree oil, lavender oil **Natural Hair Oils** Olive oil, grapeseed oil **Will my hair grow back?** Hair loss can be permanent if not treated promptly **Is the hair loss permanent?** Can be permanent if not managed early **Can I prevent it?** Regular scalp care, anti-inflammatory treatments **What treatments are effective?** Corticosteroids, anti-inflammatory medications **General Nutrients** Anti-inflammatory foods (turmeric, ginger) **Specific Foods** Berries, fatty fish, nuts.

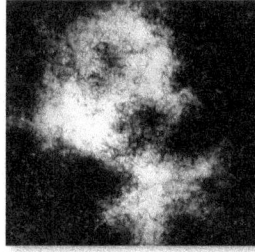

Androgenetic Alopecia

Causes Genetic predisposition, hormonal changes **Mechanics** Miniaturization of hair follicles **Herbal Remedies** Saw palmetto, green tea extract **Natural Hair Oils** Jojoba oil, argan oil **Will my hair grow back?** Varies, can slow progression but not fully reverse **Is the hair loss permanent?** Progressive but can be managed **Can I prevent it?** Regular check-ups, manage hormones **What treatments are effective?** Minoxidil, anti-androgens **General Nutrients** Protein, Zinc, Biotin **Specific Foods** Eggs, lean meats, beans.

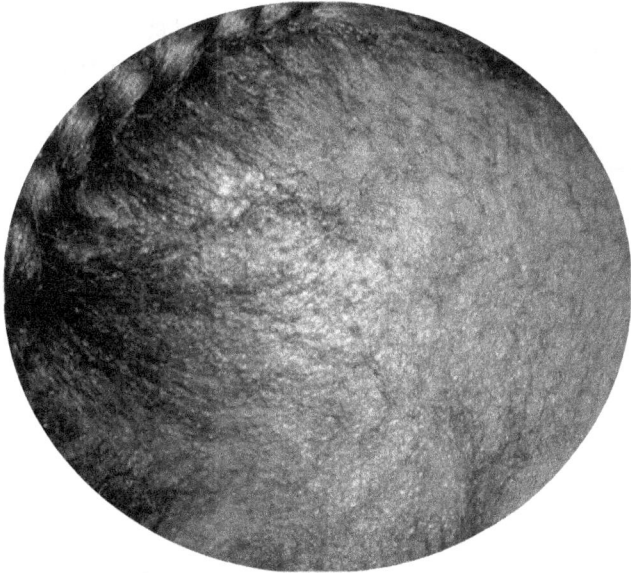

HERBAL HAIR AND SCALP TREATMENTS

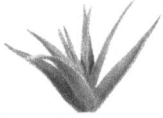

Aloe Vera

Aloe vera soothes the scalp, reduces inflammation, and promotes hair growth. Applying fresh aloe vera gel to the scalp can help maintain a healthy environment for hair follicles.

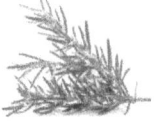

Rosemary Oil

Rosemary oil is known to stimulate blood circulation in the scalp, promoting hair growth and preventing hair loss. Mixing a few drops of rosemary oil with a carrier oil and massaging it into the scalp can be beneficial.

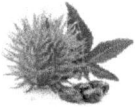

Castor Oil

Castor oil is rich in ricinoleic acid, which helps improve blood circulation to the scalp and strengthen hair roots. Applying castor oil to the scalp and hair can enhance hair growth and reduce breakage.

Onion Juice

Onion juice contains sulfur, which boosts collagen production and helps with hair growth. Applying onion juice to the scalp and leaving it for 15-30 minutes before washing it off can stimulate hair follicles.

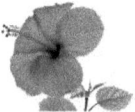

Hibiscus

Hibiscus flowers and leaves are rich in vitamins and antioxidants that promote hair growth. Making a paste of hibiscus leaves and flowers and applying it to the scalp can nourish the hair and prevent hair loss.

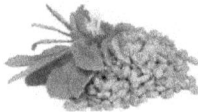

Fenugreek

Fenugreek seeds are a good source of protein and nicotinic acid, which strengthen hair follicles and encourage hair growth. Soaking fenugreek seeds overnight, grinding them into a paste, and applying it to the scalp can help reduce hair fall.

Natural Hair Growth Syrup

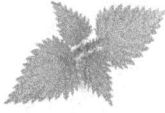

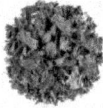

1 cup nettle leaf (dried)

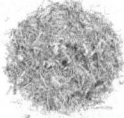

1 cup horsetail (dried)

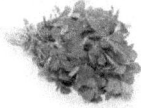

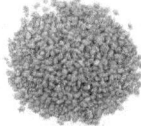

1 cup fenugreek seeds

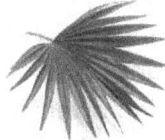

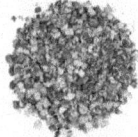

1 cup saw palmetto berries (dried)

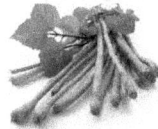

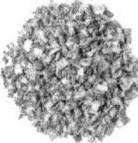

1 cup burdock root (dried)

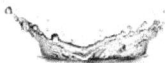

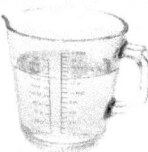

10 cups water

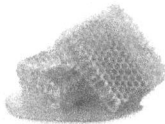

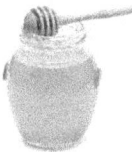

4 cups raw honey
(or vegetable glycerin
for a vegan option)

Benefits and Uses

Nettle Leaf: Rich in vitamins A, C, K, and several B vitamins, as well as minerals like iron, calcium, magnesium, and silica. Promotes hair growth by strengthening hair follicles and improving scalp health.

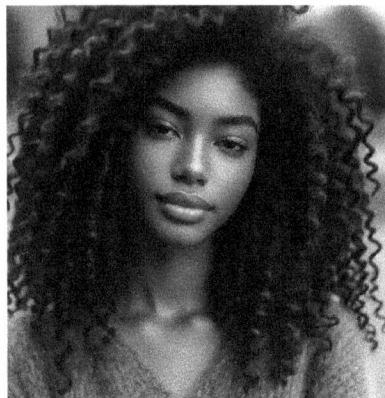

Horsetail: Contains high levels of silica and selenium, essential for hair strength and growth. Helps improve hair texture and reduces hair loss.

Fenugreek Seeds: High in protein and nicotinic acid, which are known to strengthen hair shafts, prevent breakage, and promote hair growth. Also helps in moisturizing the scalp.

Saw Palmetto Berries: Known to inhibit DHT, a hormone linked to hair loss. Supports healthy hair growth by balancing hormone levels. **Burdock Root:** Contains vitamin A, which is important for nourishing the scalp and strengthening hair. Promotes healthy hair growth and reduces scalp irritation.

Precautions

Consult a healthcare provider before use, especially if pregnant, nursing, or on medication. Do not exceed the recommended dosage. Keep out of reach of children.

FDA Disclaimer

These statements have not been evaluated by the Food and Drug Administration. This product is not intended to diagnose, treat, cure, or prevent any disease.

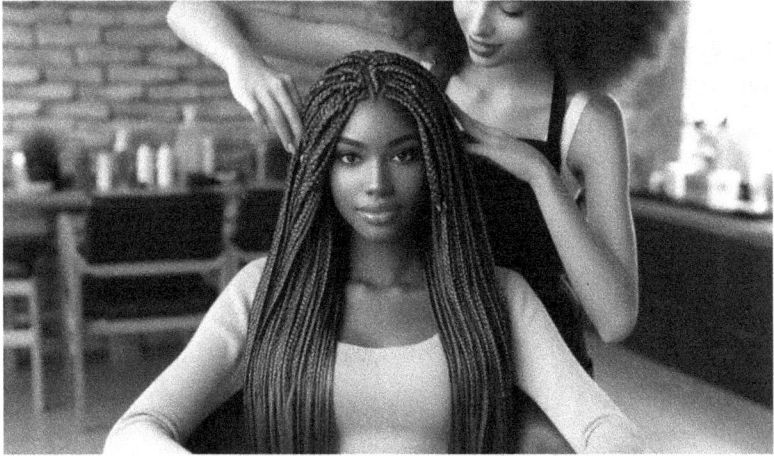

Human Hair Wigs and Weaves: Health, Hygiene, and Spiritual Implications

The popularity of human hair wigs, weaves, and extensions continues to grow as they offer versatility in styling, a natural look, and can help those experiencing hair loss. However, these products often undergo chemical treatments, and concerns have arisen over their potential health effects, as well as the spiritual implications of wearing hair that once belonged to someone else.

Chemical Concerns and Potential Scalp Issues

Human hair wigs and weaves are often treated with various chemicals to sanitize, bleach, dye, and style them before they reach consumers. Some of the common chemicals used include: **Ammonia and Bleach**: Used to strip color and lighten hair. This process can leave residual chemicals that, when in contact with the scalp, may cause irritation. **Silicone**: Often added to give the hair a smooth, shiny appearance, but can create a buildup on both the weave and the scalp. **Formaldehyde**: Occasionally used to disinfect hair, this preservative is a known irritant and allergen.

Chemically Treated Hair Health Issues

Long-term use of chemically treated hair extensions can lead to issues such as: **Scalp Irritation**: Redness, itching, and sensitivity due to chemical residues in the hair. **Hair Breakage**: Especially around the edges where the extensions are attached, as chemicals and added weight can weaken natural hair. **Allergic Reactions**: Symptoms such as itching, burning, or scalp dryness can indicate a sensitivity to one or more chemicals.

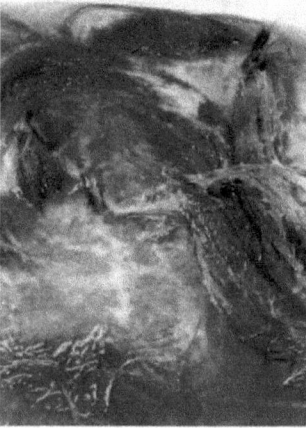

Proper Cleaning Tips for Wigs and Extensions

To reduce potential irritation, it's important to cleanse hair extensions or wigs before the first wear. Here are some effective cleaning methods: **Apple Cider Vinegar (ACV) Soak**: Fill a basin with warm water, add 1/4 cup of ACV, and soak the hair for 15-30 minutes. Apple cider vinegar helps remove chemical residues, balances pH levels, and kills bacteria.

Gentle Shampoo and Conditioning: Wash the hair thoroughly with a gentle, sulfate-free shampoo, followed by a light conditioner. Rinse well to ensure no residue remains. **Natural Oils**: After drying, applying light natural oils such as coconut or jojoba oil can help maintain softness and shine. Avoid using oils near the scalp to prevent pore-clogging buildup. **Air Drying**: Allow the hair to air dry instead of using heat, as this reduces damage and prevents the release of any residual fumes from chemical treatments.

Spiritual Implications of Wearing Human Hair

Hair holds symbolic significance in many cultures, and it's believed to carry the essence, memories, and experiences of its original owner. When hair is donated or sold, it may come from individuals in a variety of life circumstances, including deceased persons, and is sometimes obtained under conditions that are not fully disclosed to buyers. For many people, wearing hair extensions made from unknown sources can have spiritual and emotional implications.

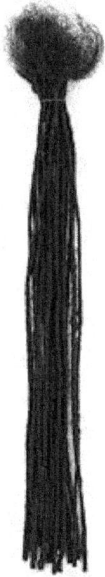

Mood and Energy Transfer Some believe that wearing hair from another person, especially if it was sourced under distressing circumstances, could transfer the previous owner's emotional or spiritual energy to the wearer. This transfer is thought to impact mood, focus, or even spiritual well-being.

Health Implications While not scientifically proven, some people report feeling different after wearing human hair sourced from unknown individuals, suggesting a perceived energetic or psychosomatic connection.

Protective Practices To minimize these effects, it's common to cleanse extensions and wigs using sage, incense, or even an ACV rinse with the intention of removing any residual energy and making the hair "neutral" before wearing it.

In particular, **locs** carry an especially strong significance, as they represent years of growth and personal connection. In various spiritual beliefs, locs may also symbolize dedication, wisdom, and strength. Using human locs, therefore, can feel like connecting with another's spiritual journey. Some individuals prefer synthetic hair or human hair that they are certain is ethically sourced to avoid these concerns.

With mindful preparation and cleaning, as well as a conscious awareness of the energy and origins of the hair, wearers can make informed choices that support their physical and emotional well-being.

Chapter 11
Journey into Eye and Mouth Health

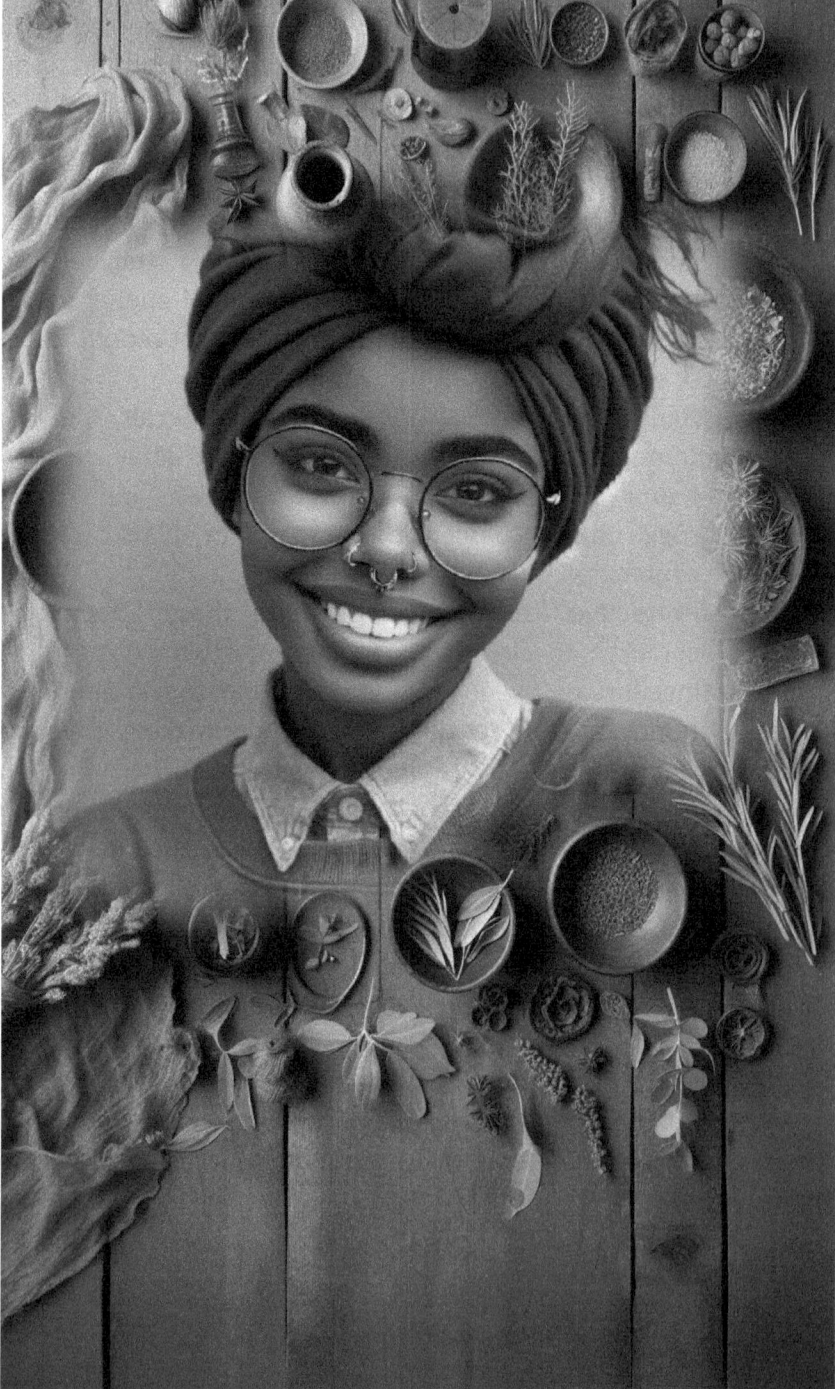

Understanding Eye Health
Cataracts

Cataracts involve the clouding of the eye's lens, leading to vision impairment. Symptoms include difficulty seeing at night, halos around lights, and fading colors. Prevention and management may include a diet rich in antioxidants, which help protect the eyes from oxidative stress. Foods like leafy greens, carrots, and berries are excellent sources of vitamins A and C, known for their eye health benefits. Additionally, bilberry extract, often used in natural medicine, has been shown to improve night vision and slow the progression of cataracts. Regular eye exams are crucial for early detection and management of cataracts.

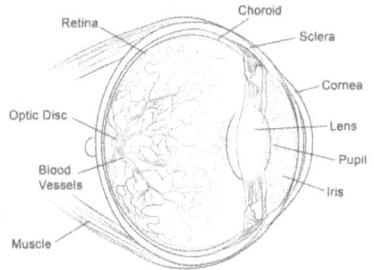

Glaucoma

Glaucoma is characterized by increased intraocular pressure, which can lead to optic nerve damage if untreated. A holistic approach to managing glaucoma includes reducing stress, as high-stress levels can exacerbate the condition. Mindfulness practices such as yoga and meditation can help lower stress and support overall eye health. Supplementing with omega-3 fatty acids, found in flaxseeds and walnuts, may also help reduce intraocular pressure. Early detection is key, so regular screenings are essential.

Diabetic Retinopathy

Diabetic retinopathy is a complication of diabetes that affects the blood vessels in the retina. Controlling blood sugar levels through a balanced diet and regular exercise is crucial. Herbal remedies like cinnamon and fenugreek can aid in stabilizing blood sugar levels. Additionally, ginkgo biloba, known for its circulatory benefits, can improve blood flow to the eyes, potentially reducing the risk of retinopathy. Managing blood sugar levels is critical in preventing this condition.

Natural Pain Management

For natural pain management, especially in cases of eye strain or discomfort, applying a warm chamomile tea compress can provide soothing relief. Chamomile's anti-inflammatory properties help relax the eye muscles and reduce redness.

Jimerito Honey Benefits to the Eyes

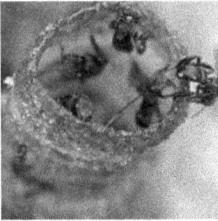

Jimerito honey, also known as "Jimieíto" honey, is a unique and potent variety of honey harvested from the wildflowers and medicinal plants of the Caribbean and South America. Renowned for its therapeutic properties, Jimerito honey has been used traditionally in holistic medicine to treat a wide range of ailments. Its rich nutrient profile and natural bioactive compounds make it particularly beneficial for eye health and general wellness.

Benefits of Jimerito Honey for Eye Health

Jimerito honey is rich in antioxidants, vitamins, and minerals that can significantly benefit eye health. These components help protect the eyes from oxidative stress, inflammation, and infections.

Antioxidant Protection

Jimerito honey contains high levels of antioxidants such as flavonoids, phenolic acids, and ascorbic acid (vitamin C). These antioxidants help neutralize free radicals, which can damage eye cells and lead to conditions such as cataracts and age-related macular degeneration (AMD).

Anti-Inflammatory Properties

The anti-inflammatory compounds in Jimerito honey, including flavonoids and polyphenols, can help reduce inflammation in the eyes. This is particularly beneficial for conditions such as conjunctivitis (pink eye) and dry eye syndrome, which are common among people of all ages.

Antibacterial Effects

Jimerito honey has natural antibacterial properties that can help prevent and treat bacterial infections of the eye. Its application can soothe irritation and promote healing, making it an effective remedy for minor eye infections and irritations.

Moisturizing and Healing

For individuals experiencing dry eye syndrome or other forms of eye discomfort, Jimerito honey's natural humectant properties can provide relief. It helps retain moisture and promotes healing of the delicate tissues around the eyes.

Nutrient-Rich Composition

Jimerito honey is packed with essential nutrients, including vitamins A, E, and C, as well as minerals like zinc. These nutrients are crucial for maintaining healthy vision and protecting the eyes from damage.

How to Use Jimerito Honey for Eye Health

Eye Drops: A diluted solution of Jimerito honey can be used as natural eye drops. Mix one part Jimerito honey with three parts sterile water and apply a few drops to each eye using a sterile dropper. This can help soothe irritation and reduce inflammation. Eye Compress: For a soothing eye compress, mix Jimerito honey with warm water and soak a clean cloth in the solution. Place the cloth over closed eyes for 10-15 minutes to reduce redness and inflammation. Several other herbal remedies can support eye health: Bilberry is rich in anthocyanins, which are potent antioxidants that support eye health.

Consuming bilberry supplements or tea can improve night vision and reduce the risk of cataracts and AMD. Eyebright (Euphrasia officinalis) has been traditionally used to treat eye infections and inflammation. It can be used as an eye wash or in compress form to soothe irritated eyes.

Ginkgo Biloba enhances blood circulation, including in the eyes, which can help improve vision and reduce the risk of glaucoma and AMD. Ginkgo biloba supplements or tea can be incorporated into a daily routine. Turmeric's anti-inflammatory properties, due to its active ingredient curcumin, can help reduce eye inflammation. Adding turmeric to meals or taking turmeric supplements can support overall eye health. Aloe Vera gel can be used to soothe and moisturize the eyes. Ensure the gel is free from additives and gently apply it around the eyes to reduce puffiness and irritation.

Natural Solutions for Chapped Lips and Dry Mouth

Chapped lips and dry mouth can be uncomfortable and lead to further oral health issues. Natural remedies can provide relief and promote hydration. Coconut Oil: Apply a thin layer of coconut oil to chapped lips for its moisturizing and healing properties. Aloe Vera Gel: Use aloe vera gel to soothe and hydrate dry lips. Hydration: Drink plenty of water throughout the day to keep the mouth and lips hydrated. Humidifier: Using a humidifier in your living space can add moisture to the air, helping to alleviate dry mouth. Herbal Teas: Drinking herbal teas like chamomile or licorice root can help stimulate saliva production and soothe dry mouth.

Dental Hygiene and Oral Health

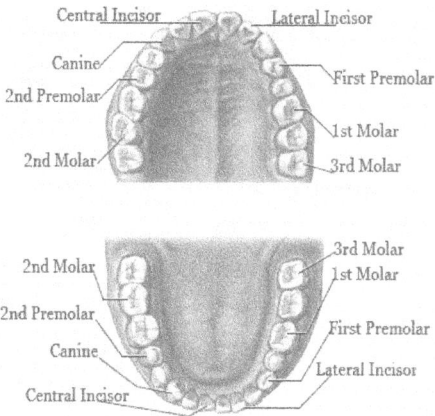

Central Incisor
Lateral Incisor
Canine
First Premolar
2nd Premolar
1st Molar
2nd Molar
3rd Molar

3rd Molar
2nd Molar
1st Molar
2nd Premolar
First Premolar
Canine
Lateral Incisor
Central Incisor

Dental hygiene encompasses daily practices aimed at preventing oral diseases and maintaining a healthy mouth. For Black women, it's crucial to prioritize regular brushing and flossing to remove plaque and food particles, reducing the risk of tooth decay and gum disease. Additionally, scheduling regular dental check-ups and cleanings is essential for early detection and treatment of any oral health issues.

Herbal Remedies

Incorporating herbal remedies into dental care routines can provide additional benefits for oral health. Herbs like neem, clove, and peppermint have antimicrobial properties that help combat bacteria and promote gum health. Natural remedies such as aloe vera gel can soothe gum inflammation, and coconut oil pulling can aid in oral detoxification. Additionally, the use of a miswak stick, a traditional teeth-cleaning tool, can help reduce plaque, whiten teeth, and improve overall oral hygiene due to its natural antibacterial properties.

Common Dental Issues

Black women may face specific dental challenges, including tooth decay, cavities, chapped lips, cracked corners of the mouth, and dry mouth. Tooth decay and cavities can result from poor oral hygiene, sugary diets, or genetic factors. Chapped lips and cracked corners of the mouth may be exacerbated by environmental factors or nutritional deficiencies. Dry mouth, also known as xerostomia, can be caused by medications, hormonal changes, or systemic diseases.

Causes of Tooth Decay and Cavities

Cavities are not directly caused by sugar but by the acid produced when bacteria in the mouth consume sugar. The bacteria feed on sugars and carbohydrates, producing acid as a byproduct. This acid softens the enamel, leading to the formation of cavities over time. Consistent exposure to acid, whether from bacterial activity or acidic foods and beverages, weakens the enamel and results in dental erosion and decay. **Symptoms and Effects:** Symptoms of tooth decay and cavities include tooth sensitivity, visible holes or pits, persistent toothache, and discoloration. Addressing these symptoms promptly is essential to prevent further complications.

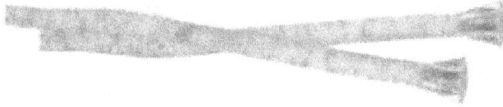

Miswak Stick A Natural Toothbrush

Natural Remedies and Preventive Measures

Natural remedies and preventive measures can help manage and prevent tooth decay and cavities: **Oil Pulling:** Swishing coconut or sesame oil in the mouth for 15-20 minutes can help reduce bacteria and plaque buildup, improving oral hygiene and detoxifying the mouth. **Calcium and Phosphorus-Rich Foods:** Consuming leafy greens, nuts, seeds, and dairy alternatives rich in calcium and phosphorus can help strengthen enamel and prevent decay. **Clove Oil:** Applying diluted clove oil to a cotton ball and placing it on the affected tooth can provide relief from toothache due to its natural analgesic and antibacterial properties. **Green Tea:** Drinking green tea can reduce bacteria in the mouth and prevent cavities, as it contains catechins with antimicrobial properties. **Miswak Stick:** Using a miswak stick can naturally clean teeth, reduce plaque, and improve oral hygiene.

Nutrient Deficiency and Its Impact on Dental Health

Nutrient deficiencies can significantly affect dental health, leading to problems such as tooth decay, gum disease, and other oral health issues. Ensuring a well-balanced diet rich in essential vitamins and minerals is vital for maintaining strong teeth and healthy gums.

Key Nutrients for Dental Health

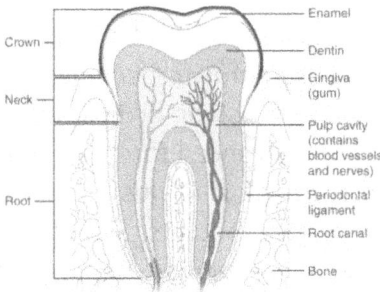

Vitamin D: Essential for calcium absorption, which is crucial for strong teeth and bones. Sources include fortified plant-based milk, exposure to sunlight, and supplements if necessary. **Calcium:** Vital for maintaining tooth structure and bone density. Sources include fortified plant-based milk, leafy green vegetables, nuts, and seeds. **Vitamin C:** Important for healthy gums and connective tissues. Sources include citrus fruits, berries, bell peppers, and broccoli.

Vitamin A: Supports the maintenance of mucous membranes in the mouth and promotes saliva production. Sources include carrots, sweet potatoes, and dark leafy greens. **B Vitamins:** Necessary for overall oral health, particularly for preventing mouth sores and inflammation. Sources include whole grains, legumes, nuts, and seeds. **Iron:** Crucial for maintaining healthy tissues in the mouth. Sources include legumes, tofu, spinach, and fortified cereals. **Calcium Carbonate:** Often used in toothpaste to help remove surface stains and polish teeth without damaging the enamel.

Gum Disease

Gum disease, or periodontal disease, is a common oral health issue characterized by inflammation of the gums and damage to the surrounding tissues and bones. Black women may be at higher risk for gum disease due to factors such as hormonal fluctuations, genetics, and socioeconomic disparities. Maintaining good oral hygiene, avoiding tobacco use, and managing underlying health conditions can help prevent gum disease.

Types of Gum Disease

Gingivitis: The mildest form of gum disease, gingivitis is often caused by poor oral hygiene and can cause gums to become red, swollen, and bleed easily, especially when brushing or flossing. If left untreated, gingivitis can lead to more advanced forms of gum disease. *Periodontitis:* An advanced form of gingivitis that can affect the gums, teeth, jawbone, and gingival pockets. Symptoms include chronic bad breath and receding gums. *Aggressive Periodontitis:* A rapid progression of periodontitis. *Chronic Periodontitis:* The most common form of periodontitis, which cannot be completely cured because the supportive tissue cannot be rebuilt. However, a dentist can use scaling and root planning procedures, antimicrobial treatments, or surgery to halt the disease's progression.

Overall Wellness Tips for Dental Health

In addition to the above remedies and preventive measures, maintaining overall wellness is key to dental health: Balanced Diet: Eat a balanced diet rich in vitamins and minerals to support oral health. Stress Management: Practice stress management techniques like meditation, yoga, or deep breathing exercises, as stress can negatively impact oral health. Regular Exercise: Engage in regular physical activity to promote overall health, which can indirectly benefit dental health. Adequate Sleep: Ensure you get enough sleep each night, as sleep is essential for overall health and well-being. By incorporating these natural remedies, preventive measures, and wellness tips into your daily routine, you can effectively manage and prevent common dental issues and maintain optimal oral health.

Oral Sex Dangers and Hygiene

Practicing safe oral sex is essential for protecting both oral and overall health. Black women should be aware of the risks associated with oral sex, including the transmission of sexually transmitted infections (STIs) such as herpes, gonorrhea, and human papillomavirus (HPV). Using barrier methods like dental dams or condoms during oral sex can reduce the risk of STI transmission. Additionally, maintaining good oral hygiene and regular dental check-ups is crucial for overall oral health, regardless of sexual activity.

Risk Factors

STI Transmission Oral sex can transmit various STIs including herpes, gonorrhea, chlamydia, syphilis, HPV (human papillomavirus), and HIV.- Risks increase with unprotected oral-genital contact

Preventive Measures

Use condoms or dental dams (barriers) during oral sex to reduce risk.- Get tested regularly for STIs and encourage partners to do the same.- Limit the number of sexual partners.- Communicate openly with partners about sexual health and history.

Oral Health Risks Bacteria and viruses can be transmitted between partners, leading to oral infections.- Poor oral hygiene can increase risks of infections and oral health issues.- Cuts or sores in the mouth can provide entry points for infections.

Preventive Measures

Maintain good oral hygiene, including regular brushing and flossing.- Avoid oral sex if either partner has oral sores, cuts, or infections.- Use mouthwash or rinse with water before and after oral sex.

HPV and Oral Cancer HPV transmitted through oral sex can increase the risk of oral cancers, including throat cancer.- Certain strains of HPV are linked to oral cancer development.

Preventive Measures

HPV vaccination (available for both males and females) can reduce the risk of HPV-related cancers.- Practice safer sex practices and get regular medical check-ups.- Discuss HPV vaccination with healthcare providers.

Allergic Reactions

Some individuals may experience allergic reactions to proteins in semen or vaginal fluids.- Symptoms can include itching, swelling, or redness of the lips, tongue, or throat

Risk Factors

Preventive Measures

Discuss any known allergies with sexual partners.- Seek medical attention if severe allergic reactions (anaphylaxis) occur.- Consider allergy testing if reactions are severe or persistent.

Risk of HIV Transmission Although lower risk compared to unprotected vaginal or anal sex, HIV can still be transmitted through oral sex, particularly if there are cuts or sores in the mouth or genitals.- Risk increases if ejaculation occurs in the mouth or if the person performing oral sex has gum disease.

Preventive Measures

Use condoms or dental dams during oral sex.- Limit the number of sexual partners and get tested regularly for HIV.- Consider pre-exposure prophylaxis (PrEP) for individuals at high risk of HIV infection.

Syphilis and Gonorrhea Risks Syphilis and gonorrhea can be transmitted through oral-genital contact.- Symptoms may not always be present, leading to undiagnosed infections and potential complications.

Preventive Measures

Use condoms or dental dams to reduce the risk of transmission.- Get tested for STIs regularly, especially after unprotected sexual contact.- Encourage partners to get tested and treated for STIs.

Note: Communication with sexual partners about sexual health and STI history is crucial. Regular testing and safer sex practices can reduce the risk of STI transmission during oral sex. Seeking medical advice if any symptoms or concerns arise is important for early detection and treatment. Remember if you are suffering don't be embarrassed or ashamed medical professionals have seen cases like this before you will not be the first or the last to need treatment. Choose your health!

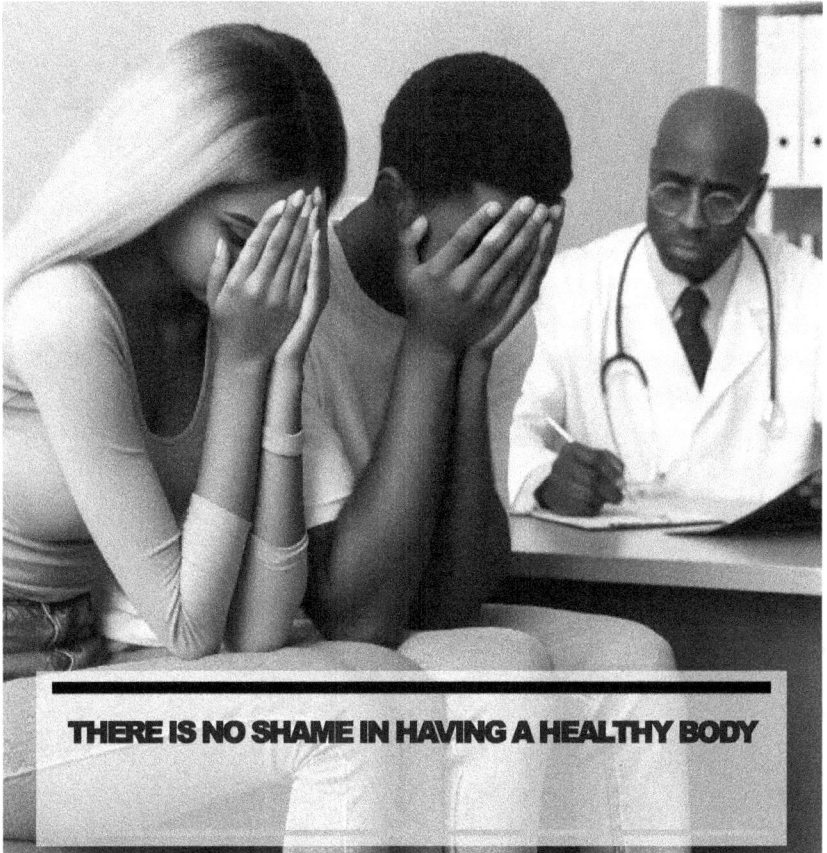

THERE IS NO SHAME IN HAVING A HEALTHY BODY

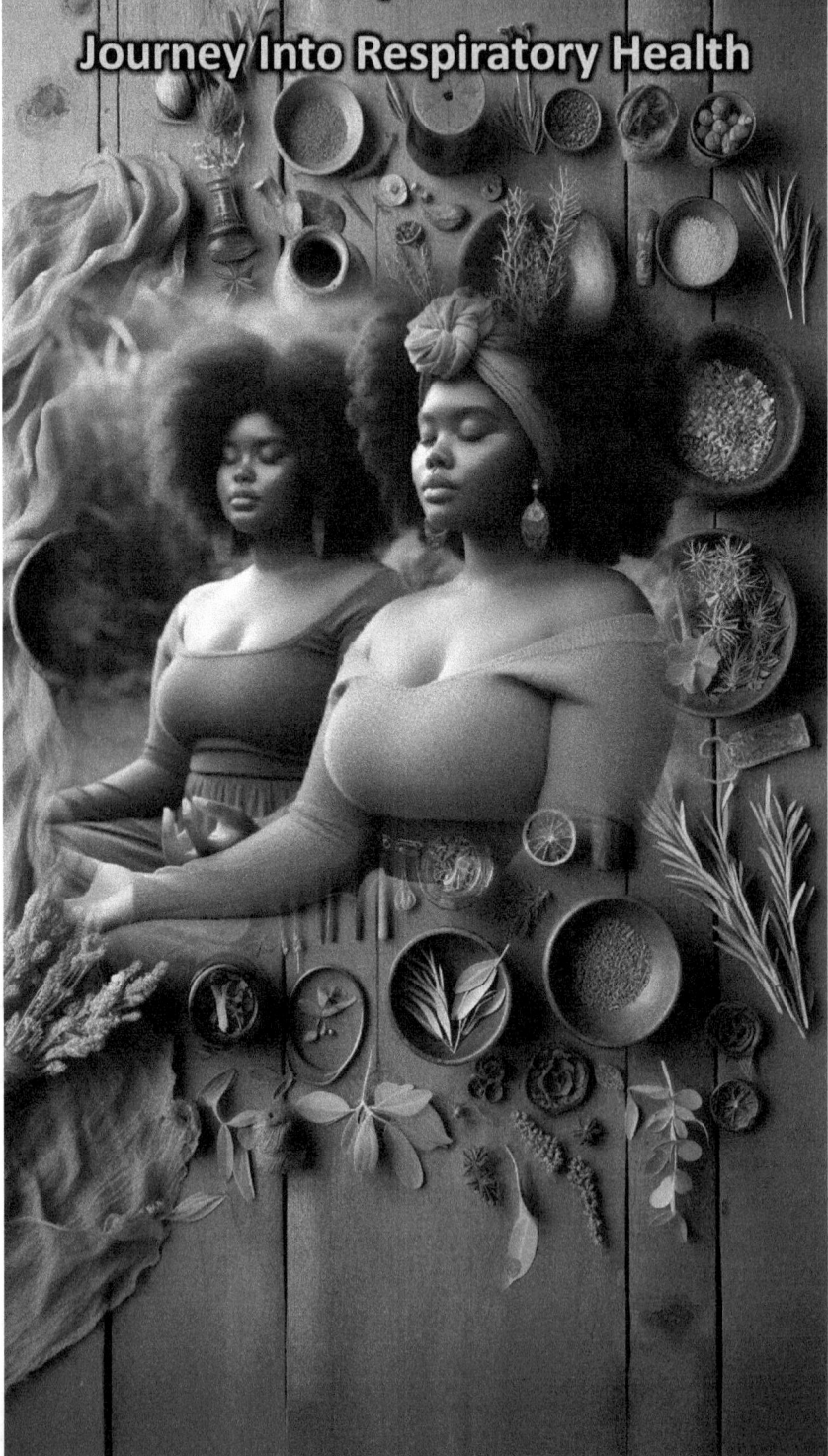

Chapter 12
Journey Into Respiratory Health

Respiratory System
LUNGS TRACHEA BRONCHI NASAL PASSAGES MUSCLES OF BREATHING

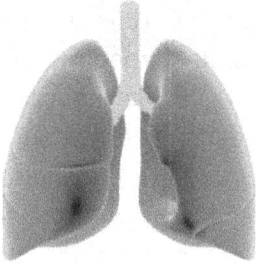

The respiratory system is a complex network of organs and tissues that facilitate breathing. It includes the lungs, trachea, bronchi, nasal passages, and the muscles involved in breathing. Understanding the structure and function of each component is essential for comprehending how this system supports life.

The lungs are the primary organs of the respiratory system, situated in the chest cavity on either side of the heart. The right lung is composed of three lobes, whereas the left lung consists of two lobes. This asymmetry accommodates the heart, which lies slightly to the left of the midline. The lungs are responsible for the critical exchange of oxygen and carbon dioxide, a process vital for cellular respiration and overall metabolic function.

The trachea, commonly known as the windpipe, is a hollow tube supported by cartilage rings that prevent it from collapsing. It serves as the main passage for air to travel from the nasal and oral cavities to the lungs. The trachea bifurcates into two main bronchi, which are the large tubes that lead into each lung. These bronchi further divide into smaller tubes called bronchioles, which branch out extensively within the lungs, resembling the branches of a tree. At the end of these bronchioles are tiny air sacs known as alveoli, where the actual exchange of oxygen and carbon dioxide occurs.

The muscles of breathing, including the diaphragm, intercostal muscles, and abdominal muscles, play a crucial role in the mechanics of respiration. The diaphragm is a dome-shaped muscle located beneath the lungs. When it contracts, it flattens and increases the thoracic cavity's volume, causing air to be drawn into the lungs. The intercostal muscles, situated between the ribs, also assist by expanding and contracting the chest cavity. The abdominal muscles aid in forced exhalation, such as when coughing or exercising.

The nasal passages are responsible for warming, humidifying, and filtering the air we inhale. This process is vital for protecting the delicate tissues within the respiratory system from cold, dry air and airborne particles. Additionally, the respiratory system includes the mouth, sinuses, and pharynx (throat), which also contribute to the process of breathing, as well as functions like speech production and sensing odors.

Respiration is the primary function of the respiratory system, involving the intake of oxygen and the expulsion of carbon dioxide. This gas exchange is essential for maintaining the body's acid-base balance, which is crucial for normal cellular functions and metabolic processes. The respiratory system also plays a significant role in speech production, as the flow of air from the lungs passes through the vocal cords, enabling the formation of sounds. Moreover, the ability to sense odors is facilitated by the old factory receptors in the nasal passages.

Maintaining the health of the respiratory system can be supported by holistic and natural remedies. For instance, herbal syrups, elixirs, and salves can be used to alleviate respiratory conditions and enhance lung function. These natural treatments often contain ingredients known for their anti-inflammatory, expectorant, and soothing properties.

Respiratory Issues

Respiratory health is a critical aspect of overall well-being, and certain respiratory conditions disproportionately affect Black women. Understanding these conditions, their symptoms, and the available treatments can help in managing and improving respiratory health.

Common Respiratory Issues

Black women are more prone to several respiratory conditions due to a combination of genetic, environmental, and socioeconomic factors. Some of the most common respiratory issues include asthma, chronic obstructive pulmonary disease (COPD), and allergies.

Asthma

Asthma is a chronic condition characterized by inflammation and narrowing of the airways, causing difficulty in breathing. Black women have higher rates of asthma and asthma-related complications, partly due to genetic predispositions and environmental triggers.

Chronic Obstructive Pulmonary Disease (COPD)

COPD is a group of lung diseases, including emphysema and chronic bronchitis, which cause airflow blockage and breathing-related problems. Black women who smoke or have long-term exposure to pollutants are at a higher risk of developing COPD.

Allergies

Allergies occur when the immune system reacts to a foreign substance, such as pollen, dust, or pet dander. Allergic reactions can cause respiratory symptoms like sneezing, coughing, and wheezing, which can exacerbate asthma or other respiratory conditions.

Symptoms and Causes

The symptoms of respiratory issues can vary depending on the condition but commonly include: Shortness of breath, Wheezing, Chronic cough, Chest tightness, and Increased mucus production.

The causes of respiratory issues can include: **Genetic factors**: Family history of asthma or allergies. **Environmental factors**: Exposure to air pollution, tobacco smoke, and occupational hazards. **Socioeconomic factors**: Limited access to healthcare and higher rates of stress and poor living conditions. **Lifestyle factors**: Smoking and sedentary lifestyle.

? QUESTIONS TO ASK YOUR DOCTOR ?

What is the cause of my respiratory symptoms?
What tests do I need to diagnose my condition?
How can I manage my symptoms at home?
Are there lifestyle changes that could improve my respiratory health?
What treatments are available for my condition?

!TESTS TO REQUEST!

Pulmonary function tests (PFTs)
Chest X-ray or CT scan
Allergy testing
Blood tests for immune function
Spirometry to measure airflow obstruction

Respiratory Issue	Description	Natural Remedies
Asthma	Chronic inflammation of the airways	Ginger, turmeric, eucalyptus oil
COPD	Chronic obstructive pulmonary disease	Peppermint, ginseng, licorice root
Allergies	Immune system reaction to allergens	Quercetin, stinging nettle, butterbur
Bronchitis	Inflammation of the bronchial tubes	Thyme, honey, mullein
Pneumonia	Infection causing lung inflammation	Garlic, echinacea, elderberry

Cleansing the Respiratory System

Cleansing the respiratory system can improve lung function and overall respiratory health. Here are some natural ingredients and methods to consider: Steam Inhalation: Use essential oils like eucalyptus or peppermint in hot water. Inhale the steam to open up the airways and clear mucus. Herbal Teas: Drink teas made from herbs like ginger, thyme, mullein, and peppermint to soothe the respiratory tract and reduce inflammation. Hydration: Drink plenty of water to keep the mucous membranes hydrated and thin mucus for easier expulsion. Diet: Include foods rich in antioxidants, such as berries, citrus fruits, and leafy greens, to support lung health and reduce inflammation. Honey and Lemon: A mixture of honey and lemon in warm water can soothe the throat and act as a natural cough suppressant. Garlic and Ginger: Consuming garlic and ginger can help reduce inflammation and fight infections due to their antimicrobial properties.

Airway Inflammation

Chronic airway inflammation is a hallmark of conditions like asthma and COPD. It leads to increased mucus production and airway narrowing, making breathing difficult. Managing inflammation through medication and lifestyle changes is crucial.

Increased Metabolic Demand

Respiratory issues often increase the body's metabolic demand as the respiratory muscles work harder to facilitate breathing. Adequate nutrition and rest are important to meet these increased demands. While blood type has not been definitively linked to respiratory conditions, individual variations in immune response and susceptibility to infections can play a role. Blood type may influence inflammation levels, metabolic demands, and overall respiratory health.

Heat Relations and Prevention

Heat can exacerbate respiratory symptoms, especially in individuals with asthma. Staying cool, avoiding outdoor activities during high pollution days, and using air conditioning can help prevent flare-ups.

Smokers it is imperative that you cleanse your respiratory system

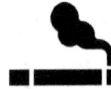

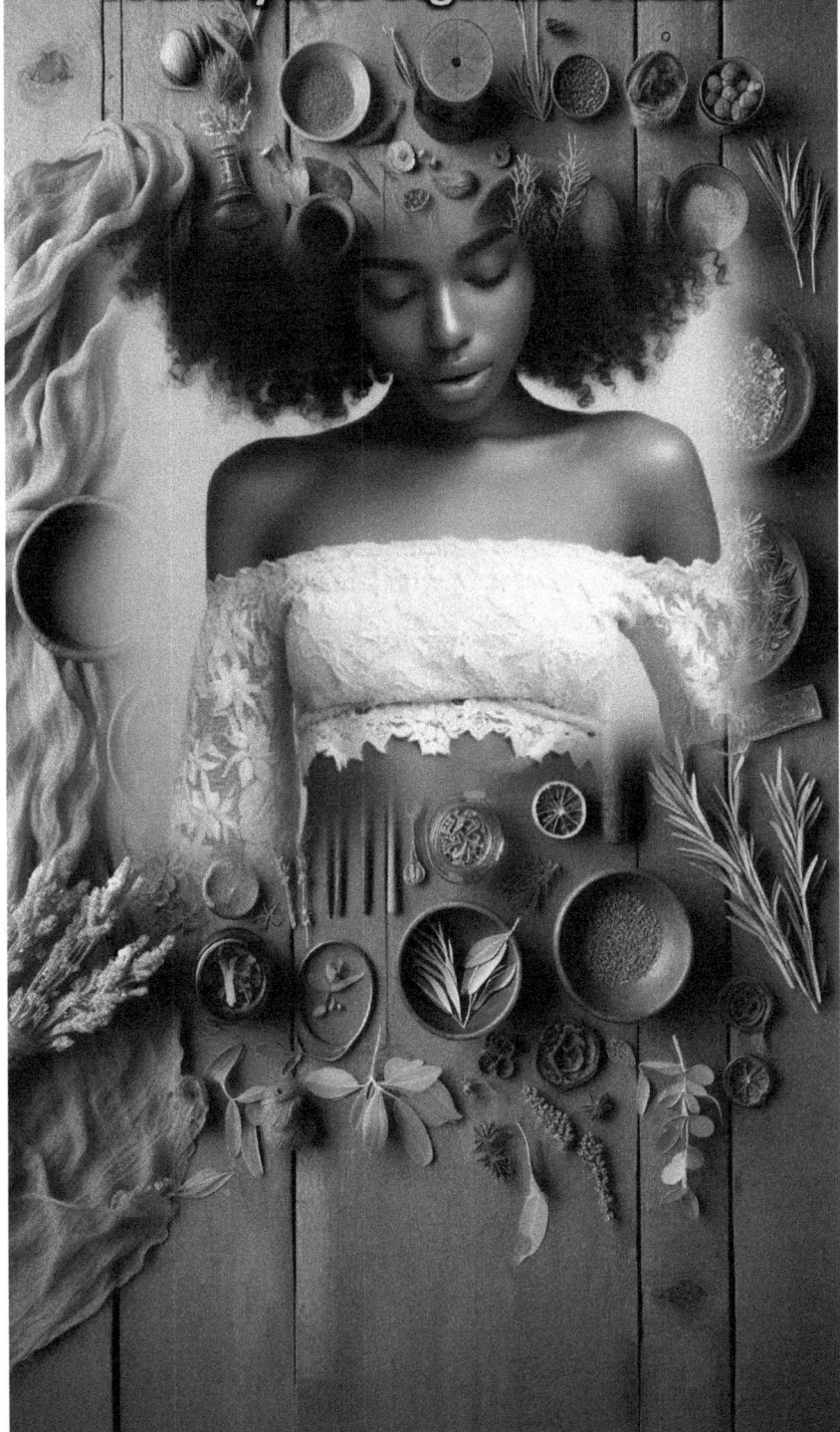

Chapter 13
Journey Into Digestive Health

Digestive System
STOMACH SMALL INTESTINE LARGE INTESTINE

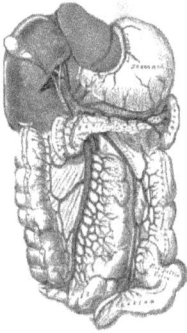

The digestive system, also known as the alimentary canal or gastrointestinal tract, is a complex network of organs responsible for breaking down food into nutrients and fuel for the body. This system includes the mouth, esophagus, stomach, small intestine, and large intestine, each playing a crucial role in the digestion process.

The process begins in the mouth, where food is chewed and mixed with saliva, which contains enzymes that start breaking down carbohydrates. The food then travels down the esophagus, a muscular tube in the chest, which uses rhythmic contractions to move the food into the stomach.

The stomach is a hollow organ with strong muscular walls. It holds the ingested food and mixes it with gastric acid and digestive enzymes, breaking it down into a liquid or paste. This mixture, called chyme, is then gradually released into the small intestine. The small intestine is a long, muscular tube about 22 feet in length, divided into three segments: the duodenum, jejunum, and ileum. In the duodenum, enzymes from the pancreas and bile from the liver further break down the food. The jejunum and ileum primarily absorb nutrients and water into the bloodstream through their walls. The extensive surface area provided by the villi and microvilli in the small intestine maximizes nutrient absorption.

The large intestine, or colon, is the largest part of the digestive tract, measuring about five feet in length. It absorbs water and salts from the remaining undigested food matter, transforming it into solid waste. This waste is then stored in the rectum until it is expelled from the body during defecation.

Maintaining a healthy digestive system is essential due to higher prevalence rates of certain disorders, such as irritable bowel syndrome (IBS) and colorectal cancer. Incorporating holistic and natural remedies can support digestive health, offering alternatives to conventional medications.

Gut Bacteria and Digestive Health

Black women may experience digestive issues due to differences in their gut bacteria and other contributing factors. Research indicates that Black women have different compositions of gut bacteria compared to white women. These differences in microbiota can play a significant role in metabolic processes, potentially contributing to insulin resistance and other metabolic conditions. The gut microbiome is a complex community of microorganisms that influences many aspects of health, including digestion, immunity, and even mood. Variations in gut bacteria can affect the efficiency of nutrient absorption, the immune response to pathogens, and the regulation of inflammation, which are all critical components of overall health.

Maintaining a balanced gut microbiome can be supported by incorporating herbs like ginger, which aids in digestion and reduces inflammation, and turmeric, known for its anti-inflammatory properties. Consuming probiotics from natural sources like fermented foods can also help restore and maintain healthy gut bacteria.

Good Gut Bacteria

From an herbalist's viewpoint, fostering and maintaining a healthy balance of gut bacteria is essential for overall well-being. The gut microbiome, a diverse community of microorganisms residing in the digestive tract, plays a critical role in digestion, immunity, and overall health. The approach to supporting good gut bacteria emphasizes natural, plant-based remedies and dietary practices that align with health principles.

The Role of Gut Bacteria

Good gut bacteria are crucial for breaking down food, synthesizing vitamins, and protecting against harmful pathogens. These beneficial microorganisms help maintain the integrity of the gut lining, reduce inflammation, and support a robust immune system. An imbalance in the gut microbiome, often referred to as dysbiosis, can lead to various health issues, including digestive disorders, weakened immunity, and metabolic conditions.

Herbal and Natural Remedies for Gut Health

From an herbalist perspective, the focus is on natural, plant-based approaches to enhance and maintain gut health. Here are several key strategies: *Prebiotic-Rich Foods* Prebiotics are non-digestible fibers that promote the growth of beneficial gut bacteria. Incorporating prebiotic-rich foods into the diet is essential for nourishing the microbiome. Foods such as chicory root, dandelion greens, garlic, onions, and asparagus are excellent sources of prebiotics. These foods provide the necessary nutrients to support the proliferation of good gut bacteria.

Probiotic Foods and Fermented Products

Probiotics are live beneficial bacteria that can be consumed through certain foods. Fermented foods are a rich source of probiotics and have been used for centuries to promote gut health. Incorporating foods like sauerkraut, kimchi, miso, tempeh, and fermented vegetables into the diet can introduce beneficial bacteria to the gut. Homemade fermented beverages like kombucha and water kefir are also excellent sources of probiotics.

Herbal Support for Gut Health

Several herbs are particularly beneficial for supporting gut health and promoting a balanced microbiome. These include: ***Ginger:*** Known for its anti-inflammatory and digestive properties, ginger helps soothe the digestive tract and can promote the growth of beneficial bacteria. ***Turmeric:*** With its powerful anti-inflammatory and antioxidant properties, turmeric supports gut health by reducing inflammation and promoting a healthy microbiome. ***Slippery Elm:*** This herb can soothe the digestive tract and support the mucosal lining of the gut, creating a favorable environment for beneficial bacteria. ***Licorice Root:*** Known for its soothing and healing properties, licorice root can help protect the gut lining and support overall digestive health. ***Aloe Vera:*** Aloe vera juice can aid digestion and support gut health by soothing the intestinal lining and promoting a balanced microbiome.

Alkaline Diet for Gut Health

An alkaline diet, which focuses on consuming foods that maintain the body's pH balance, is another key aspect of supporting gut health. This dietary approach emphasizes the consumption of fresh fruits, vegetables, nuts, and seeds while avoiding processed foods, refined sugars, and animal products. An alkaline diet helps reduce inflammation, supports detoxification, and creates an environment conducive to the growth of beneficial gut bacteria.

Fasting and Detoxification

Periodic fasting and detoxification can also support gut health by giving the digestive system a rest and allowing the body to eliminate toxins. Herbal teas and natural detox drinks, such as those made with dandelion root or burdock root, can assist in this process. Fasting can help reset the gut microbiome, promoting the growth of beneficial bacteria and improving overall digestive health.

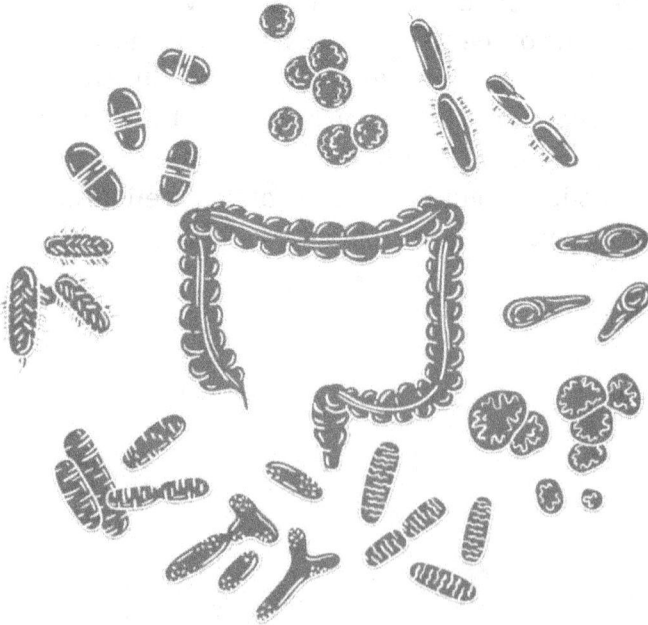

Ridding Parasites Naturally

Parasites can disrupt the balance of the gut microbiome, leading to a variety of health issues such as digestive problems, fatigue, and weakened immunity. Herbal remedies can effectively help rid the body of these unwanted organisms. **Wormwood**: Known for its potent anti-parasitic properties, wormwood can be used to expel intestinal worms. **Black Walnut Hulls**: This herb is renowned for its ability to cleanse the body of parasites.

Insomnia

Post Meal Bloating

Body Odor

Intense Sugar Cravings

Mood Changes

Nightly Teeth Grinding

Bumps on Skin

Anal Itching

Halitosis or Thrush

In Toilet

Clove: Clove has powerful antimicrobial properties and can kill parasite eggs, preventing the infestation from reoccurring. Symptoms of parasitic infections can include bloating, gas, abdominal pain, diarrhea, fatigue, and unexplained weight loss. Regular detoxification and the use of anti-parasitic herbs can help maintain a parasite-free gut environment.

Remedies for Constipation

Constipation can be a sign of an imbalance in the gut microbiome or a lack of fiber in the diet. Addressing constipation naturally involves dietary adjustments and the use of herbal remedies. **Psyllium Husk:** A natural source of soluble fiber, psyllium husk can help bulk up stool and promote regular bowel movements. **Flaxseeds:** High in fiber and omega-3 fatty acids, flaxseeds can help alleviate constipation. **Senna Leaf:** Senna is a natural laxative that stimulates bowel movements and can provide relief from constipation. **Hydration:** Adequate water intake is crucial for preventing and relieving constipation. Herbal teas can also support hydration and digestive health. Symptoms of constipation include infrequent bowel movements, difficulty passing stool, abdominal discomfort, and bloating. Incorporating high-fiber foods, staying hydrated, and using gentle herbal laxatives can help maintain regular bowel movements and overall digestive health.

Good Gut Bacteria

Fostering and maintaining a healthy balance of gut bacteria is essential for overall well-being. The gut microbiome, a diverse community of microorganisms residing in the digestive tract, plays a critical role in digestion, immunity, and overall health. The approach to supporting good gut bacteria emphasizes natural, plant-based remedies and dietary practices that align with health principles.

The Role of Gut Bacteria

Good gut bacteria are crucial for breaking down food, synthesizing vitamins, and protecting against harmful pathogens. These beneficial microorganisms help maintain the integrity of the gut lining, reduce inflammation, and support a robust immune system. An imbalance in the gut microbiome, often referred to as dysbiosis, can lead to various health issues, including digestive disorders, weakened immunity, and metabolic conditions.

Herbal and Natural Remedies for Gut Health

The focus is on natural, plant-based approaches to enhance and maintain gut health. Here are several key strategies: ***Prebiotic-Rich Foods*** Prebiotics are non-digestible fibers that promote the growth of beneficial gut bacteria. Incorporating prebiotic-rich foods into the diet is essential for nourishing the microbiome. Foods such as chicory root, dandelion greens, garlic, onions, and asparagus are excellent sources of prebiotics. These foods provide the necessary nutrients to support the proliferation of good gut bacteria.

Probiotic Foods and Fermented Products Probiotics are live beneficial bacteria that can be consumed through certain foods. Fermented foods are a rich source of probiotics and have been used for centuries to promote gut health. Incorporating foods like sauerkraut, kimchi, miso, tempeh, and fermented vegetables into the diet can introduce beneficial bacteria to the gut. Homemade fermented beverages like kombucha and water kefir are also excellent sources of probiotics.

Herbal Support for Gut Health

Several herbs are particularly beneficial for supporting gut health and promoting a balanced microbiome. These include: *Ginger*: Known for its anti-inflammatory and digestive properties, ginger helps soothe the digestive tract and can promote the growth of beneficial bacteria. *Turmeric*: With its powerful anti-inflammatory and antioxidant properties, turmeric supports gut health by reducing inflammation and promoting a healthy microbiome.

Slippery Elm: This herb can soothe the digestive tract and support the mucosal lining of the gut, creating a favorable environment for beneficial bacteria. *Licorice Root:* Known for its soothing and healing properties, licorice root can help protect the gut lining and support overall digestive health. *Aloe Vera*: Aloe vera juice can aid digestion and support gut health by soothing the intestinal lining and promoting a balanced microbiome.

Alkaline Diet for Gut Health

An alkaline diet, which focuses on consuming foods that maintain the body's pH balance, is another key aspect of supporting gut health. This dietary approach emphasizes the consumption of fresh fruits, vegetables, nuts, and seeds while avoiding processed foods, refined sugars, and animal products. An alkaline diet helps reduce inflammation, supports detoxification, and creates an environment conducive to the growth of beneficial gut bacteria.

Fasting and Detoxification

Periodic fasting and detoxification can also support gut health by giving the digestive system a rest and allowing the body to eliminate toxins. Herbal teas and natural detox drinks, such as those made with dandelion root or burdock root, can assist in this process. Fasting can help reset the gut microbiome, promoting the growth of beneficial bacteria and improving overall digestive health.

Ridding Parasites Naturally

Parasites can disrupt the balance of the gut microbiome, leading to a variety of health issues such as digestive problems, fatigue, and weakened immunity. Herbal remedies can effectively help rid the body of these unwanted organisms. **Wormwood**: Known for its potent anti-parasitic properties, wormwood can be used to expel intestinal worms.

Black Walnut Hulls: This herb is renowned for its ability to cleanse the body of parasites. *Clove:* Clove has powerful antimicrobial properties and can kill parasite eggs, preventing the infestation from reoccurring. Symptoms of parasitic infections can include bloating, gas, abdominal pain, diarrhea, fatigue, and unexplained weight loss. Regular detoxification and the use of anti-parasitic herbs can help maintain a parasite-free gut environment.

Remedies for Constipation

Constipation can be a sign of an imbalance in the gut microbiome or a lack of fiber in the diet. Addressing constipation naturally involves dietary adjustments and the use of herbal remedies. *Psyllium Husk*: A natural source of soluble fiber, psyllium husk can help bulk up stool and promote regular bowel movements. *Flaxseeds:* High in fiber and omega-3 fatty acids, flaxseeds can help alleviate constipation. *Senna Leaf:* Senna is a natural laxative that stimulates bowel movements and can provide relief from constipation. *Hydration:* Adequate water intake is crucial for preventing and relieving constipation. Herbal teas can also support hydration and digestive health. Symptoms of constipation include infrequent bowel movements, difficulty passing stool, abdominal discomfort, and bloating. Incorporating high-fiber foods, staying hydrated, and using gentle herbal laxatives can help maintain regular bowel movements and overall digestive health.

Remedies for Nausea

Nausea can be caused by various factors, including digestive disturbances, motion sickness, or stress. Herbal remedies can provide natural relief from nausea without the side effects associated with conventional medications. *Ginger:* Ginger is a well-known remedy for nausea. Consuming ginger tea or ginger chews can help soothe the stomach and reduce nausea. *Peppermint:* Peppermint tea or essential oil can provide relief from nausea by relaxing the muscles of the gastrointestinal tract. *Chamomile:* Chamomile tea has calming properties that can help alleviate nausea and settle the stomach. *Fennel:* Fennel seeds or tea can help reduce nausea and aid digestion by relaxing the muscles of the gastrointestinal tract. Symptoms of nausea include a queasy or unsettled feeling in the stomach, an urge to vomit, and sometimes dizziness or sweating. Using herbal teas and essential oils can provide quick and effective relief from nausea.

Helicobacter Pylori (HP) Infection and Herbal Remedies

Black individuals have a higher risk of Helicobacter pylori (HP) infection. This bacterium can cause chronic inflammation of the stomach lining, known as gastritis, and is a major risk factor for the development of dyspepsia (indigestion), peptic ulcers, and other gastrointestinal issues. HP infection is more prevalent in populations with limited access to healthcare and those experiencing socio-economic challenges, contributing to disparities in gastrointestinal health outcomes. The presence of HP can lead to symptoms such as abdominal pain, bloating, nausea, and loss of appetite. Natural remedies for managing HP infection include mastic gum, which has been shown to combat the bacterium, and herbal teas made from licorice root or slippery elm to soothe and protect the stomach lining. Incorporating these natural treatments can help alleviate symptoms and support overall digestive health.

Managing Digestive Functions Naturally

Changes in digestive functions can manifest as various symptoms, including bloating, gas, and constipation. These symptoms may arise from alterations in the gut microbiota, dietary habits, stress, or other health conditions. The digestive system's ability to process food efficiently and absorb nutrients is vital for maintaining health, and disruptions can lead to discomfort and other complications.
Herbal remedies such as peppermint tea can help relieve bloating and gas, while aloe vera juice may assist with constipation. Including high-fiber foods and staying hydrated are also essential for promoting healthy digestion.

Cancer Risks and Herbal Approaches
Stomach Cancer

Black women are twice as likely to be diagnosed with stomach cancer and 2.3 times more likely to die from it than white women. Symptoms of stomach cancer can include unintentional weight loss, persistent stomach pain, nausea, and vomiting. Herbal approaches to support stomach health include consuming a diet rich in antioxidant foods such as berries, leafy greens, and herbs like dandelion root, which can detoxify the and improve digestion.

Colorectal Cancer

Colorectal cancer also shows a significant disparity, with Black Americans being 20% more likely to be diagnosed and 40% more likely to die from the disease than their white counterparts. This type of cancer can cause symptoms such as changes in bowel habits, blood in the stool, abdominal discomfort, and unexplained weight loss. To reduce the risk of colorectal cancer, incorporating herbs like burdock root, which has purifying properties, and consuming foods high in fiber can help maintain a healthy colon.

Pancreatic Cancer

Pancreatic cancer rates are at least 30% higher in Black men and women than in other racial groups. Pancreatic cancer symptoms may include jaundice, weight loss, diabetes, and upper abdominal pain that radiates to the back. Herbal remedies such as milk thistle can support liver and pancreas health, and consuming bitter melon, known for its anti-cancer properties, can be beneficial.

Gallbladder Issues and Herbal Solutions

Gallbladder issues are another concern, often presenting as gallstones or inflammation of the gallbladder (cholecystitis). Symptoms of gallbladder problems can include severe abdominal pain, nausea, vomiting, and jaundice. To support gallbladder health, herbal remedies such as artichoke extract can stimulate bile production, and dandelion tea can help detoxify the liver and promote bile flow. Maintaining a diet low in unhealthy fats and high in fresh fruits and vegetables is also essential.

Diagnostic Tests and Herbal Recommendations

For the diagnosis of these conditions, it is essential to consult a healthcare provider who may recommend specific tests. For stomach and colorectal cancer, endoscopic procedures such as gastroscopy and colonoscopy are standard. Imaging tests like CT scans and MRIs can help diagnose pancreatic cancer. Gallbladder issues are often evaluated using ultrasound and HIDA scans. Blood tests may also be conducted to check for markers indicative of these diseases.

Herbalist Holistic Liver Detox

The liver is one of the most vital organs in the body, responsible for filtering toxins from the blood, producing bile for digestion, and storing essential nutrients. Given its critical role, maintaining liver health is essential for overall well-being. A holistic liver detox aims to support and enhance the liver's natural detoxification processes using natural herbs, dietary adjustments, and lifestyle changes.

Critical Importance of Maintaining Liver Health		
Efficient detoxification of harmful substances	Metabolism and storage of nutrients	Regulation of blood sugar levels
Production of bile for fat digestion	Synthesis of essential proteins and clotting factors	

The Importance of Liver Health

Maintaining liver health is crucial for the body's overall well-being and functionality. The liver plays a vital role in several essential bodily processes, making its proper function indispensable. One of the primary responsibilities of the liver is the efficient detoxification of harmful substances. This organ filters toxins from the blood, converting them into less harmful compounds that can be excreted from the body. Additionally, the liver is integral to the metabolism and storage of nutrients. It helps in breaking down nutrients from the food we eat, storing vitamins and minerals, and releasing them into the bloodstream as needed.

The liver also plays a key role in the regulation of blood sugar levels. By storing glucose as glycogen and releasing it when necessary, the liver helps maintain stable blood sugar levels, which is critical for energy balance. Moreover, the production of bile, a substance necessary for the digestion and absorption of fats, is another essential function of the liver. Bile helps emulsify fats in the digestive tract, making them easier to absorb. Lastly, the liver is responsible for the synthesis of essential proteins and clotting factors. These proteins are crucial for various bodily functions, including blood clotting and maintaining fluid balance within the circulatory system.

Common Causes of Liver Stress

Several factors can contribute to liver stress and compromise its function. One of the most well-known causes is excessive alcohol consumption. Alcohol is metabolized in the liver, and excessive intake can lead to liver damage and conditions such as fatty liver disease, hepatitis, and cirrhosis. A poor diet high in processed foods and sugars can also strain the liver. Processed foods often contain high levels of unhealthy fats, sugars, and additives, which can contribute to liver fat accumulation and inflammation. Exposure to environmental toxins and pollutants is another significant cause of liver stress. The liver works to detoxify these substances, but prolonged or excessive exposure can overwhelm its capacity and lead to damage. Chronic stress has also been identified as a factor that can negatively affect liver health. Stress hormones can influence liver function and contribute to the development of liver diseases. Certain medications and drug use can also pose a risk to liver health. Many drugs are processed by the liver, and overuse or misuse can lead to liver toxicity and damage.

Common Causes of Liver Stress		
Excessive alcohol consumption	Poor diet high in processed foods and sugars	Exposure to environmental toxins and pollutants
Chronic stress	Certain medications and drug use	

Symptoms of Liver Dysfunction

When the liver is not functioning properly, it can manifest in various symptoms that indicate underlying issues. Fatigue and weakness are common signs of liver dysfunction, as the liver is crucial for energy metabolism. Jaundice, characterized by the yellowing of the skin and eyes, is a clear indication of liver problems. This occurs when there is an accumulation of bilirubin, a byproduct of red blood cell breakdown, due to impaired liver function. Abdominal pain and swelling can also suggest liver dysfunction. The liver may become enlarged or inflamed, causing discomfort and distention in the abdominal area. Changes in urine and stool color are other indicators. Dark urine and pale stools can result from problems with bile production or excretion. Chronic itching is another symptom associated with liver dysfunction. It can occur due to the buildup of bile acids in the skin. Unexplained weight loss is also a concerning symptom that may be related to liver problems, reflecting the body's inability to properly process and utilize nutrients.

Symptoms of Liver Dysfunction		
Fatigue and weakness	Dark urine and pale stools	Abdominal pain and swelling
Chronic itching	Unexplained weight loss	Jaundice (yellowing of the skin and eyes)

Liver Detox Methods

Certain herbs are renowned for their liver-supporting properties. Here are some effective herbs for liver detoxification: **Milk Thistle** Contains silymarin, which has antioxidant and anti-inflammatory properties that protect liver cells and promote regeneration. **Dandelion Root** Acts as a diuretic, promoting the elimination of toxins through urine and supporting liver function. **Turmeric** Contains curcumin, known for its anti-inflammatory and antioxidant effects, aiding in liver detoxification. **Burdock Root** Purifies the blood by removing toxins and supports liver health through its antioxidant properties.

Artichoke Leaf Stimulates bile production, improving digestion and assisting in the elimination of toxins. **Schisandra** Boosts liver detoxification enzymes and offers protective effects against liver damage. **Yarrow** Enhances bile flow and has anti-inflammatory properties that support liver health. **Black Seed Oil** Contains thymoquinone, which has antioxidant and anti-inflammatory properties beneficial for liver function. **Plantain** Supports liver health through its anti-inflammatory and wound-healing properties.

Gaia-Grown Nettle Acts as a natural diuretic, helping to flush toxins from the body and supporting liver function. **Oil of Oregano** Has antimicrobial properties that can help reduce liver inflammation caused by infections. **Mullein Flower** Known for its soothing properties and ability to support overall liver health. **Elecampane Root** Promotes liver function by stimulating bile production and supporting overall liver health. **Marshmallow Root and Leaf** Provides mucilage, which soothes and protects the liver tissues. **Common Mallow** Known for its anti-inflammatory properties that support liver health. **White Horehound** The stimulant action of white horehound works on mucus production in the body, helping the body get rid of it. Contains antimicrobial properties.

Dietary Changes
Emphasizing an alkaline diet can significantly support liver health. This includes consuming alkaline-forming foods such as fresh fruits and vegetables, including leafy greens, berries, and citrus fruits. Whole grains like quinoa and brown rice, as well as nuts and seeds, are also beneficial. It is important to minimize the intake of toxins by reducing the consumption of alcohol, caffeine, processed foods, and refined sugars. Adequate hydration is crucial, so drinking plenty of water helps to flush out toxins from the body. Incorporating healthy fats, such as those found in avocados, nuts, and olive oil, can further promote liver health.

Lifestyle Modifications

Regular exercise is essential as it promotes blood circulation and aids in the detoxification process. Managing stress through techniques such as meditation, yoga, and deep breathing exercises can help reduce stress, which can negatively impact liver health. Ensuring adequate sleep is also important, as sufficient rest supports overall health and liver function.

Natural Detox Protocol

Starting the day with a glass of warm water and lemon can stimulate liver function, setting a positive tone for the day. Herbal teas made from liver-supportive herbs such as dandelion root, milk thistle, or turmeric can be included in the daily routine. Incorporating liver-friendly ingredients like beets, leafy greens, and turmeric into smoothies is another effective strategy. Focusing on a plant-based, alkaline diet rich in fresh vegetables, fruits, whole grains, and healthy fats for meals is recommended. Additionally, considering natural supplements that contain liver-supportive herbs can further enhance liver health.

? QUESTIONS TO ASK YOUR DOCTOR ?

What is the current state of my liver health based on tests?

Are there any specific liver function tests you recommend?

What dietary or lifestyle changes would you suggest to support my liver health?

Are there any potential interactions between my current medications and liver detox herbs?

How often should I monitor my liver function if I start a detox regimen?.

Liver Detoxification

The liver is one of the most vital organs in the body, responsible for filtering toxins from the blood, producing bile for digestion, and storing essential nutrients. Given its critical role, maintaining liver health is essential for overall well-being. A holistic liver detox aims to support and enhance the liver's natural detoxification processes using natural herbs, dietary adjustments, and lifestyle changes.

The Importance of Liver Health

Maintaining liver health is crucial for: Efficient detoxification of harmful substances, Metabolism and storage of nutrients, Regulation of blood sugar levels, Production of bile for fat digestion and Synthesis of essential proteins and clotting factors.

Common Causes of Liver Stress

Excessive alcohol consumption, Poor diet high in processed foods and sugars, Exposure to environmental toxins and pollutants, Chronic stress, and Certain medications and drug use

Symptoms of Liver Dysfunction

Fatigue and weakness, Jaundice (yellowing of the skin and eyes), Abdominal pain and swelling, Dark urine and pale stools, Chronic itching, and Unexplained weight loss

Liver Detox Methods

A thorough liver detox involves several key components: herbal remedies, dietary changes, and lifestyle modifications.

Alkaline Diet: Emphasizing alkaline-forming foods can support liver health. This includes: Fresh fruits and vegetables (e.g., leafy greens, berries, citrus fruits), Whole grains (e.g., quinoa, brown rice), Nuts and seeds. **Avoiding Toxins**: Minimize intake of alcohol, caffeine, processed foods, and refined sugars. **Hydration**: Drinking plenty of water to assist in flushing out toxins. **Healthy Fats**: Incorporating healthy fats such as those found in avocados, nuts, and olive oil.

Lifestyle Modifications

Regular Exercise: Promotes blood circulation and aids in the detoxification process. **Stress Management**: Techniques such as meditation, yoga, and deep breathing exercises help reduce stress, which can negatively impact liver health. **Adequate Sleep**: Ensuring sufficient rest supports overall health and liver function.

Natural Detox Protocol

Morning Routine: Start the day with a glass of warm water and lemon to stimulate liver function. **Herbal Tea**: Drink herbal teas made from liver-supportive herbs such as dandelion root, milk thistle, or turmeric. **Smoothies**: Incorporate liver-friendly ingredients like beets, leafy greens, and turmeric into daily smoothies. **Meals**: Focus on a plant-based, alkaline diet rich in fresh vegetables, fruits, whole grains, and healthy fats. **Supplementation**: Consider natural supplements that contain liver-supportive herbs.

? QUESTIONS TO ASK YOUR DOCTOR ?

What is the current state of my liver health based on tests?

Are there any specific liver function tests you recommend?

What dietary or lifestyle changes would you suggest to support my liver health?

Are there any potential interactions between my current medications and liver detox herbs?

How often should I monitor my liver function if I start a detox regimen?

Detoxification Methods to Help the Liver

Herb	Treatment
Milk Thistle	Contains silymarin, which has antioxidant and anti-inflammatory properties that protect liver cells and promote regeneration.
Dandelion Root	Acts as a diuretic, promoting the elimination of toxins through urine and supporting liver function.
Turmeric	Contains curcumin, known for its anti-inflammatory and antioxidant effects, aiding in liver detoxification.
Burdock Root	Purifies the blood by removing toxins and supports liver health through its antioxidant properties.
Artichoke Leaf	Stimulates bile production, improving digestion and assisting in the elimination of toxins.
Schisandra	Boosts liver detoxification enzymes and offers protective effects against liver damage.
Yarrow	Enhances bile flow and has anti-inflammatory properties that support liver health.
Black Seed Oil	Contains thymoquinone, which has antioxidant and anti-inflammatory properties beneficial for liver function.
Plantain	Supports liver health through its anti-inflammatory and wound-healing properties.
Gaia-Grown Nettle	Acts as a natural diuretic, helping to flush toxins from the body and supporting liver function.
Oil of Oregano	Has antimicrobial properties that can help reduce liver inflammation caused by infections.
Mullein Flower	Known for its soothing properties and ability to support overall liver health.
Elecampane Root	Promotes liver function by stimulating bile production and supporting overall liver health.
Marshmallow Root and Leaf	Provides mucilage, which soothes and protects the liver tissues.
Common Mallow	Known for its anti-inflammatory properties that support liver health.
White Horehound	The stimulant action of white horehound works on mucus production in the body, helping the body get rid of it. Contains antimicrobial properties.

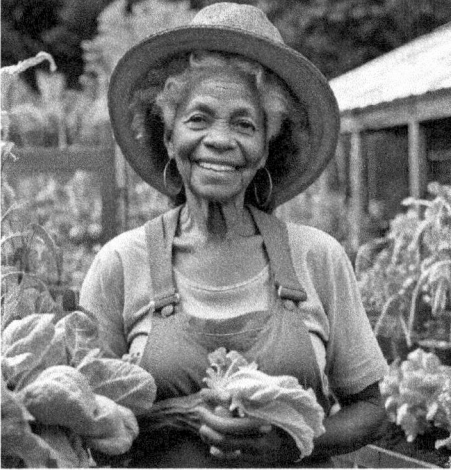

Nutrition and Dietary Needs

Macronutrients and Micronutrients Black women have unique nutritional needs that must be addressed for optimal health. Key nutrients include: **Protein**: Essential for muscle repair and growth. Sources include lean meats, legumes, and nuts. **Healthy Fats**: Important for brain health and hormone balance. Sources include avocados, olive oil, and fatty fish. **Vitamins and Minerals**: Focus on calcium, vitamin D, iron, and B vitamins to prevent common deficiencies.

Common Nutritional Deficiencies Many Black women are at risk for deficiencies in vitamin D, iron, and calcium due to genetic factors and dietary patterns. Addressing these deficiencies is crucial: **Vitamin D**: Sun exposure and fortified foods. **Iron**: Leafy greens, lean meats, and iron supplements if needed. **Calcium**: fortified non-dairy milks, and leafy greens.

Dietary Recommendations and Meal Planning Creating balanced meals that cater to the unique needs of Black women involves: **Diverse Diet**: Incorporating a variety of fruits, vegetables, whole grains, and proteins. **Hydration**: Drinking adequate water to support overall health. **Cultural Foods**: Integrating traditional African and Caribbean foods into a healthy diet.

Dietary Requirements and Traditional Diet The traditional Diet is inherently rich in nutrients and tailored to the physiological needs of people of African descent. This section outlines the key differences in dietary needs between Black and Caucasian populations, emphasizing the importance of a nutrient-dense diet for optimal health. The traditional Diet emphasizes significantly higher fiber intake compared to the typical processed food diet commonly consumed by Caucasians. Fiber is crucial for digestive health, helping to maintain regular bowel movements, reducing the risk of colon cancer, and aiding in weight management.

This dietary fiber intake should be eight times higher in the traditional Diet, reflecting its reliance on whole, plant-based foods. In contrast to the high sodium levels found in processed foods, the traditional Diet requires only one-sixth of this amount. Lowering sodium intake is vital for reducing the risk of hypertension, a common precursor to heart disease and stroke. By consuming less sodium, individuals can maintain healthier blood pressure levels and reduce cardiovascular risk.

Calcium Intake
Calcium is another critical nutrient that is needed in significantly higher amounts—seven times more—within the traditional Diet. Calcium is essential for strong bones and teeth, muscle function, and nerve signaling. Given that many African populations have higher rates of lactose intolerance, alternative calcium sources such as leafy greens, nuts, and seeds are crucial.

Phosphorus Intake

Phosphorus intake should be five to eight times higher in the traditional Diet compared to a processed food diet. Phosphorus works closely with calcium to build strong bones and teeth, and it is also important for the body's energy production and storage.

Vitamin Intake

Vitamin intake, both water-soluble and fat-soluble, is significantly higher in the traditional Diet. Water-soluble vitamins, such as vitamin C and the B vitamins, are necessary for energy production, immune function, and skin health. Fat-soluble vitamins, such as vitamins A, D, E, and K, are vital for vision, bone health, antioxidant protection, and blood clotting. These vitamins are often found in higher quantities in fresh fruits, vegetables, and whole foods.

Sunlight Exposure

Sunlight exposure is another crucial aspect, as it is necessary for the synthesis of vitamin D. The traditional Diet and lifestyle require 80% more sunlight stimulation for the pineal organ, which plays a role in regulating circadian rhythms and overall health. This increased need for sunlight highlights the importance of spending time outdoors and ensuring adequate exposure to natural light.

Water intake

Water intake is also markedly higher in the traditional Diet, requiring 90% more than the typical processed food diet. Adequate hydration is essential for maintaining body temperature, lubricating joints, protecting sensitive tissues, and eliminating waste. Higher water consumption supports overall health and helps prevent dehydration.

A diet rich in organic vegetables and fruits is a cornerstone of the traditional Diet, requiring an 85% higher intake than that found in processed food diets. These foods provide essential vitamins, minerals, and antioxidants that help prevent chronic diseases, support immune function, and maintain overall health.

Meat consumption in the traditional Diet is limited to about 15% of the diet, and it includes organic animal flesh, often consumed during times of cultural and health decline. This moderate intake of meat, which can include insects, ensures a balanced intake of protein and other nutrients without the health risks associated with high meat consumption, such as cardiovascular disease and certain cancers.

Cow's milk is generally avoided in the traditional Diet due to its indigestibility for many individuals of African descent. Consuming cow's milk can lead to colds, allergies, diseases, and mood swings. Instead, alternatives such as plant-based milks are preferred, which are easier to digest and do not cause the adverse effects associated with cow's milk.

The traditional Diet is tailored to meet the specific nutritional needs of people of African descent, emphasizing higher intake of fiber, calcium, phosphorus, vitamins, water, and organic vegetables and fruits, while reducing sodium and cow's milk consumption and moderating meat intake.

Nutrient/ Food Item	Traditional Diet (Black Population)	Processed Food Diet (Caucasian Population)
Fiber	8 times higher	Low
Sodium	1/6th of processed food diet	High
Calcium	7 times higher of processed food diet	Low
Phosphorus	5-8 times higher of processed food diet	Low
Water-soluble Vitamins	Higher levels	Often deficient
Fat-soluble Vitamins	Higher levels	Often deficient
Sunlight Exposure	80% more for the Pineal Organ	Less emphasis
Water Intake	90% higher	Often inadequate
Vegetables and Fruits	85% higher and organic	Low
Meat	15% organic meats eaten thru cultural/health decline	High
Cow's Milk	Indigestible = colds, allergies, diseases, and mood swings	Commonly consumed

Health Implications of Dietary Differences

Higher Fiber Intake: Promotes digestive health, reduces the risk of chronic diseases such as heart disease and diabetes, and aids in weight management. **Reduced Sodium Intake**: Lowers blood pressure and reduces the risk of cardiovascular diseases. **Increased Calcium and Phosphorus**: Supports bone health and prevents osteoporosis and other bone-related disorders. **Adequate Vitamin Levels**: Essential for overall health, including immune function, skin health, and preventing deficiencies that can lead to diseases. **Sunlight Exposure**: Crucial for vitamin D synthesis, which is important for bone health, immune function, and overall well-being. ***Higher Water Intake***: Ensures proper hydration, supports bodily functions, and aids in detoxification. ***Higher Intake of Organic Vegetables and Fruits***: Provides essential vitamins, minerals, and antioxidants, which are vital for preventing diseases and maintaining health. ***Moderate Meat Consumption:*** Reduces the risk of chronic diseases associated with high meat intake, such as heart disease and certain cancers. ***Avoidance of Cow's Milk:*** Prevents digestive issues, allergies, and other health problems associated with lactose intolerance and milk proteins.

Protein	Healthy Fats	Vitamin D	Iron	Calcium
Walnut	Avocados	Eggs	Leafy greens	Non-dairy milks
Legumes	Olive oil	Mushrooms	Kidney Beans	Broccoli
Chickpeas	Fatty fish	Sea Moss	Almonds	Mustard collard greens

Drinking Water and Herbal Infusions

By incorporating these natural infusions into your daily routine, you can enjoy the added benefits of hydration and nutrients, making water consumption more enjoyable and beneficial for your overall health.

The Importance of Drinking Water

Water is essential for life and maintaining overall health. It plays several critical roles in the body, including: **Hydration:** Water is crucial for maintaining fluid balance in the body, which is essential for all bodily functions. **Temperature Regulation:** It helps regulate body temperature through sweating and respiration. **Digestion:** Water aids digestion by helping break down food so that nutrients can be absorbed. **Detoxification:** It assists in flushing out toxins and waste products from the body through urine and sweat. **Joint Lubrication:** Water keeps the joints lubricated, which is important for mobility and preventing joint pain. **Skin Health:** Adequate hydration keeps the skin moisturized and can improve its appearance and elasticity. **Cognitive Function:** Proper hydration is linked to better concentration, alertness, and short-term memory.

Effects of Herbal Infusions

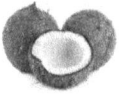

Coconut Water

Hydration: Coconut water is rich in electrolytes, making it excellent for rehydration, especially after exercise. Nutrient Boost: It provides essential minerals like potassium, magnesium, and calcium. Antioxidants: Contains antioxidants that help combat oxidative stress.

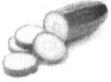

Cucumber Water

Hydration: Cucumber adds extra hydration due to its high water content. Skin Health: It contains silica, which is beneficial for skin health. Detoxification: Helps in detoxifying the body and promoting kidney health.

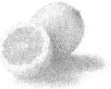

Lemon Water

Vitamin C: Lemons are rich in vitamin C, which boosts the immune system. Digestion: Lemon water can aid in digestion and act as a natural diuretic, helping to cleanse the liver. Alkalizing Effect: Despite being acidic, lemon has an alkalizing effect on the body, which can help balance pH levels.

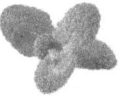

Mint Water

Digestion: Mint is known for its digestive benefits and can help alleviate indigestion and bloating. Cooling Effect: It provides a refreshing and cooling sensation, which is particularly enjoyable in hot weather. Breath Freshener: Mint can help freshen breath naturally.

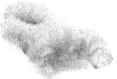

Ginger Water

Anti-Inflammatory: Ginger has powerful anti-inflammatory properties that can help reduce inflammation and pain. Digestive Health: It promotes healthy digestion and can alleviate nausea. Immune Boost: Ginger helps strengthen the immune system due to its antioxidant properties.

Tips for Making Herbal Infused Water

Preparation: Wash all ingredients thoroughly before use. ***Cutting:*** Slice fruits and vegetables thinly to release more flavor. ***Infusion Time:*** Allow the water to infuse for at least 2-4 hours in the refrigerator for maximum flavor. ***Storage:*** Store infused water in a glass container to preserve its freshness. ***Consumption:*** Drink the infused water within 24-48 hours for the best taste and nutritional benefits.

Natural Healing Through Diet and Herbs

An alkaline diet and plant-based nutrition is foundational principles for achieving optimal health. This section delves into these principles and how they contribute to overall well-being, particularly for Black women.

Alkaline Diet

An alkaline diet focuses on consuming foods that help maintain a balanced pH level in the body, ideally keeping it slightly alkaline. An alkaline diet emphasizes natural, plant-based foods such as leafy greens, fruits, nuts, seeds, and certain grains, while avoiding acidic foods like meat, dairy, refined sugars, and processed foods. The primary goal is to create an internal environment that discourages the development of diseases and supports overall health. The benefits of an alkaline diet are significant. Black women are statistically more likely to suffer from chronic conditions such as hypertension, diabetes, and heart disease, all of which can be mitigated through diet. By following an alkaline diet, Black women can reduce inflammation, which is a common underlying factor in many chronic diseases. Additionally, this diet can help maintain a healthy weight, support digestive health, and improve energy levels. The focus on nutrient-rich, whole foods ensures that Black women receive essential vitamins and minerals that may be lacking in a typical Western diet, thereby enhancing overall well-being and reducing the risk of nutrient deficiencies.

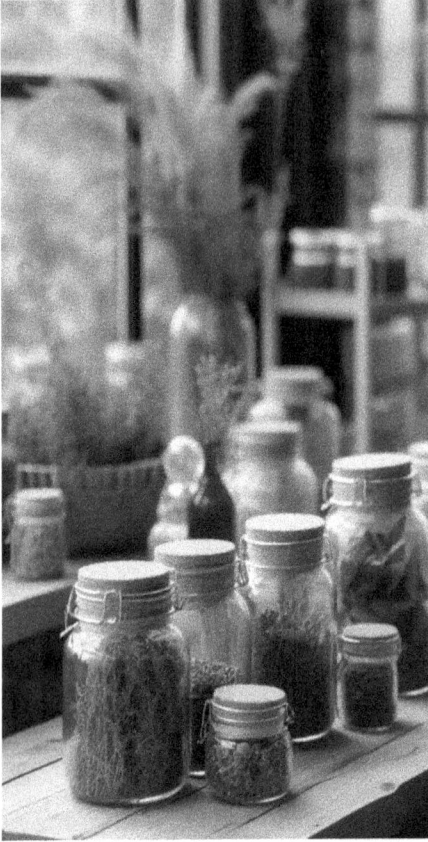

Natural Herbs

Using natural herbs to detoxify and support overall health is a cornerstone of holistic healing. It is recommended that specific herbs are known for their cleansing and health-promoting properties. Herbs such as burdock root, sarsaparilla, and yellow dock are lauded for their ability to purify the blood, detoxify the liver, and support the body's natural elimination processes. These herbs are often consumed in teas or taken as supplements to harness their full benefits. For women, who may face unique health challenges related to systemic inequalities and higher exposure to environmental toxins, incorporating these natural herbs can be particularly beneficial.

Herbs that support detoxification can help counteract the effects of pollutants and toxins that disproportionately affect Black communities. Furthermore, these herbs can provide relief from menstrual and reproductive health issues such as fibroids and endometriosis, conditions that Black women are more likely to experience. By using natural herbs as part of a regular health regimen, Black women can enhance their body's ability to heal and maintain health naturally.

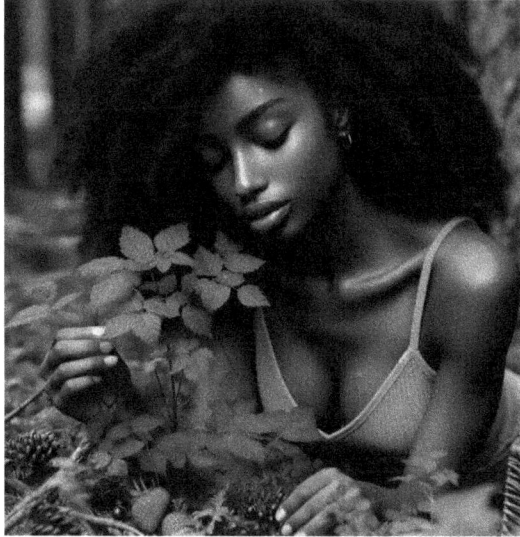

Plant-Based Nutrition

Plant-based nutrition, which emphasizes a diet rich in fruits, vegetables, nuts, and seeds, is central to health practices. This approach to eating ensures a high intake of fiber, antioxidants, and essential nutrients, which are vital for maintaining good health. Plant-based diets are associated with lower risks of chronic diseases, improved digestion, and better overall health outcomes. For Black women, a plant-based diet can offer numerous health benefits. Many Black women face higher rates of obesity and related health conditions such as diabetes and cardiovascular disease.

A plant-based diet can aid in weight management by providing nutrient-dense, low-calorie foods that promote satiety and reduce overeating. Additionally, the high fiber content in a plant-based diet supports digestive health, which can help alleviate issues like constipation and improve nutrient absorption. By reducing the intake of animal products and processed foods, Black women can decrease their risk of chronic diseases and enjoy a more balanced, energized lifestyle.

Herbal Remedies and Natural Therapies

Incorporating natural remedies and therapies into daily routines can enhance health and well-being. The use of herbal teas, essential oils, and regular detoxification practices should be a part of a health regimen. Herbal teas, such as chamomile and ginger, can provide relaxation and aid digestion, while essential oils like lavender and tea tree offer benefits for stress relief and skin care. For Black women, who may experience higher levels of stress due to societal and cultural pressures, incorporating these natural remedies can be particularly advantageous. Herbal teas can serve as a soothing ritual that promotes mental calmness and physical relaxation, helping to manage stress and anxiety. Essential oils, used in aromatherapy or skincare, can provide a natural way to enhance mood and address skin concerns without the harsh chemicals often found in commercial products. Regular detoxification practices, supported by herbs like burdock root and sarsaparilla, can help Black women cleanse their bodies of toxins, improve skin health, and boost overall vitality.

Healthy Body Detoxification

Detoxification is an essential aspect of health practices. A healthy body detox involves using natural methods to cleanse the body and support the organs responsible for detoxification, such as the liver, kidneys, and lymphatic system. Methods such as periodic fasting, hydration, and the use of specific detoxifying herbs help to eliminate toxins and rejuvenate the body. Detoxification can play a crucial role in maintaining health and preventing disease. Due to higher exposure to environmental toxins and the stress of systemic inequalities, detoxification can help mitigate these adverse effects by promoting efficient elimination of harmful substances. Regular detox routines can also support reproductive health, reduce symptoms of PMS, and enhance overall energy levels.

How to Heal the Body Naturally

Natural approaches to health emphasize the use of plant-based diets and herbal remedies to maintain an alkaline environment in the body. Here's a comprehensive guide on detoxifying the body, healing the gut, and regulating the nervous system using natural methods.

Detoxify the Body

Alkaline Diet: Consuming alkaline foods helps cleanse and detoxify the body. Foods like leafy greens, fruits, vegetables, nuts, and seeds are essential. **Avoid Acidic Foods** It is recommended to avoid processed foods, sugars, dairy, and meat, which can contribute to acidity and toxin buildup in the body. **Herbal Teas and Supplements** *Burdock Root:* Known for its blood-purifying properties, burdock root helps detoxify the liver and promote healthy skin. *Sarsaparilla:* This herb is renowned for its high iron content and blood-purifying abilities, helping to cleanse the body. *Dandelion Root:* Acts as a diuretic to aid in the elimination of toxins through urine. *Hydration:* Drinking plenty of natural spring water helps flush out toxins effectively.

Heal Your Gut

A Mucus-Free Diet eliminates foods that cause excess mucus production in the body. Excess mucus can lead to inflammation and digestive issues. *Benefits:* Helps reduce inflammation, supports healthy digestion, and promotes a balanced gut flora.

Probiotic Foods: Naturally, fermented foods can introduce beneficial bacteria to the gut. *Herbal Infusions:* Herbs like ginger and chamomile can soothe the digestive tract and reduce inflammation. *Sea Moss:* Rich in minerals and nutrients, sea moss supports digestive health and helps heal the gut lining.

Regulate Your Nervous System

Diet and Lifestyle: *Alkaline Diet* Maintaining an alkaline diet supports overall health, including the nervous system. *Mineral-Rich Foods:* Foods rich in magnesium, potassium, and other essential minerals help in nerve function and relaxation.

Approved Foods & Foods to Avoid

To support a balanced, nerve-friendly diet, it is best to avoid: **Refined Sugars and Sweeteners**: Including agave syrup, date sugar, and artificial sweeteners. **Processed Oils**: Such as hydrogenated oils, margarine, and butter. By highlighting nutrient-dense, alkaline foods and minimizing inflammatory, processed items, you can help maintain optimal nerve function and overall well-being.

Recommended **Vegetables**: Leafy greens, cucumbers, zucchini Vegetables to Limit or Avoid: Potatoes, corn, beans Recommended **Fruits**: Berries, apples, pears Fruits to Limit or Avoid: Bananas, avocados, oranges **Grains** Recommended: Quinoa, wild rice, amaranth Grains to Limit or Avoid: Wheat, barley, oats **Nuts & Seeds** Recommended: Almonds, chia seeds, flax seeds Nuts & Seeds to Limit or Avoid: Peanuts, cashews, sunflower seeds **Beverages** Recommended: Herbal teas, spring water Beverages to Limit or Avoid: Coffee, soda, dairy milk **Oils & Fats** Recommended: Olive oil, coconut oil Oils & Fats to Limit or Avoid: Butter, margarine, processed oils.

Herbal Remedies

Valerian Root: Known for its calming properties, valerian root can help reduce anxiety and promote restful sleep. Passionflower: This herb is often used to treat anxiety and insomnia, helping to soothe the nervous system. Linden Flower: Acts as a natural sedative to help calm the mind and body. Hydration and Rest: Hydration: Drinking adequate water is essential for nervous system health. Adequate Sleep: Ensuring sufficient rest and sleep supports nervous system regulation and overall mental health.

Mucus-Free Diet Chart

Detoxifying the Body

Alkaline diet, hydration, and specific herbs (burdock root, sarsaparilla, dandelion root). Methods: Avoid acidic foods, drink herbal teas, and consume alkaline foods.

Healing the Gut

Mucus-Free Diet, high-fiber alkaline foods, and natural herbal remedies. Methods: Eliminate mucus-forming foods, use ginger, chamomile, and sea moss for gut health.

Regulating the Nervous System

Alkaline diet, mineral-rich foods, and calming herbs. Methods: Use valerian root, passionflower, linden flower, maintain hydration, and ensure adequate sleep.

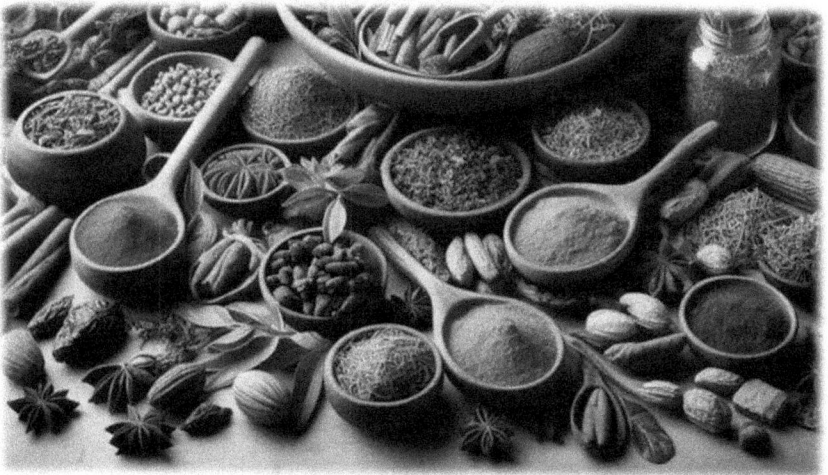

Blood Type O Menu

TY
PE
O

Breakfast: Smoothie: Spinach, kale, cucumber, green apple, and chia seeds.
Herbal Tea: Burdock root tea.
Lunch: Quinoa salad with avocado, cherry tomatoes, red onions, and lemon-tahini dressing. Side of steamed broccoli with a sprinkle of sea salt.
Dinner: Baked sweet potato with a side of sautéed collard greens and garlic.
Mixed greens salad with pumpkin seeds, cucumbers, and a balsamic vinegar dressing. **Snack:** Almonds and fresh berries.

Blood Type A Menu

TY
PE
A

Breakfast:
Fresh fruit salad: Oranges, strawberries, kiwi, and blueberries.
Herbal Tea: Sarsaparilla tea.
Lunch:
Brown rice bowl with sautéed zucchini, bell peppers, and black beans.
Mixed greens with a light vinaigrette.
Dinner: Grilled portobello mushrooms with a side of steamed asparagus. Quinoa and roasted beet salad with walnuts. **Snack:** Sliced apples with almond butter.

TYPE B

Blood Type B Menu

Breakfast: Buckwheat pancakes topped with fresh blueberries and a drizzle of agave syrup. Herbal Tea: Yellow dock tea.

Lunch: Lentil and vegetable soup (carrots, celery, onions, garlic).

Side of mixed greens with sunflower seeds and lemon dressing.

Dinner: Stir-fried tofu with bok choy, carrots, and snap peas over a bed of quinoa. Steamed kale with a touch of olive oil and garlic. **Snack:** Celery sticks with hummus.

TYPE AB

Blood Type AB Menu

Breakfast: Smoothie: Spinach, banana, almond milk, flax seeds. Herbal Tea: Red clover tea.

Lunch: Chickpea and avocado salad with mixed greens, cucumbers, and cherry tomatoes.

Side of roasted Brussels sprouts.

Dinner Stuffed bell peppers with quinoa, black beans, and corn. Mixed greens salad with sliced almonds and a lemon vinaigrette. **Snack:** Handful of dried apricots and raw cashews.

For Women Under 30

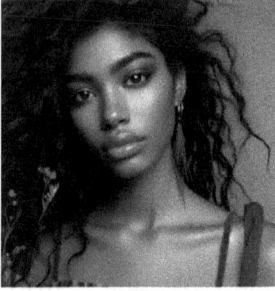

Breakfast: Acai bowl topped with banana slices, granola, and hemp seeds. **Herbal Tea:** Chamomile tea. **Lunch:** Spelt grain salad with mixed vegetables, chickpeas, and tahini dressing. Side of cucumber and tomato salad. **Dinner:** Grilled vegetable skewers (zucchini, bell peppers, mushrooms) over wild rice. Kale and avocado salad with sesame seeds. **Snack:** Fresh fruit (grapes, apples).

For Women Over 30

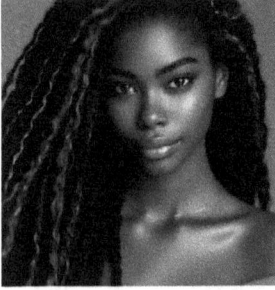

Breakfast: Warm oatmeal with chia seeds, fresh berries, and a drizzle of maple syrup. **Herbal Tea:** Ginger tea.
Lunch: Mixed greens with quinoa, roasted sweet potatoes, and a citrus vinaigrette. Side of steamed broccoli.
Dinner: Baked butternut squash with sautéed spinach and garlic. Lentil and vegetable stew. **Snack:** Walnuts and sliced pears.

For Women Over 50

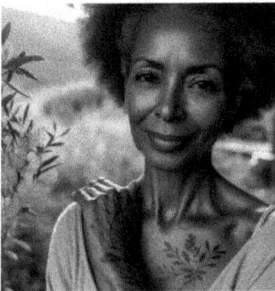

Breakfast: Millet porridge with almond milk, flax seeds, and sliced strawberries. **Herbal Tea:** Dandelion root tea. **Lunch:** Arugula salad with roasted beets, walnuts, and a light balsamic dressing. Side of roasted carrots and parsnips. **Dinner:** Cauliflower and chickpea curry over brown rice. Steamed greens with a dash of olive oil and lemon juice. **Snack:** Mixed nuts and dried figs.

The Role of Mucus and Acidity in Disease

Traditional medical science attributes pathogens such as bacteria and viruses to the causes of many diseases. However, there is a growing body of thought that suggests mucus and acidity within the body might be fundamental contributors to the development and progression of diseases. This perspective emphasizes the importance of maintaining an alkaline environment to promote overall health and prevent illness.

Mucus and Acidity as Disease Causes

Mucus and acidity cause disease posits that the body's internal environment plays a critical role in health. Proponents of this theory argue that an excess buildup of mucus and a high level of acidity in the body can create conditions that are conducive to disease.

Mucus in Disease

Mucus is a slippery secretion produced by and covering mucous membranes. It serves as a protective layer to keep tissues moist and to trap foreign particles and pathogens. However, when the body produces excessive mucus, it can obstruct normal bodily functions and create an environment that promotes disease. For example: **Bronchitis**: Excess mucus in the bronchial tubes can lead to chronic inflammation and infection, causing bronchitis. **Pneumonia**: Mucus accumulation in the lungs can trap bacteria and viruses, leading to pneumonia. **Diabetes**: Mucus in the pancreatic ducts can impair insulin secretion, contributing to the development of diabetes.

Acidity in Disease

Acidity in the body is often measured by pH levels, with lower pH indicating higher acidity. The theory posits that high levels of acidity can lead to an imbalance that disrupts normal cellular functions and promotes disease. Acidic environments are thought to: *Damage Tissues*: Acidic conditions can erode tissues and cells, leading to inflammation and chronic disease. *Promote Pathogens*: Many harmful bacteria and viruses thrive in acidic environments, which can exacerbate infections and diseases. **Weaken the Immune System**: High acidity can compromise the immune system, making the body more susceptible to infections and illnesses.

Supporting Evidence

While mainstream medical research typically focuses on pathogens as primary disease causes, there is evidence supporting the role of mucus and acidity in disease: *Inflammation:* Chronic inflammation is a well-documented response to excessive mucus and high acidity, contributing to a variety of diseases, including cardiovascular diseases, arthritis, and certain cancers. *Gut Health*: Studies show that an alkaline diet can promote better gut health by reducing inflammation and balancing gut microbiota, which are crucial for a robust immune system. *Cellular Health:* Research indicates that maintaining an alkaline environment helps protect cells from oxidative stress and damage, which are precursors to chronic diseases.

Diet and Lifestyle Interventions

Proponents of the mucus and acidity theory often recommend dietary and lifestyle changes to reduce mucus production and acidity levels. Key recommendations include: *Alkaline Diet:* Consuming a diet rich in alkaline foods such as fruits, vegetables, nuts, and seeds helps balance the body's pH levels. *Hydration:* Drinking plenty of water, particularly spring water, helps flush out toxins and maintain a healthy pH balance. *Avoiding Acidic Foods:* Reducing intake of processed foods, animal products, and caffeine can lower body acidity. *Regular Exercise:* Physical activity helps improve circulation and reduce inflammation, contributing to overall pH balance and mucus reduction. The theory that mucus and acidity cause disease offers an alternative perspective to the traditional pathogen-centered model.

By focusing on the body's internal environment and emphasizing the importance of maintaining an alkaline state, this approach advocates for health practices. While more research is needed to fully validate this theory, adopting a diet and lifestyle that promotes alkalinity and reduces mucus buildup can contribute to overall health and potentially prevent various diseases.

The Mucus-Reducing Alkaline Diet

The mucus-reducing alkaline diet is a plant-based dietary regimen designed to control acid levels in the body. It is believed that regulating these levels protects cells against harmful mucus buildup, which can affect various organs and lead to diseases. This diet posits that excess mucus in specific areas of the body causes different health issues: for example, mucus in the bronchial tubes leads to bronchitis, mucus in the lungs leads to pneumonia, and mucus in the pancreatic ducts leads to diabetes. This diet is designed to reduce mucus by maintaining an alkaline environment within the body. It comprises mainly natural, plant-based foods that are believed to balance the body's pH and prevent disease.

Nutritional Guide Compliance

Only consume foods listed in the nutritional guide, including approved fruits, vegetables, grains, nuts, and seeds.

Hydration Drink 1 gallon (3.8 liters) of spring water daily. Adequate hydration is crucial for maintaining bodily functions and flushing out toxins.

Supplementation Take supplements an hour before any medications. These supplements are designed to provide additional nutrients that support overall health.

No Animal The diet strictly prohibits the consumption of animal products. This rule aligns with the diet's plant-based focus, which is believed to promote better health.

No Alcohol Alcohol consumption is not allowed as it can disrupt the body's natural balance and hinder the detoxification process.

Avoid Wheat Only consume "natural-growing grains" listed in the guide, avoiding wheat products that are often heavily processed.

No Microwave Avoid using a microwave to heat food to prevent nutrient degradation.

No Canned

or Seedless Fruits Consume fresh, whole fruits with seeds to ensure maximum nutritional benefit.

Fruits Most fruits are allowed as long as they are not canned or hybrid varieties. This ensures the consumption of fresh, natural fruits that provide essential vitamins and minerals.

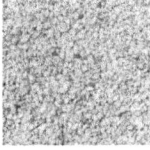

Raw Sesame Seeds Tiny seeds that are often used in cooking and baking. They have a nutty flavor and are rich in nutrients. *Nutritional Benefits* High in healthy fats, protein, and fiber; rich in calcium, magnesium, and iron; contains antioxidants such as sesamin and sesamol that support heart health and reduce inflammation

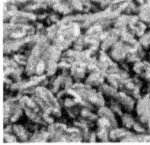

Walnuts A type of tree nut that has a rich, slightly bitter flavor. They are known for their high omega-3 fatty acid content. *Nutritional Benefits* High in omega-3 fatty acids, protein, and fiber; rich in antioxidants, vitamins (such as vitamin E), and minerals (such as magnesium and phosphorus); supports brain health and reduces inflammation.

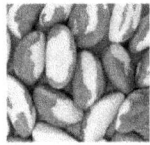

Brazil Nuts Large nuts native to the Amazon rainforest, known for their high selenium content. *Nutritional Benefits* Extremely high in selenium, a mineral important for thyroid function and immune health; rich in healthy fats, protein, and fiber; contains antioxidants that support heart health.

Alkaline Grains The consumption of specific grains is encouraged:

Quinoa A gluten-free grain that contains all nine essential amino acids, making it a complete protein. It is also rich in fiber, vitamins, and minerals. *Nutritional Benefits* High in protein and fiber; rich in magnesium, iron, potassium, and antioxidants; supports heart health and helps regulate blood sugar levels.

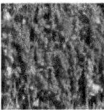

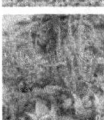

Amaranth An ancient grain known for its high protein content and complete amino acid profile. It is gluten-free and rich in fiber, vitamins, and minerals. *Nutritional Benefits* High in protein and fiber; rich in magnesium, iron, and calcium; contains antioxidants and anti-inflammatory properties.

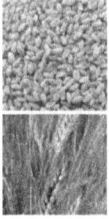

Kamut An ancient variety of wheat that is higher in protein and essential fatty acids than modern wheat. It has a nutty flavor and is easily digestible. *Nutritional Benefits* High in protein, selenium, and zinc; good source of dietary fiber; rich in polyphenols and antioxidants that support immune health.

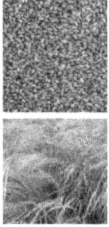

Spelt An ancient grain that is a distant cousin to modern wheat. It has a slightly sweet and nutty flavor and is more easily digestible than regular wheat. *Nutritional Benefits* High in protein, fiber, and B vitamins; rich in manganese, phosphorus, and magnesium; supports heart health and may aid in reducing cholesterol levels.

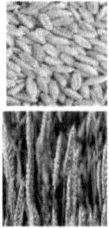

Rye A grain that is often used in bread and other baked goods. It is high in fiber and has a distinctive, hearty flavor. *Nutritional Benefits* High in dietary fiber; rich in manganese, phosphorus, and magnesium; supports digestive health and helps maintain healthy blood sugar levels.

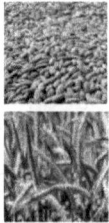

Teff A tiny grain from Ethiopia that is naturally gluten-free and packed with nutrients. It has a mild, nutty flavor and is often used in traditional Ethiopian dishes. *Nutritional Benefits* High in protein, fiber, and iron; rich in calcium and vitamin C; contains resistant starch that supports healthy blood sugar levels and promotes gut health.

Oils All plant-based oils are allowed, supporting a diet rich in healthy fats.

Approved Foods in the Mucus-Reducing Alkaline Diet

Vegetables The diet emphasizes the consumption of natural alkaline vegetables, which help maintain the body's pH balance:

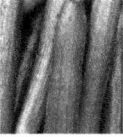

Cucumber: A type of squash with a mild flavor and crisp texture. It is often used in Latin American cuisine. *Nutritional Benefits* Low in calories; high in fiber, vitamin C, and antioxidants; supports digestive health and boosts immune function.

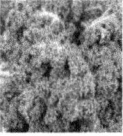

Kale: A nutrient-dense leafy green with a slightly bitter taste, often used in salads and smoothies. *Nutritional Benefits* High in vitamins A, C, and K; rich in calcium, iron, and antioxidants; supports bone health, immune function, and reduces inflammation.

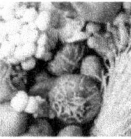

Mushrooms (all, except shiitake) Various types of mushrooms that add umami flavor to dishes and are rich in nutrients. *Nutritional Benefits* Low in calories; high in B vitamins, selenium, and antioxidants; supports immune health and provides anti-inflammatory benefits.

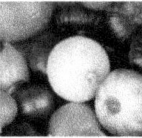

Onions A common vegetable with a pungent flavor used in a variety of cuisines. *Nutritional Benefits* Low in calories; high in vitamin C, B vitamins, and antioxidants; supports immune health and contains anti-inflammatory properties.

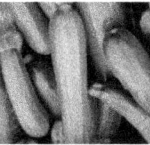

Zucchini A type of summer squash with a mild flavor and high water content. *Nutritional Benefits* Low in calories; high in vitamins A, C, and potassium; rich in antioxidants; supports digestive health and hydration.

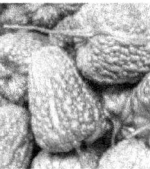

Chayote (Mexican squash) A type of squash with a mild flavor and crisp texture. It is often used in Latin American cuisine. *Nutritional Benefits* Low in calories; high in fiber, vitamin C, and antioxidants; supports digestive health and boosts immune function.

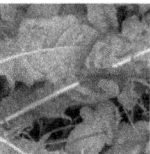

Dandelion greens Leafy greens with a slightly bitter taste, often used in salads and herbal remedies. *Nutritional Benefits* High in vitamins A, C, and K; rich in calcium, iron, and antioxidants; supports liver health and detoxification.

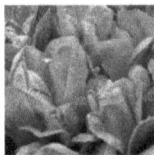

Lettuce (all, except iceberg) Various types of lettuce, each with a unique flavor and texture, except for iceberg which is less nutrient-dense. *Nutritional Benefits* Low in calories; high in vitamins A, C, and K; rich in fiber and antioxidants; supports digestive health and provides essential nutrients.

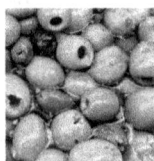

Olives Small fruits that are often cured and used in Mediterranean cuisine, known for their healthy fats. *Nutritional Benefits* High in monounsaturated fats and vitamin E; contains antioxidants and anti-inflammatory compounds; supports heart health and reduces oxidative stress.

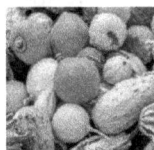

Squash A versatile vegetable with a sweet, mild flavor, available in many varieties. *Nutritional Benefits* Low in calories; high in vitamins A, C, and B6; rich in fiber and antioxidants; supports eye health and immune function.

Health Implications for Black Women
Black women face unique health challenges, including higher rates of certain chronic diseases such as diabetes and hypertension. Adopting a diet that emphasizes natural, unprocessed foods could potentially help mitigate these risks. The emphasis on hydration and nutrient-dense, plant-based foods supports overall wellness and may contribute to better health outcomes.

Understanding Mucus and Disease

The mucus-reducing alkaline diet is centered on the idea that mucus buildup is a primary cause of many diseases. Here is how excess mucus is linked to specific health conditions: **Bronchitis:** Excess mucus in the bronchial tubes can obstruct airways, leading to inflammation and infection. **Pneumonia:** Mucus accumulation in the lungs can create an environment conducive to bacterial and viral infections, causing pneumonia. **Diabetes:** Mucus in the pancreatic ducts can interfere with the pancreas's ability to produce insulin, contributing to diabetes.

Nutritional Components of the Diet

The diet includes a variety of foods that are alkaline-forming and nutrient-rich. These include: **Fruits:** Berries, melons, and tropical fruits that are high in vitamins, minerals, and antioxidants. **Vegetables:** Leafy greens, sea vegetables, and other alkaline-forming veggies that support cellular health. **Grains:** Quinoa, amaranth, and spelt, which are considered "natural-growing" grains and are less processed. **Nuts and Seeds:** Almonds, walnuts, and hemp seeds, providing healthy fats and proteins.

The mucus-reducing alkaline diet offers a holistic approach to health by focusing on plant-based, natural foods to maintain an alkaline environment in the body. By adhering to its strict guidelines, individuals, particularly Black women who face higher risks for certain diseases, may experience improved health outcomes. Hydration, natural food choices, and the avoidance of processed products are key components of this dietary regimen, aiming to reduce mucus buildup and promote overall wellness.

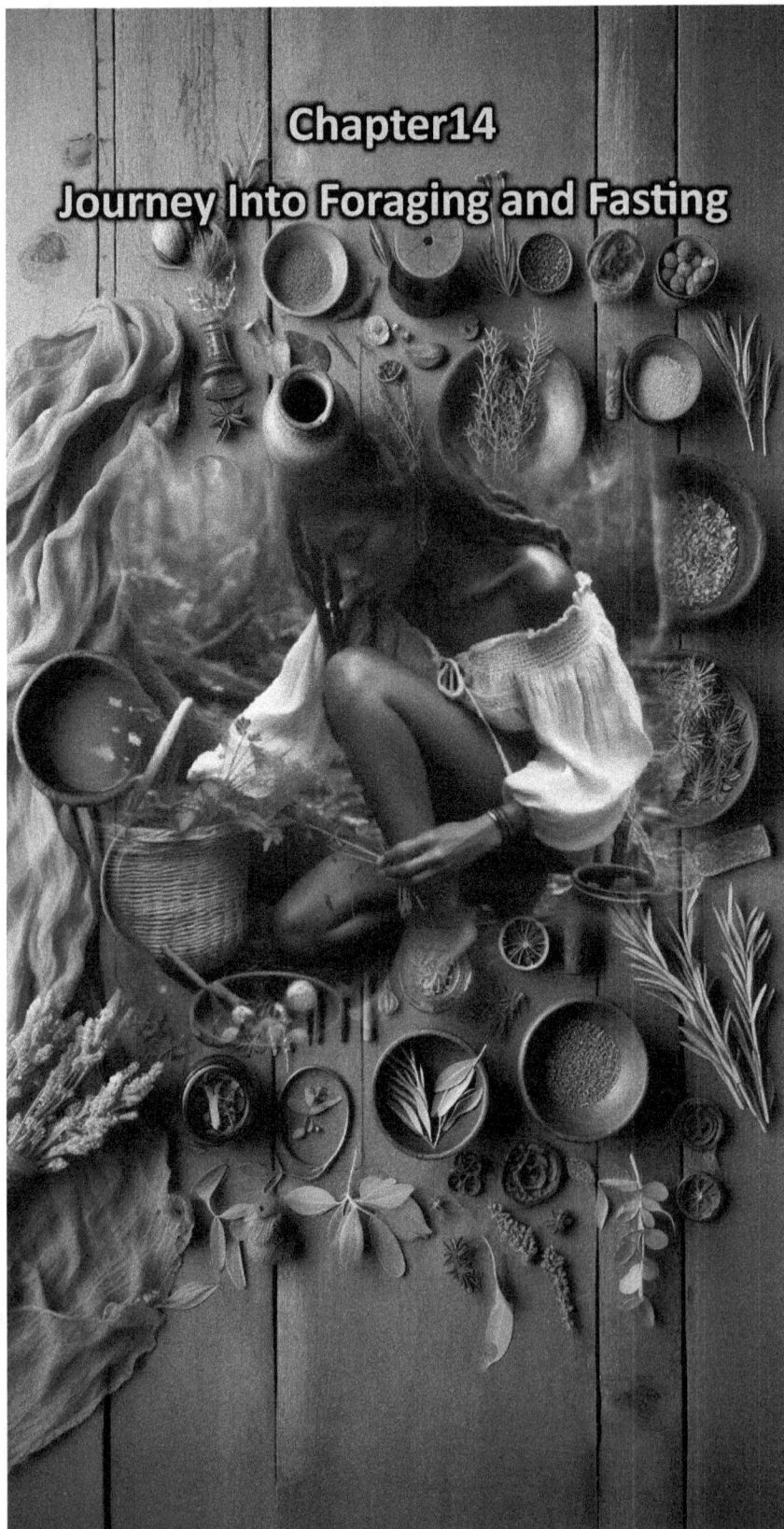

Chapter14
Journey Into Foraging and Fasting

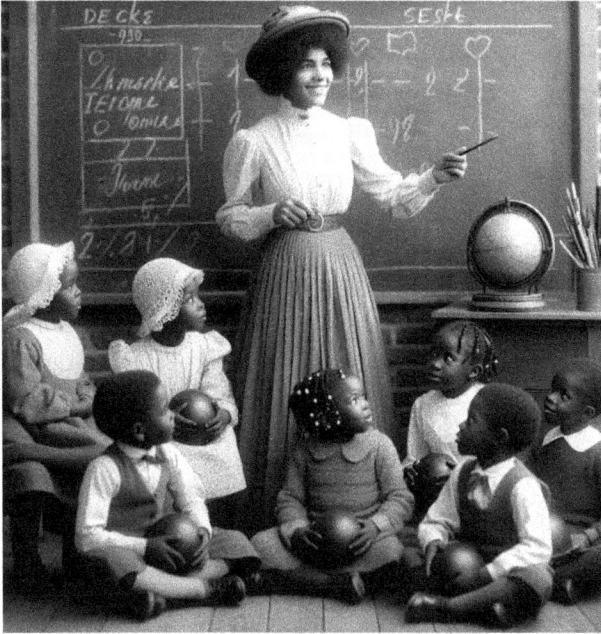

Fruits and Vegetables Pre-1920s

Before the 1920s and the rise of modern agriculture, many fruits and vegetables were very different in appearance and nutritional profile compared to what we see today. The public education system, which influenced dietary standards in America, started to adopt more systematic views on nutrition, often driven by industrial agriculture and food processing advances. This has led to changes in how fruits and vegetables are grown, harvested, and consumed.

In terms of whether there are "true" vegetables, botanically speaking, vegetables are a bit of a misnomer because most of what we call vegetables are parts of plants, including leaves (lettuce, spinach), roots (carrots, beets), stems (celery, asparagus), and flowers (broccoli, cauliflower). Technically, the term "vegetable" is more culinary than botanical.

Fruits

Apples: The apples grown before the 20th century were far more diverse and less sweet than many modern varieties. Heirloom varieties were more common, and apples were often smaller, more tart, and hardier. **Bananas**: Wild bananas contained seeds and had tougher flesh compared to today's seedless varieties like the Cavendish, which became popular in the 20th century. **Tomatoes**: Originally viewed with suspicion (due to their association with the nightshade family), tomatoes were smaller and more varied in color. They hadn't undergone the large-scale selective breeding that has created the uniform, large varieties of today. **Berries**: Many berries, such as strawberries and blueberries, were smaller and wild varieties were common. They had a more complex flavor profile compared to the cultivated varieties we eat now.

Vegetables (Culinary definition):

Carrots: Carrots were originally purple, white, or yellow before selective breeding produced the orange varieties we commonly see today. **Potatoes**: Potatoes were more diverse and closer to their wild ancestors in South America. Today's varieties have been cultivated for uniformity and size. **Cabbage, Kale, and Broccoli**: These are all from the same plant species (*Brassica oleracea*), but in the pre-modern era, they were less hybridized and exhibited more diversity in appearance and taste. **Corn**: Corn (maize) used to be smaller and less sweet. The modern hybridized varieties we consume now were not available until the early 20th century. **Squash**: Native Americans grew various types of squashes long before modern agriculture, with many being smaller, tougher, and less sweet than the squashes we are familiar with today.

Are There "True" Vegetables?

From a botanical perspective: **Fruits** are the mature ovary of a plant and contain seeds. Examples include tomatoes, cucumbers, and squash, which we commonly refer to as vegetables in culinary terms. **Vegetables** *(culinary)* include other plant parts like roots (carrots), stems (celery), leaves (lettuce), and flowers (broccoli). However, botanically, most of these don't fall under the category of "fruits." Some plants like spinach, lettuce, and kale are considered true vegetables since they don't bear seeds or develop from the flower's ovary—they are simply parts of the plant used for food.

Impact of Modern Agriculture

Selective Breeding: After the 1920s, many fruits and vegetables underwent selective breeding to improve characteristics like size, taste, yield, and resistance to pests and diseases. While this led to larger, more uniform, and more visually appealing produce, it also came with trade-offs. Many fruits and vegetables were bred to be sweeter (as a consumer preference shifted toward sweeter foods), but in the process, they often lost their original flavor complexity and some of their nutritional value. **Genetic Diversity Loss:** One of the most significant impacts of modern agriculture is the reduction in genetic diversity. Heirloom varieties, which were traditionally grown by smaller farms and local communities, were often replaced by high-yield, uniform crops suitable for large-scale industrial farming. This shift led to the disappearance of many wild and heirloom varieties that were naturally more resilient to climate and pests.

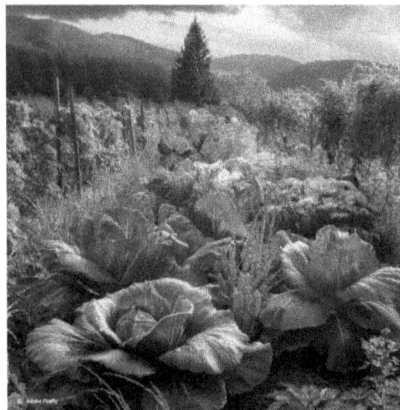

With fewer varieties being cultivated, plants became more vulnerable to diseases and pests because of the reduced genetic pool, leading to increased use of pesticides and herbicides. *Nutritional Changes:* Modern fruits and vegetables generally contain more sugar and fewer micronutrients than their pre-1920s counterparts. Studies have shown that industrial farming practices, soil depletion, and selective breeding for traits like sweetness and size have contributed to a reduction in the levels of key vitamins and minerals in many crops.

Nutrient Content Changes Over Time

A study published in the *Journal of the American College of Nutrition* (2004) compared nutrient data for 43 garden crops between 1950 and 1999 and found significant declines in several nutrients, including: **Protein**: 6% decline **Calcium**: 16% decline **Iron**: 15% decline **Riboflavin (Vitamin B2)**: 38% decline **Vitamin C**: 20% decline.

The decline in nutrients is largely due to breeding crops for traits like yield, size, and pest resistance, which often come at the expense of nutrient density. The increase in sugar content, for instance, makes fruits more appealing but decreases their overall nutritional value.

Nutrient Change from 1950 to 1999

Protein	-6%
Calcium	-16%
Iron	-15%
Riboflavin (B2)	-38%
Vitamin C	-20%

Are Modern Fruits and Vegetables Healthy?

While fruits and vegetables today are still considered healthy and vital for a balanced diet, they may not be as nutrient-dense as they once were. However, even with their reduced nutrient content, consuming modern fruits and vegetables still offers numerous health benefits, such as fiber, vitamins, and antioxidants that are essential for overall health.

Root Vegetables

Root vegetables, such as carrots, beets, and sweet potatoes, are still considered healthy. However, they too have been impacted by selective breeding. For instance, carrots were originally purple or white, and their orange color was bred for consumer preference. Modern root vegetables may have a higher sugar content but still provide essential nutrients like potassium, fiber, and vitamins A and C.

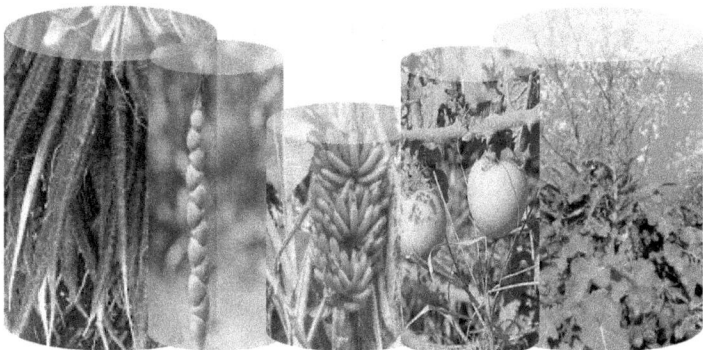

Actions that Reduced Wild

The shift toward industrial farming and the commodification of agriculture in the 20th century had a significant impact on the decline of wild-growing fruits and vegetables. Several factors contributed to this.

Land Development and Deforestation

The expansion of cities, highways, and large-scale farms led to the destruction of habitats where wild fruits and vegetables naturally grew. Wild ecosystems that supported indigenous plants were often cleared for monoculture crops. Monoculture Farming: The adoption of monoculture (growing one type of crop in large areas) replaced the diversity of wild-growing plants. Monoculture farming depleted the soil and made the land unsuitable for many wild plants to thrive naturally.

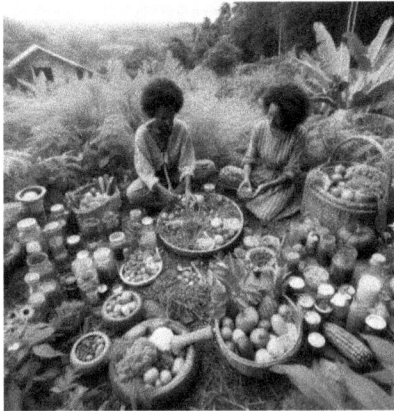

Chemical Pesticides and Herbicides

The widespread use of chemical fertilizers, pesticides, and herbicides in modern agriculture also had a devastating impact on the growth of wild plants. These chemicals not only affect pests but can also harm wild plants and soil health, further reducing the potential for natural growth of wild fruits and vegetables.

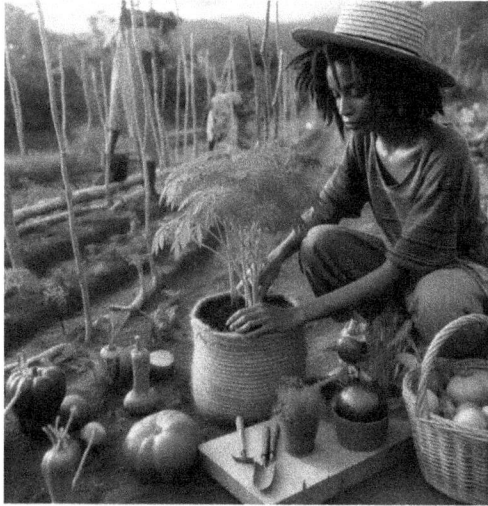

Agricultural Policies

U.S. agricultural policies and subsidies have traditionally favored large-scale farming of certain crops (like corn, soybeans, and wheat) over others, reducing the space and resources available for the cultivation of more diverse plant species. Government regulations and the industrialization of farming have further led to the loss of wild-growing food sources.

What Can Be Done to Restore Wild Food Growth?

One way to encourage the growth of wild fruits and vegetables is through the adoption of agroecology or permaculture practices. These approaches focus on creating self-sustaining ecosystems that mimic natural processes, allowing for a greater diversity of plants to grow in harmony with the environment. ***Community and Urban Gardens:*** Creating more community gardens and supporting urban gardening initiatives can reintroduce heirloom and wild varieties of fruits and vegetables. These gardens help foster biodiversity and allow individuals to grow nutrient-dense, local food.

Seed Saving and Heirloom Varieties: Promoting heirloom seed saving can help preserve the genetic diversity of fruits and vegetables. Seed banks and organizations that focus on conserving wild and heirloom varieties play an essential role in protecting these plants from extinction. *Land Conservation:* Protecting natural habitats through land conservation efforts can support the re-establishment of wild-growing fruits and vegetables. Programs that focus on rewilding, such as restoring natural ecosystems, can help bring back native plants that were once abundant. *Sustainable Agricultural Practices:* Encouraging farmers to adopt sustainable farming techniques that prioritize soil health and biodiversity can create environments where wild plants can grow alongside cultivated crops.

Identification Protocols of Foraging

Visual Characteristics: Detailed descriptions of size, shape, color, and texture. *Habitat:* Typical environments and geographical regions. *Seasonality:* Best times of year for harvesting. *Edibility Tests:* Steps to ensure the plant or mushroom is safe to consume. *Look-Alikes:* Information on common poisonous or inedible look-alikes and how to differentiate them.

Foraging Basics

Safety First: Always ensure positive identification before consuming wild foods. *Sustainable Practices:* Harvest responsibly to ensure plant populations remain healthy. *Rotation:* Harvest different areas in rotation to prevent over-foraging. *Minimal Impact:* Take only a small percentage of available plants or mushrooms. *Leave No Trace:* Respect the environment and leave it as you found it.

What is a Raw Diet?

A raw diet primarily consists of uncooked and unprocessed foods. The idea behind this diet is that cooking can destroy essential nutrients and enzymes in food, which are vital for digestion and overall health. Raw foodists focus on consuming raw fruits, vegetables, nuts, seeds, and sometimes sprouted grains and legumes. This diet is rich in vitamins, minerals, and fiber, which can support overall health, including gut health, which is particularly important for addressing issues like anemia and low iron levels.

Benefits of a Raw Diet

Nutrient-Rich: Raw foods are packed with essential nutrients, including vitamins, minerals, and antioxidants, which can support energy levels, skin health, and overall wellness. **Digestive Health:** A raw diet is high in fiber, which can promote healthy digestion and gut health. This is particularly beneficial for African American women, who may be more prone to certain digestive issues. **Natural Detoxification:** The abundance of fresh fruits and vegetables in a raw diet can help the body naturally detoxify, potentially improving liver function and overall metabolic health. **Weight Management:** Raw foods are generally lower in calories and higher in fiber, making them satisfying and supportive of healthy weight management.

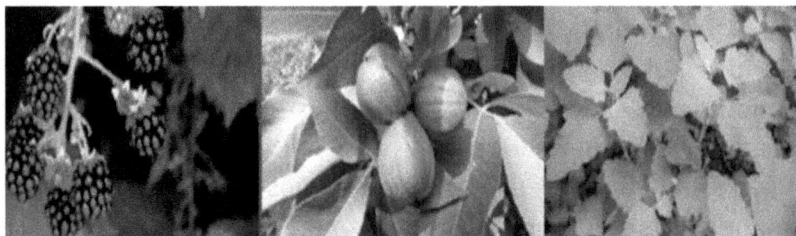

Raw Diet Recipe: Foraging and Creating Your Own

One of the empowering aspects of a raw diet is the opportunity to connect with nature by foraging for your own ingredients. This not only enhances the nutritional value of your meals but also deepens your relationship with the environment and the foods you consume.

Challenge: Get to Know Your Local Edible Plants

To truly embrace the raw food lifestyle, challenge yourself to learn about the edible plants in your area. Take time to explore local parks, forests, or even your backyard, and identify safe and nutritious wild foods. This practice not only enhances your diet but also empowers you to create unique and personalized raw recipes that are deeply connected to your environment and cultural heritage.

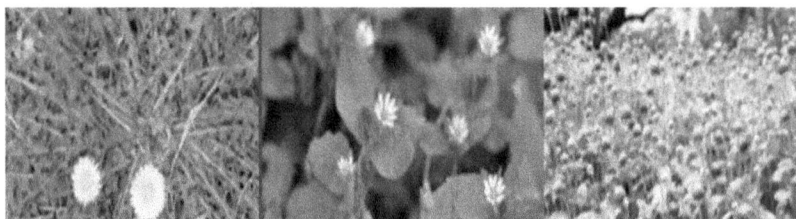

Simple Foraged Raw Salad Recipe

Ingredients:

2 cups of foraged greens (e.g., dandelion greens, chickweed, wild spinach)

1 cup of wild berries (e.g., blackberries, mulberries, or any edible local berries)

1/4 cup of foraged nuts (e.g., acorns or hickory nuts, if available)

1 avocado, diced

1 lemon, juiced

1 tablespoon of cold-pressed olive oil

A pinch of sea salt

Optional: edible flowers like violets or nasturtiums for garnish

Instructions:

Thoroughly wash and dry your foraged greens, berries, and nuts.

In a large bowl, combine the greens, wild berries, and diced avocado.

Crush the foraged nuts into smaller pieces and sprinkle them over the salad.

In a small bowl, mix the lemon juice, olive oil, and sea salt to create a simple dressing.

Pour the dressing over the salad and toss gently to combine.

Garnish with edible flowers if available.

This salad is a perfect introduction to a raw diet, combining the freshness of locally foraged ingredients with the simplicity of raw preparation. Not only does it provide a nutrient-dense meal, but it also connects you to your surroundings and the natural abundance available in your environment.

Raw Honey: A Natural Sweetener

Raw honey is honey that has not been heated, pasteurized, or processed in any way. It is collected straight from the beehive, filtered to remove impurities like beeswax and bee parts, and then packaged. Because it is unprocessed, raw honey retains all of its natural enzymes, vitamins, minerals, and antioxidants, which are often lost during the pasteurization process.

Benefits of Raw Honey

Rich in Antioxidants: Raw honey contains various antioxidants, including phenolic compounds, which help combat free radicals in the body. This can reduce oxidative stress and support overall health. *Enzymes and Nutrients*: Raw honey is a source of enzymes like glucose oxidase, which can support digestive health. It also contains small amounts of vitamins and minerals, such as vitamin C, calcium, and iron. *Antibacterial and Antifungal Properties*: Raw honey has natural antibacterial and antifungal properties, making it a traditional remedy for wound healing and infection prevention. *Supports Digestive Health:* Raw honey can act as a prebiotic, feeding the beneficial bacteria in your gut, which supports digestive health and overall well-being. *Natural Energy Source:* Due to its natural sugars (glucose and fructose), raw honey provides a quick energy boost, making it a healthier alternative to processed sugars.

How to Use Raw Honey in a Raw Diet

Sweetener: Use raw honey as a natural sweetener in smoothies, raw desserts, or salad dressings. *Spread:* Enjoy raw honey on raw bread or crackers made from sprouted grains or seeds. *Marinades and Sauces:* Combine raw honey with lemon juice, olive oil, and herbs to create a delicious raw marinade or sauce. *Immune Support:* Add a spoonful of raw honey to herbal teas or warm (not hot) water with lemon for an immune-boosting drink.

Note: While raw honey has many health benefits, it should be consumed in moderation due to its high natural sugar content. Additionally, it is important to avoid giving raw honey to infants under one year old, as it can contain spores of the bacterium Clostridium botulinum, which can be harmful to young children.

Harvesting Raw Honey in the Wild for Beginner Foragers

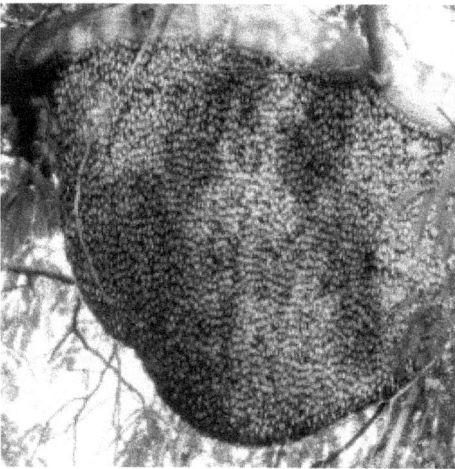

Harvesting raw honey from wild bees can be an enriching experience, but it also requires caution and respect for the bees and their environment. Here's a guide to help beginner foragers approach this task safely. **Respect the Bees: *Approach with Care:*** Bees are generally not aggressive if they don't feel threatened. Move slowly, avoid sudden movements, and wear light-colored clothing, as bees are attracted to dark colors. *Use Smoke:* A gentle puff of smoke can calm bees, making them less likely to sting. You can create smoke using a bee smoker or by burning natural materials like dried grass or pine needles.

Protective Gear

Bee Suit: If possible, wear a beekeeping suit with a veil to protect your face and body from stings. *Gloves:* Wear gloves, but be aware that they can reduce dexterity. Some experienced foragers opt for thin gloves or even go without, relying on calm movements to avoid stings.

Bee Stinger Dangers and Remedies

Remove the Stinger: If you are stung, remove the stinger as quickly as possible to reduce the amount of venom released. Use a flat object like a credit card to scrape it out, rather than pinching it, which can inject more venom. *Clean the Area:* Wash the sting site with soap and water to prevent infection.

Natural Remedies for Bee Stings

Ice Pack: Apply an ice pack or cold compress to reduce swelling and numb the area. *Baking Soda Paste:* Mix baking soda with water to form a paste and apply it to the sting site. This can help neutralize the venom and reduce pain. *Raw Honey:* Interestingly, raw honey itself can be applied to the sting. It has anti-inflammatory and antibacterial properties that can soothe the skin. *Aloe Vera:* Apply fresh aloe vera gel to the sting to help reduce inflammation and provide relief.

Anaphylactic Shock: Symptoms and Remedies

Anaphylactic shock is a severe, potentially life-threatening allergic reaction that can occur in some people after a bee sting. It requires immediate medical attention.

Symptoms of Anaphylactic Shock

Difficulty Breathing: Tightness in the chest, wheezing, or shortness of breath. ***Swelling:*** Rapid swelling of the face, lips, tongue, or throat. ***Hives:*** Widespread hives or rash, often accompanied by itching. ***Nausea or Vomiting:*** Feeling nauseous, vomiting, or having diarrhea. ***Dizziness or Fainting:*** A feeling of lightheadedness or loss of consciousness. ***Rapid or Weak Pulse:*** A noticeable change in heart rate.

Immediate Actions

Use an Epinephrine Auto-Injector: If the person has a known allergy, use an epinephrine auto-injector (EpiPen) immediately. This is the most effective treatment for anaphylaxis. ***Call Emergency Services:*** Even if the symptoms seem to improve after using an EpiPen, call emergency services immediately, as further medical treatment may be necessary.

Lie Down with Legs Elevated: If the person is conscious, have them lie down with their legs elevated to improve blood flow to vital organs. ***Monitor Breathing:*** If the person loses consciousness or stops breathing, perform CPR if you are trained to do so until help arrives.

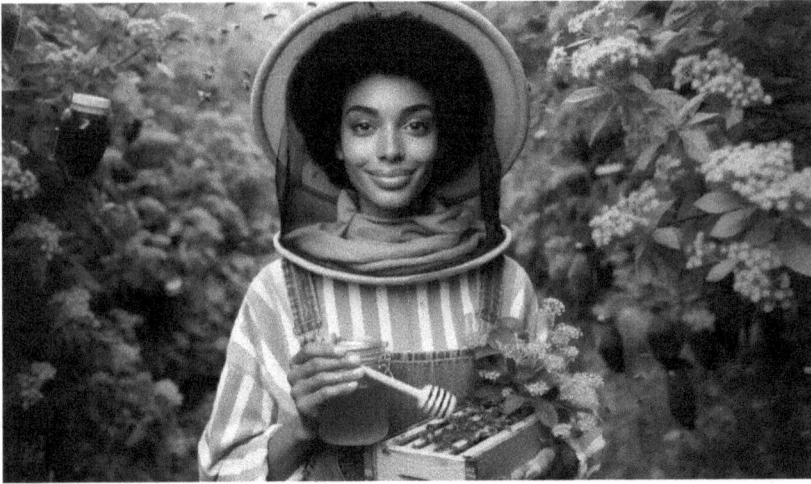

Additional Information

Practice Sustainable Foraging: Only take a small amount of honey, leaving enough for the bees to survive, especially during colder months. Harvesting responsibly ensures the bees can continue to thrive and produce honey. ***Learn from Experienced Foragers:*** If you are new to foraging honey, consider joining an experienced beekeeper or forager to learn the skills and techniques needed to harvest honey safely and sustainably.

Harvesting raw honey in the wild can be a rewarding experience, but it's essential to prioritize safety, both for yourself and the bees. With the right preparation and knowledge, you can enjoy the benefits of wild honey while respecting the natural environment.

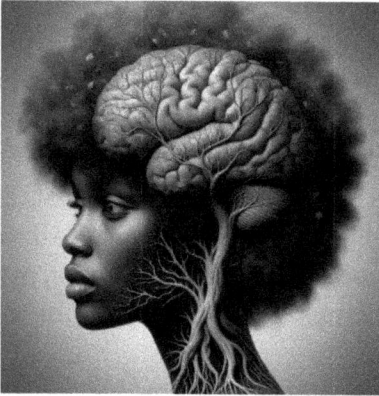

Fasting for Health and Wellness

Fasting is an ancient practice that has been utilized for spiritual, mental, and physical well-being across various cultures. For Black women, fasting can offer numerous health benefits, including cellular rejuvenation, improved metabolic health, and enhanced mental clarity. This section explores the health benefits of fasting, different fasting methods, and how to fast safely and effectively. Emphasis is placed on natural, animal-free, and holistic approaches influenced by traditional wisdom and modern science.

Cellular Rejuvenation

One of the key benefits of fasting is the process of autophagy, where the body cleans out damaged cells and regenerates new ones. This cellular rejuvenation can lead to improved function of various organs, enhanced skin health, and a reduced risk of chronic diseases. **Metabolic Health** Fasting can improve insulin sensitivity, lower blood sugar levels, and reduce inflammation. These benefits are particularly important for Black women who may be at a higher risk of conditions like diabetes and metabolic syndrome. Fasting helps in regulating hormones and supports weight management by promoting fat loss while preserving lean muscle mass.

Mental Clarity and Emotional Health

Fasting can enhance mental clarity and cognitive function. It has been shown to improve mood and reduce symptoms of depression and anxiety. The discipline and mindfulness required for fasting can also lead to a greater sense of control and emotional resilience. **Detoxification** Fasting allows the digestive system to rest and detoxify. This process can help eliminate toxins from the body, improve digestion, and promote overall gut health. A cleaner, more efficient digestive system can enhance nutrient absorption and energy levels.

Different Fasting Methods

Intermittent Fasting Intermittent fasting (IF) involves cycling between periods of eating and fasting. Common methods include: **16:8 Method:** Fasting for 16 hours and eating during an 8-hour window. For example, you might eat between 12 PM and 8 PM. **5:2 Method:** Eating normally for five days of the week and restricting calories to 500-600 on the other two days. **Alternate-Day Fasting:** Fasting every other day, with some variations allowing for a small meal on fasting days. **Extended Fasting** Extended fasting involves fasting for longer periods, typically 24 hours or more. This type of fasting should be approached with caution and ideally under medical supervision, especially for beginners. **24-Hour Fast:** Also known as a "full day fast," where you fast from dinner to dinner or lunch to lunch. **48-Hour Fast:** A more extended fast that can provide deeper detoxification and cellular benefits.

Preparation

Gradual Introduction: Start with shorter fasting periods and gradually increase the duration as your body adapts. **Hydration:** Drink plenty of water before, during, and after fasting. Herbal teas and infused water can also help maintain hydration and provide additional health benefits. **During the Fast: Mindful Eating:** During eating windows, focus on consuming nutrient-dense, plant-based foods such as fruits, vegetables, whole grains, nuts, seeds, and legumes. **Avoid Processed Foods:** Steer clear of processed and refined foods that can hinder the benefits of fasting. **Breaking the Fast: Ease Back into Eating:** Break your fast with light, easily digestible foods such as fruits, smoothies, or vegetable soups. Gradually reintroduce more substantial meals. **Continue Hydration:** Keep drinking water and herbal teas to support digestion and detoxification.

Fasting Safety and Considerations

Listen to Your Body: Pay attention to how your body responds to fasting. If you experience dizziness, extreme fatigue, or other concerning symptoms, break your fast and consult a healthcare professional. **Medical Conditions:** If you have any underlying medical conditions or are pregnant, nursing, or taking medications, consult with a healthcare provider before starting a fasting regimen. **Nutritional Balance:** Ensure that your diet during eating windows is balanced and provides all necessary nutrients to support overall health.

Practices to Enhance Fasting

Herbal Teas and Infusions: **Ginger Tea:** Supports digestion and reduces nausea. **Peppermint Tea:** Helps with bloating and digestive discomfort. **Dandelion Tea:** Acts as a natural detoxifier and supports liver function.

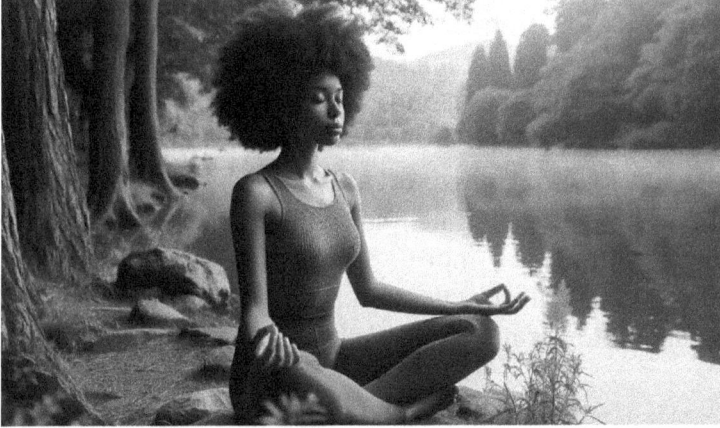

Mindfulness and Meditation

Incorporate mindfulness practices such as meditation, deep breathing, or yoga to enhance the mental and emotional benefits of fasting. These practices can help reduce stress, improve focus, and foster a deeper connection with your body. **Physical Activity** Engage in light physical activity such as walking, stretching, or gentle yoga during fasting periods. This can help maintain energy levels and support overall well-being.

30-Day Fasting Calendar

Day 1
Fasting: 8 PM - 12 PM **Eating:** 12 PM - 8 PM
Tip: Start with plenty of water. Aim for 2L today.

Day 2
Fasting: 8 PM - 12 PM **Eating:** 12 PM - 8 PM
Tip: Include a walk today. Stay hydrated.

Day 3
Fasting: 8 PM - 12 PM **Eating:** 12 PM - 8 PM
Tip: Focus on whole foods. Avoid processed snacks.

Day 4
Fasting: 8 PM - 12 PM **Eating:** 12 PM - 8 PM
Tip: Try a new herbal tea. Peppermint or ginger is great.

Day 5
Fasting: 8 PM - 12 PM **Eating:** 12 PM - 8 PM
Tip: Practice mindfulness or meditation for 10 minutes.

Day 6
Fasting: 8 PM - 12 PM **Eating:** 12 PM - 8 PM
Tip: Break your fast with a smoothie. Add greens.

Day 7
Fasting: 8 PM - 12 PM **Eating:** 12 PM - 8 PM
Tip: 24-hour fast. Eat 8 PM - 8 PM next day.

Day 8
Fasting: 8 PM - 12 PM **Eating:** 12 PM - 8 PM
Tip: Hydrate well after extended fast.

Day 9
Fasting: 8 PM - 12 PM **Eating:** 12 PM - 8 PM
Tip: Light yoga or stretching today.

Day 10
Fasting: 8 PM - 12 PM **Eating:** 12 PM - 8 PM
Tip: Include vitamin-rich fruits in your meals.

Day 11
Fasting: 8 PM - 12 PM **Eating:** 12 PM - 8 PM
Tip: Drink herbal tea to support digestion.

Day 12
Fasting: 8 PM - 12 PM **Eating:** 12 PM - 8 PM
Tip: Focus on gratitude. Write down 3 things you're grateful for.

Day 13
Fasting: 8 PM - 12 PM **Eating:** 12 PM - 8 PM
Tip: Avoid sugar-laden foods. Opt for natural sweeteners.

Day 14
Fasting: 8 PM - 12 PM **Eating:** 12 PM - 8 PM
Tip: 24-hour fast. Eat 8 PM - 8 PM next day.

30-Day Fasting Calendar

Day 15
Fasting: 8 PM - 12 PM **Eating:** 12 PM - 8 PM
Tip: Enjoy a balanced meal with proteins and veggies.

Day 16
Fasting: 8 PM - 12 PM **Eating:** 12 PM - 8 PM
Tip: Practice deep breathing exercises.

Day 17
Fasting: 8 PM - 12 PM **Eating:** 12 PM - 8 PM
Tip: Add nuts and seeds to your meals for healthy fats.

Day 18
Fasting: 8 PM - 12 PM **Eating:** 12 PM - 8 PM
Tip: Include a colorful salad in your diet.

Day 19
Fasting: 8 PM - 12 PM **Eating:** 12 PM - 8 PM
Tip: Stay active. Try a light exercise routine.

Day 20
Fasting: 8 PM - 12 PM **Eating:** 12 PM - 8 PM
Tip: Hydrate well. Aim for 2.5L of water today.

Day 21
Fasting: 8 PM - 12 PM **Eating:** 12 PM - 8 PM
Tip: 24-hour fast. Eat 8 PM - 8 PM next day.

Day 22
Fasting: 8 PM - 12 PM **Eating:** 12 PM - 8 PM
Tip: Incorporate legumes for added protein.

Day 23
Fasting: 8 PM - 12 PM **Eating:** 12 PM - 8 PM
Tip: Mindfulness meditation for 15 minutes.

Day 24
Fasting: 8 PM - 12 PM **Eating:** 12 PM - 8 PM
Tip: Drink a smoothie with greens and fruits.

Day 25
Fasting: 8 PM - 12 PM **Eating:** 12 PM - 8 PM
Tip: Light walk or yoga session.

Day 26
Fasting: 8 PM - 12 PM **Eating:** 12 PM - 8 PM
Tip: Consume a variety of colorful vegetables.

Day 27
Fasting: 8 PM - 12 PM **Eating:** 12 PM - 8 PM
Tip: Drink herbal teas like chamomile or peppermint.

Day 28
Fasting: 8 PM - 12 PM **Eating:** 12 PM - 8 PM
Tip: 24-hour fast. Eat 8 PM - 8 PM next day.

Day 29
Fasting: 8 PM - 12 PM **Eating:** 12 PM - 8 PM
Tip: Reflect on your progress. Write down your thoughts.

Day 30
Fasting: 8 PM - 12 PM **Eating:** 12 PM - 8 PM
Tip: Think about your finish line reward.

Day 31
Fasting: 8 PM - 12 PM **Eating:** 12 PM - 8 PM
Tip: Celebrate your achievements. Plan for future goals.

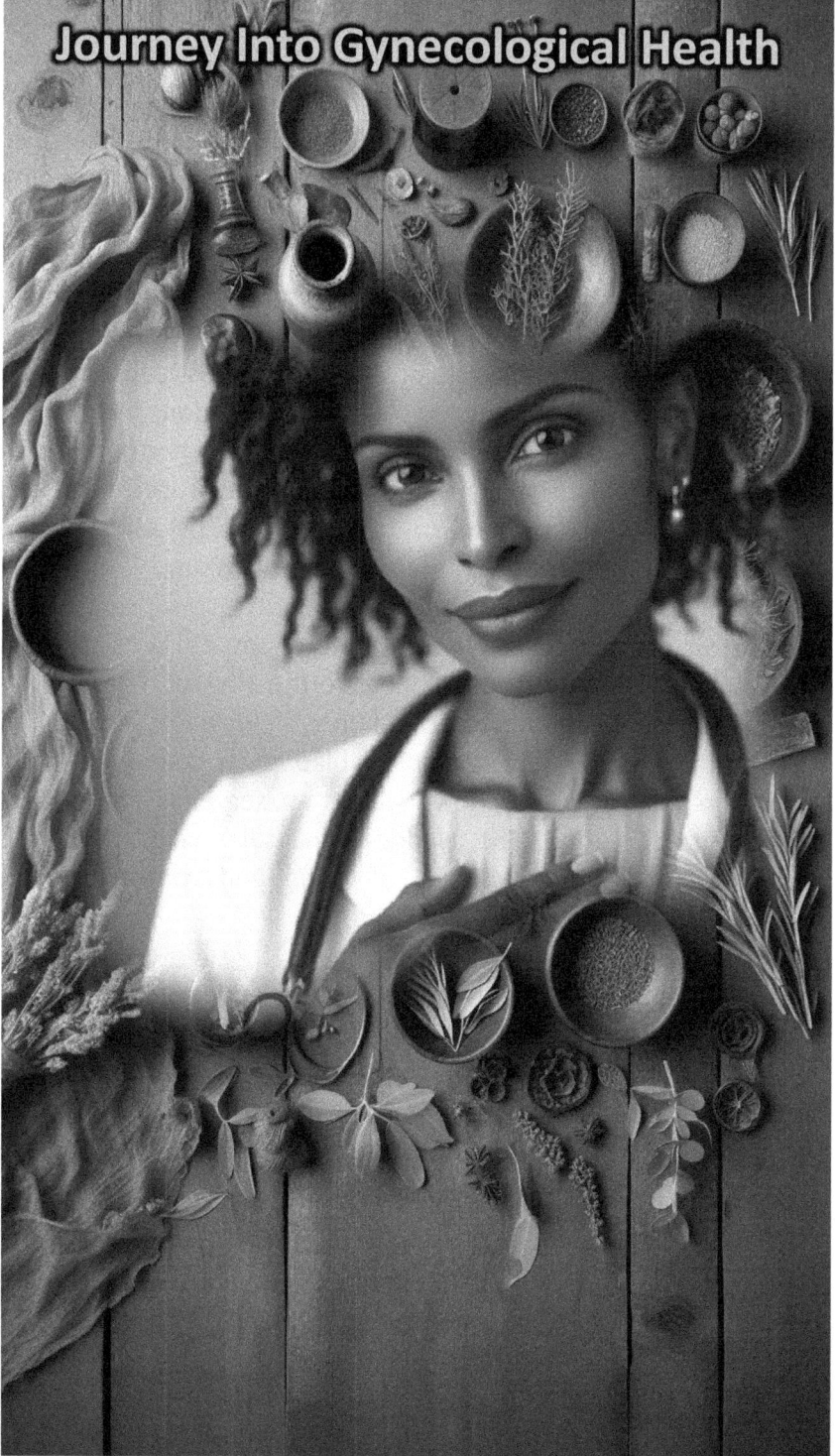

Chapter 15
Journey Into Gynecological Health

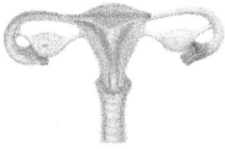

Urinary System
KIDNEYS URETERS BLADDER URETHRA

The urinary system, also referred to as the urinary tract or renal system, comprises the kidneys, ureters, bladder, and urethra. This system plays a crucial role in removing waste from the body, regulating blood pressure, maintaining pH balance, and controlling electrolyte and metabolite levels.

The kidneys, located in the middle back just below the ribs, contain thousands of tiny filtering units called nephrons. These nephrons filter the blood, removing waste products and excess substances to produce urine. In addition to their filtration function, the kidneys help regulate blood pressure through the release of hormones such as renin, maintain pH balance by excreting hydrogen ions and reabsorbing bicarbonate, and control salt levels by adjusting the excretion and reabsorption of sodium and potassium.

The ureters are narrow tubes composed of smooth muscle fibers that transport urine from the kidneys to the bladder. These tubes use peristaltic movements to propel urine downwards, ensuring it reaches the bladder efficiently. The bladder, a hollow, triangle-shaped organ located in the lower abdomen, serves as a temporary storage site for urine. The bladder's muscular walls stretch to accommodate varying volumes of urine and contract during urination to expel the stored fluid.

The urethra is a small tube that connects the bladder to the outside of the body, allowing urine to be expelled. When it is time to urinate, the brain sends signals to the sphincters, causing them to relax while the bladder wall tightens. This coordinated action forces urine out of the bladder and through the urethra, completing the process of urination.

Maintaining the health of the urinary system can be supported by holistic and natural remedies. For instance, natural syrups, elixirs, salves, and creams can be used to manage conditions related to the urinary system and promote overall renal health. These remedies often include ingredients with diuretic, anti-inflammatory, and soothing properties, providing a natural alternative to conventional prescription drugs.

Reproductive System
OVARIES FALLOPIAN TUBES UTERUS
CERVIX PLACENTA VULVA

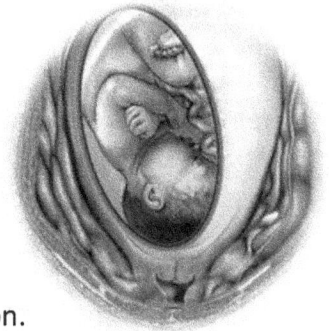

The female reproductive system is a complex network of organs that work together to create life. This system includes the uterus, fallopian tubes, ovaries, and vulva, each playing a critical role in reproductive health and function. Understanding these organs and their functions is essential for comprehending the reproductive process and maintaining overall reproductive health.

The uterus is a pear-shaped organ located in the pelvis. It is responsible for receiving and supporting a fertilized egg during pregnancy. The uterus has two main parts: the cervix, which is the lower, narrow part, and the corpus, which is the main body of the uterus that expands during pregnancy. Each month, the lining of the uterus thickens with blood and other substances in preparation for a potential pregnancy. If pregnancy occurs, the fertilized egg implants in the uterine lining and grows into a fetus and then a baby. If pregnancy does not occur, the lining is shed and flows out of the body as menstrual blood, a process known as menstruation or a period.

The fallopian tubes are narrow tubes that connect the uterus to the ovaries, serving as pathways for eggs to travel from the ovaries to the uterus. Fertilization of an egg by sperm typically occurs in the fallopian tubes, specifically in the ampullary part. Once fertilized, the egg continues its journey to the uterus, where it may implant and begin the development process.

The ovaries are two small, oval-shaped glands located on either side of the uterus. They produce eggs and hormones such as estrogen and progesterone, which are vital for female development and reproductive health. These hormones regulate the menstrual cycle, support pregnancy, and influence various other bodily functions. During a woman's menstrual cycle, the ovaries release an egg in a process called ovulation.

The vulva is the collective term for the external genitalia of the female reproductive system. It includes structures such as the labia, clitoris, and vaginal opening. The vulva protects the internal reproductive organs, plays a significant role in sexual arousal and stimulation, and facilitates sexual intercourse.

Understanding Hormonal Imbalance & The Menstrual Cycle

The Menstrual Cycle is divided into several phases, each regulated by fluctuations in hormone levels: *Menstrual Phase:* This phase marks the beginning of the cycle with the shedding of the uterine lining. It typically lasts 3-7 days. *Follicular Phase:* Lasting from day 1 to day 14, the follicular phase involves the growth of follicles in the ovaries, stimulated by Follicle-Stimulating Hormone (FSH). Estrogen levels rise, thickening the uterine lining in preparation for potential pregnancy. Follicular Phase: The rise in estrogen during this phase supports the growth of the uterine lining and prepares for ovulation.

Ovulation: Occurring around day 14, ovulation is triggered by a surge in Luteinizing Hormone (LH). An egg is released from the dominant follicle, and estrogen levels peak. Ovulation: The LH surge triggers the release of an egg, with estrogen at its peak. *Luteal Phase:* This phase lasts from day 15 to day 28. After ovulation, the ruptured follicle forms the corpus luteum, which secretes progesterone to maintain the uterine lining. If pregnancy does not occur, progesterone and estrogen levels fall, leading to menstruation. Luteal Phase: Progesterone rises after ovulation to support potential pregnancy, and if pregnancy does not occur, both progesterone and estrogen levels decline, leading to menstruation.

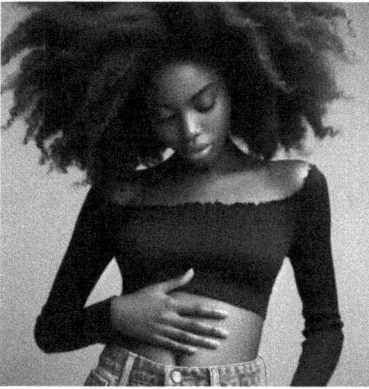

Estrogen and Progesterone

Estrogen and Progesterone are essential hormones that regulate the menstrual cycle. Estrogen is primarily involved in the development of secondary sexual characteristics and the regulation of the menstrual cycle. Progesterone prepares the uterus for pregnancy and maintains early stages of pregnancy. An imbalance, such as excess estrogen or insufficient progesterone, can disrupt the menstrual cycle and lead to various symptoms.

Impact of Feminine Products

Not all menstrual products are created equal. Some pads and tampons contain chemicals and synthetic materials that can cause irritation, allergic reactions, and even disrupt hormonal balance. Organic and natural options are preferable as they are free from harmful substances and are less likely to cause adverse reactions.

Importance of pH Balance

Maintaining a healthy vaginal pH (around 3.8-4.5) is essential for preventing infections and promoting overall feminine health. Harsh soaps and douches can disrupt this balance, so it is important to use pH-balanced feminine products and gentle, natural cleansers.

Hormonal Imbalance Heavy or Irregular Periods Symptoms
Abnormal menstrual flow or cycle length, often due to hormonal imbalances.

Fibroids Noncancerous growths in the uterus causing heavy bleeding, pelvic pain, and pressure symptoms.

Acne Hormonal fluctuations can lead to increased oil production and clogged pores, resulting in acne.

Weight Gain
Hormone imbalances can affect metabolism and appetite, leading to weight gain.

PMS Premenstrual Syndrome involves mood swings, bloating, breast tenderness, and irritability.

PCOS Polycystic Ovary Syndrome is characterized by irregular periods, cysts on the ovaries, and elevated levels of androgens.

Facial Hair Excessive hair growth, particularly on the face, due to high levels of androgens.

Cysts Fluid-filled sacs that can form on the ovaries, often associated with PCOS.

Plant-Based Diet

Emphasize whole, unprocessed foods. Avoid animal products that can contain added hormones. *Cruciferous Vegetables:* Foods like broccoli, cauliflower, and kale help balance estrogen levels. *Omega-3 Fatty Acids:* Found in flaxseeds, chia seeds, and walnuts, omega-3s help reduce inflammation and support hormonal health.

Lifestyle Changes Regular Exercise

Physical activity helps regulate hormones, improve mood, and reduce stress. *Stress Management:* Practices like yoga, meditation, and deep breathing exercises can help manage stress and balance hormones. *Sleep:* Ensuring adequate sleep is crucial for hormonal regulation and overall health.

Hysterectomy

Indications and Symptoms: A hysterectomy, the surgical removal of the uterus, may be necessary for severe cases of fibroids, endometriosis, chronic pelvic pain, or cancer. Symptoms indicating the need for a hysterectomy include severe and persistent pelvic pain, heavy bleeding, and significant pressure symptoms.

Prevention: Diet: An anti-inflammatory diet rich in fruits, vegetables, and whole grains can support uterine health. *Herbs:* Herbs like red raspberry leaf and chasteberry are known for their beneficial effects on uterine health. **Exercise:** Regular physical activity helps maintain overall health and can prevent conditions that might lead to a hysterectomy.

Prevention Strategies	Description	Benefits
Diet	Anti-inflammatory diet emphasizing fruits, vegetables, whole grains, and lean proteins.- Limiting processed foods, sugar, and saturated fats. No Animal products.	Reduces inflammation, supports overall health, and may help maintain uterine health.
Herbs	**Red Raspberry Leaf**: Contains nutrients that support uterine tone and overall reproductive health.- **Chasteberry (Vitex)**: Helps regulate hormonal balance.	Supports hormonal balance, may alleviate menstrual symptoms, and can contribute to uterine health maintenance.
Exercise	Regular physical activity, such as aerobic exercises, yoga, and strength training.- Promotes circulation and overall well-being.	Improves cardiovascular health, reduces stress, and supports hormone regulation, potentially benefiting uterine health.
Stress Management	Techniques like meditation, deep breathing, and mindfulness.- Prioritizing self-care and relaxation.	Reduces cortisol levels, supports hormone balance, and may alleviate stress-related reproductive health issues.
Supplements	Vitamin D: Supports immune function and overall health.- Omega-3 fatty acids: Anti-inflammatory properties.- Magnesium: Muscle relaxation and stress reduction.	Enhances overall health, reduces inflammation, and supports muscle relaxation, potentially benefiting uterine health.
Avoidance of Environmental Toxins	Limit exposure to endocrine disruptors such as BPA, phthalates, and pesticides.- Use of natural cleaning and personal care products.	Minimizes disruption to hormonal balance and reproductive health, potentially reducing the risk of uterine health issues.

Hormonal imbalances can cause a wide range of symptoms and conditions in Black women, significantly impacting their health and quality of life. By understanding the menstrual cycle, the role of key hormones, and the importance of maintaining pH balance, women can take proactive steps to manage these imbalances. Holistic approaches, including herbal remedies, dietary changes, and lifestyle modifications, offer effective strategies for maintaining hormonal health. Additionally, choosing safe and natural menstrual products can help reduce exposure to harmful chemicals, promoting better health outcomes.

Note: *Holistic approaches aim to support overall health and may help prevent or alleviate conditions that could lead to the need for a hysterectomy. Always consult with a healthcare provider before starting any new diet, herbal regimen, or supplement routine, especially if you have underlying health conditions or are taking medications. These preventive measures are intended to complement medical advice and treatment and should be personalized based on individual health needs and circumstances.*

Polycystic Ovary Syndrome (PCOS)

Polycystic Ovary Syndrome (PCOS) is a common endocrine disorder that affects women of reproductive age. It is characterized by a combination of symptoms related to hormonal imbalance, including irregular menstrual cycles, excess androgen levels, and polycystic ovaries. PCOS can lead to a variety of health issues such as infertility, metabolic syndrome, type 2 diabetes, and cardiovascular diseases.

Who is More Prone to PCOS?

PCOS affects women across all ethnic groups, but some studies suggest that Black women may be at a higher risk of developing the condition. The exact prevalence of PCOS in Black women is not well-documented due to variations in study populations and diagnostic criteria. However, it is known that Black women often present with more severe symptoms and are more likely to experience metabolic complications associated with PCOS.

Symptoms of PCOS

The symptoms of PCOS can vary widely but often include: ***Irregular Menstrual Cycles****:* Infrequent, prolonged, or absent periods. ***Hirsutism****:* Excessive hair growth on the face, chest, back, or other areas. ***Acne****:* Severe or persistent acne. ***Obesity or Weight Gain****:* Difficulty losing weight despite efforts. ***Acanthosis Nigricans****:* Dark, thickened patches of skin, particularly around the neck, armpits, or groin. ***Hair Thinning****:* Hair loss or thinning on the scalp. ***Infertility****:* Difficulty conceiving due to irregular ovulation. ***Mood Disorders****:* Anxiety, depression, or mood swings.

? QUESTIONS TO ASK YOUR DOCTOR ?

What tests will you perform to diagnose PCOS?
How can PCOS affect my fertility and overall health?
What lifestyle changes can help manage my symptoms?
Are there medications that can help regulate my menstrual cycle and manage other symptoms?
How does PCOS increase my risk for diabetes and heart disease?
What can I do to reduce my risk of metabolic complications?
Are there any long-term health concerns associated with PCOS?

!TESTS TO REQUEST!

When visiting a healthcare provider for PCOS, it is essential to ask the right questions and request specific tests to get a clear diagnosis and appropriate management plan. Pelvic Exam: To check for abnormalities in the reproductive organs. Ultrasound: To examine the ovaries and check for cysts. Blood Tests: To measure hormone levels (androgens, insulin, glucose, thyroid hormones, etc.). Glucose Tolerance Test: To assess insulin resistance and risk of diabetes. Lipid Profile: To evaluate cholesterol levels and cardiovascular risk

Natural Remedies for PCOS

Managing PCOS often requires a multifaceted approach, including lifestyle changes and natural remedies. Here are some holistic and natural remedies that may help alleviate PCOS symptoms: *Dietary Changes: Balanced Diet:* Focus on a diet rich in whole foods, including plenty of fruits, vegetables, whole grains, and lean proteins. *Low Glycemic Index Foods:* Helps manage blood sugar levels and insulin resistance. Examples include legumes, whole grains, and non-starchy vegetables. *Anti-Inflammatory Foods*: Include foods rich in omega-3 fatty acids, such as flaxseeds, chia seeds, and walnuts, to reduce inflammation.

Herbal Remedies

Spearmint Tea: May help reduce androgen levels and improve hirsutism. *Maca Root:* Can help balance hormones and improve fertility. *Cinnamon:* Known to improve insulin sensitivity. *Supplements: Inositol:* Aids in improving insulin resistance and ovulatory function. *Vitamin D:* Often deficient in women with PCOS and can improve metabolic and reproductive symptoms. *Chromium:* Can help with insulin resistance. **Exercise**: Regular physical activity can help manage weight, improve insulin sensitivity, and reduce symptoms of PCOS. Aim for a combination of aerobic exercises and strength training. *Stress Management*: Practices such as yoga, meditation, and mindfulness can help manage stress, which is often exacerbated by PCOS. PCOS is a chronic condition that requires long-term management. Women with PCOS should work closely with their healthcare providers to develop a personalized treatment plan that addresses their specific symptoms and health concerns. Regular monitoring and lifestyle adjustments can help manage the condition effectively and reduce the risk of complications.

Gynecological Health

Black women often face unique challenges in gynecological health. They are more likely to experience conditions such as uterine fibroids, endometriosis, and severe menstrual pain. Regular screenings and early detection are crucial in managing these conditions. Additionally, blood type can influence vaginal health, with certain blood types being more prone to specific infections. Herbal remedies, such as red raspberry leaf tea for menstrual support, and chamomile or ginger for pain relief, can be beneficial. Maintaining a balanced diet rich in iron and essential nutrients is also important to support overall reproductive health. Herbal and natural remedies offer alternative solutions for various reproductive health issues.

For menstrual pain, herbs like cramp bark and ginger can be effective. During pregnancy, red raspberry leaf tea is known to tone the uterus and prepare for labor. Postpartum, herbs such as fenugreek and blessed thistle can support breastfeeding. For menopause, black cohosh and evening primrose oil may help alleviate symptoms. Emphasizing these natural approaches can promote health and well-being for women at every stage of life.

Uterine Fibroids

Uterine fibroids are noncancerous growths that develop in the uterus. These are particularly prevalent among Black women, who often experience them more frequently and with greater severity compared to other populations. Symptoms of fibroids include heavy menstrual bleeding, prolonged periods, pelvic pain, frequent urination, and complications during pregnancy and labor. The exact cause of fibroids is unknown, but they are believed to be influenced by genetic factors and hormonal imbalances. For natural management of fibroids, herbal remedies like vitex (chaste tree berry) can help balance hormones, and green tea extract, which contains antioxidants, may reduce the growth of fibroids. Maintaining a diet rich in fruits, vegetables, and whole grains while limiting red meat and fortified plant based milks, leafy greens, and sunlight exposure can also be beneficial.

? QUESTIONS TO ASK YOUR DOCTOR ?
What are the treatment options available for fibroids?
How can I manage the symptoms naturally and through lifestyle changes?
Are there any potential side effects of the treatments?
What follow-up care will I need after treatment?

Endometriosis

Endometriosis is a condition where tissue similar to the lining of the uterus grows outside the uterus, causing severe pain, heavy periods, and sometimes infertility. This condition can be particularly debilitating and is often underdiagnosed, especially in Black women. Symptoms include pelvic pain, menstrual irregularities, pain during intercourse, and gastrointestinal issues. Herbal remedies for endometriosis include turmeric, which has anti-inflammatory properties, and ginger, which can help alleviate pain. Additionally, omega-3 fatty acids found in fish oil can reduce inflammation. A diet high in fiber and low in processed foods may also help manage symptoms.

? QUESTIONS TO ASK YOUR DOCTOR ?

How is endometriosis diagnosed, and what tests are necessary?
What are the treatment options, both medical and surgical?
How can I manage pain and other symptoms naturally?
What are the long-term implications of endometriosis on fertility and overall health?

Severe Menstrual Pain

Severe menstrual pain, or dysmenorrhea, is a common issue that significantly impacts the quality of life for many Black women. It can be caused by various underlying conditions, including fibroids and endometriosis. Symptoms include intense pelvic pain, cramping, nausea, and headaches during menstruation. To manage severe menstrual pain, herbal remedies such as cramp bark and ginger can be effective. Cramp bark acts as a muscle relaxant, while ginger reduces inflammation and pain. Drinking chamomile tea can also provide relief by soothing the nervous system and reducing cramps.

? QUESTIONS TO ASK YOUR DOCTOR ?

What could be causing my severe menstrual pain?
Are there any underlying conditions that need to be addressed?
What are the best natural remedies and lifestyle changes to alleviate pain?
How can I track my symptoms to better understand and manage my condition?

Menopause Management

Effectively managing menopause symptoms can greatly improve quality of life. Natural treatments can help relieve hot flashes and mood swings. Black cohosh and evening primrose oil are herbal remedies that may alleviate menopause symptoms. Maintaining bone health through adequate calcium and vitamin D intake is important during this stage. Hormone replacement therapy might be considered for severe symptoms but should be discussed with a healthcare provider.

Healthcare Disparities

Black women often face significant disparities in the healthcare industry, including biases that can lead to misdiagnosis and inadequate treatment. This can result in delayed diagnosis and treatment of serious conditions like endometriosis and fibroids. Black women should advocate for themselves by seeking second opinions, asking detailed questions, and ensuring they receive comprehensive care. Understanding their rights and options within the healthcare system is essential for better health outcomes.

Advocating for Better Health

Advocacy is crucial for Black women to receive proper healthcare. This includes being informed about their health conditions, understanding treatment options, and voicing their needs clearly to healthcare providers. Joining support groups and networks can provide additional resources and emotional support. Herbal and natural remedies, such as chamomile for pain relief and iron-rich foods to combat anemia, can be part of a holistic approach to health. By taking an active role in their health, Black women can work towards better outcomes and improved well-being.

Blood Types and Vaginal Health
Blood Type A

TY
PE
A

Blood type A individuals are generally more prone to bacterial infections, including bacterial vaginosis (BV). This condition occurs when there is an imbalance in the natural bacteria found in the vagina. Symptoms of BV include a thin, gray discharge with a fishy odor, itching, and burning during urination. Herbal remedies for blood type A individuals to manage BV include: *Tea tree oil:* Known for its antimicrobial properties, it can be used in diluted form as a vaginal suppository. *Garlic:* Consuming garlic can help combat bacterial infections due to its natural antibiotic properties.

? QUESTIONS TO ASK YOUR DOCTOR ?

How can I prevent bacterial infections in the vagina?
Are there specific lifestyle changes or dietary adjustments that can help maintain a healthy vaginal flora?
What are the best natural treatments for managing BV?

Blood Type B

TY
PE
B

Individuals with blood type B are more susceptible to yeast infections, caused by an overgrowth of the fungus Candida. Symptoms include thick, white, cottage cheese-like discharge, itching, and burning sensations in the vaginal area. Herbal remedies for managing yeast infections for blood type B include: *Yogurt and probiotics:* Consuming yogurt with live cultures or taking probiotic supplements can help restore the natural balance of bacteria and yeast in the vagina. *Coconut oil:* Applying coconut oil externally can help reduce yeast growth due to its antifungal properties.

How can I balance the yeast and bacteria in my vagina naturally?
Are there specific dietary recommendations to prevent yeast infections?
What natural remedies are effective for treating yeast infections?

Blood Type AB

T Y
P E
A B

Blood type AB individuals may have a combination of susceptibilities from both blood type A and B, making them prone to both bacterial vaginosis and yeast infections. Symptoms can vary depending on the infection but may include abnormal discharge, itching, burning, and odor. Herbal remedies for blood type AB include a combination of those for blood types A and B: *Tea tree oil and garlic*: For managing bacterial infections. *Probiotics and coconut oil*: For preventing and treating yeast infections.

How can I effectively manage both bacterial and yeast infections?
Are there preventative measures specific to my blood type that I should follow?
What combination of natural remedies can help maintain vaginal health?

Blood Type O

T Y
P E
O

Individuals with blood type O are more likely to experience urinary tract infections (UTIs), which can also affect vaginal health. Symptoms of UTIs include a strong urge to urinate, a burning sensation during urination, cloudy or strong-smelling urine, and pelvic pain. Herbal remedies for managing UTIs for blood type O include: *Cranberry extract*: Drinking cranberry juice or taking cranberry supplements can help prevent bacteria from adhering to the urinary tract walls. *D-mannose*: A type of sugar found in cranberries that can help flush out the urinary tract.

? QUESTIONS TO ASK YOUR DOCTOR ?

How can I prevent recurring urinary tract infections?
Are there specific lifestyle or dietary changes that can help reduce the risk of UTIs?
What are the most effective natural treatments for UTIs?

General Care for All Blood Types

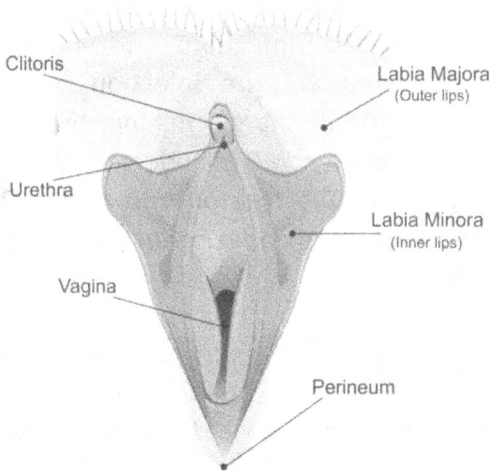

Regardless of blood type, maintaining overall vaginal health is essential. This includes practicing good hygiene, wearing breathable cotton underwear, avoiding douching, and maintaining a balanced diet rich in nutrients. Drinking plenty of water and avoiding excessive sugar intake can also help prevent infections. Regular gynecological check-ups, being proactive, and discussing symptoms with healthcare providers are crucial steps in maintaining reproductive health.

Sexual Health
Sexually Transmitted Diseases (STDs)

Sexually transmitted diseases (STDs) are infections transmitted through sexual contact. Common STDs include chlamydia, gonorrhea, syphilis, herpes, and human papillomavirus (HPV). Symptoms vary depending on the specific STD but can include unusual vaginal discharge, genital sores or warts, itching, burning during urination, and pelvic pain.

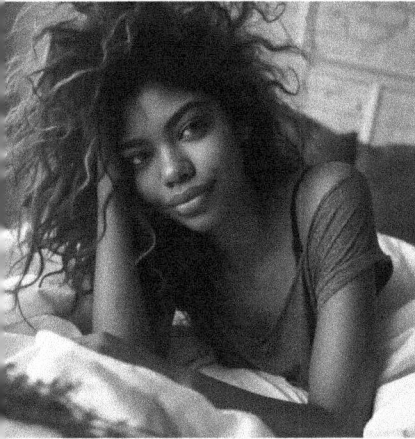

Herbal remedies and best care practices for STDs include: *Garlic:* Known for its antiviral and antibacterial properties, consuming garlic can help support the immune system in fighting infections. *Echinacea:* This herb boosts the immune system and can help the body combat viral and bacterial infections. Best care for managing STDs involves regular screening, practicing safe sex, using condoms, and maintaining open communication with sexual partners. It is crucial to follow the prescribed treatments by healthcare providers and complete the full course of medication even if symptoms subside.

? QUESTIONS TO ASK YOUR DOCTOR ?

What are the best preventive measures for avoiding STDs?
How often should I get screened for STDs?
What are the most effective treatments and natural remedies for my condition?

Sexually Transmitted Infections (STIs)

Sexually transmitted infections (STIs) often refer to the initial infection phase before symptoms develop into diseases. Common STIs include the same pathogens responsible for STDs. Symptoms might be mild or absent initially, making regular screenings essential for early detection.

Herbal remedies and best care practices for STIs include: *Goldenseal:* This herb has antimicrobial properties and can be used to support the body in fighting infections. ***Olive leaf extract****:* Known for its antiviral properties, olive leaf extract can help manage viral STIs. Preventive care involves safe sex practices, regular STI screenings, and maintaining overall health through a balanced diet and exercise. Early detection and treatment are key to preventing the progression of STIs to more serious STDs.

? QUESTIONS TO ASK YOUR DOCTOR ?

How can I detect STIs early, even if there are no symptoms?
What lifestyle changes can help prevent STIs?
Are there specific natural remedies that can support treatment?

Yeast Infections

Yeast infections, caused by the overgrowth of Candida fungus, are common and can cause significant discomfort. Symptoms include thick, white discharge resembling cottage cheese, intense itching, burning, and redness around the vaginal area. Herbal remedies and best care practices for yeast infections include: ***Probiotics****:* Taking probiotic supplements or eating yogurt with live cultures can help restore the natural balance of bacteria and yeast in the vagina. *Coconut oil:* Applying coconut oil externally can help reduce yeast growth due to its antifungal properties.

Maintaining a balanced diet low in sugar and refined carbohydrates can help prevent yeast infections. Wearing breathable cotton underwear and avoiding tight-fitting clothes can also reduce the risk.

QUESTIONS TO ASK HEALTHCARE PROVIDERS?

What are the most effective treatments for yeast infections?
How can I prevent recurrent yeast infections?
Are there any dietary changes that can help manage my symptoms?

Bacterial Vaginosis (BV)

Bacterial vaginosis (BV) occurs when there is an imbalance of the natural bacteria in the vagina, leading to an overgrowth of harmful bacteria. Symptoms include a thin, gray discharge with a fishy odor, itching, and burning during urination. Herbal remedies and best care practices for BV include: *Tea tree oil*: Known for its antimicrobial properties, it can be used in diluted form as a vaginal suppository. *Garlic*: Consuming garlic can help combat bacterial infections due to its natural antibiotic properties. Maintaining good hygiene, avoiding douching, and using mild, unscented soaps for cleaning the vaginal area can help prevent BV. Probiotics can also support the balance of healthy bacteria.

?QUESTIONS TO ASK HEALTHCARE PROVIDERS?

How can I prevent bacterial vaginosis from recurring?
What are the best natural treatments for managing BV?
Are there any lifestyle changes that can help maintain a healthy vaginal flora?

General Care for Vaginal Health

Maintaining overall vaginal health involves practicing good hygiene, wearing breathable cotton underwear, avoiding douching, and adhering to a balanced diet rich in nutrients. Drinking plenty of water and limiting sugar intake can also help prevent infections. Regular gynecological check-ups and proactive communication with healthcare providers about any symptoms are crucial for early detection and effective management of vaginal health issues.

Burdock Root: Known for its blood-purifying properties and ability to detoxify the body. **Yellow Dock:** Used for its detoxifying and anti-inflammatory properties. **Sarsaparilla:** Known for its blood-purifying and anti-inflammatory benefits. **Chaparral:** Used for its antimicrobial properties. **Elderberry:** Boosts the immune system and has antiviral properties. **Red Clover:** Known for its ability to detoxify the body and support the immune system.

Best Care Practices: Regular Screening: Ensuring regular check-ups and STD screenings to catch and treat infections early. **Safe Sex Practices:** Using condoms and having open discussions with partners about sexual health. **Complete Prescribed Treatments:** Following through with all prescribed treatments even if symptoms improve. **Maintain Hygiene:** Keeping the genital area clean and dry, using mild, unscented soaps. **Diet and Lifestyle:** Eating a balanced diet rich in nutrients, staying hydrated, managing stress, and avoiding irritants and smoking.

Chlamydia

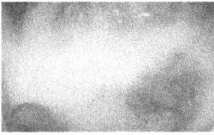

Symptoms Unusual discharge, burning during urination, pain during intercourse Herbal Remedies Elderberry: Boosts the immune system and has antiviral properties. Goldenseal: Contains berberine, which has antibacterial properties. Chaparral: Known for its antiviral and antimicrobial effects. Best Care Practices Regular screening, safe sex practices, complete prescribed treatments, maintain hygiene, avoid irritants Raw Foods: Incorporate raw fruits and vegetables to enhance nutrient intake and support the immune system. Avoid Mucus-Forming Foods: Eliminate dairy, wheat, and processed foods that can increase mucus production.

Gonorrhea

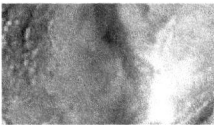

Symptoms Thick discharge, burning during urination, swollen testicles (men), pelvic pain (women) Herbal Remedies Burdock Root: Known for its blood-purifying properties, it helps cleanse the body of toxins. Sarsaparilla: Contains natural compounds that may help reduce inflammation and fight infections. Dandelion Root: Supports liver detoxification and promotes urinary tract health. Best Care Practices
Regular screening, safe sex practices, complete prescribed treatments, maintain hygiene, stay hydrated. Alkaline Diet: Focus on consuming alkaline foods such as leafy greens, fruits, and vegetables to help restore the body's pH balance. Hydration: Drink plenty of water to help flush out toxins.

Syphilis

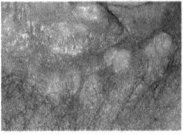

Symptoms Sores at infection site, skin rashes, swollen lymph nodes, fever Herbal Remedies Pau d'Arco: Contains lapachol, which has antimicrobial properties. Red Clover: Helps purify the blood and supports overall detoxification. Burdock Root: Assists in cleansing the blood and removing impurities. Best Care Practices Regular screening, safe sex practices, complete prescribed treatments, monitor symptoms, maintain a balanced diet. Fasting: Periodic fasting can help detoxify the body and boost the immune system. Herbal Teas: Drink teas made from recommended herbs to support detoxification and healing.

Human Papillomavirus (HPV)

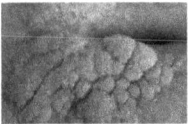

Symptoms Genital warts, abnormal Pap test results, some strains can lead to cancer Herbal Remedies Cat's Claw: Known for its immune-boosting and antiviral properties. Echinacea: Supports immune function and helps fight infections. Astragalus: Enhances immune response and helps in reducing viral loads. Best Care Practices Regular screening (Pap smears), safe sex practices, complete prescribed treatments, HPV vaccination, maintain immune health. Green Leafy Vegetables: Rich in folate and antioxidants which support the immune system. Vitamin C-Rich Foods: Citrus fruits, bell peppers, and strawberries to enhance immune function. Avoid Processed Foods: Focus on whole, nutrient-dense foods to support overall health.

Herpes

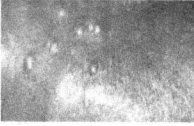

Symptoms Painful sores or blisters on genitals or mouth, itching, flu-like symptoms Herbal Remedies Lysine-Rich Foods: Consuming foods high in lysine, such as avocados and papayas, may help reduce herpes outbreaks. Sea Moss: Rich in minerals and supports immune function. Hydrangea Root: Traditionally used to treat infections and support urinary tract health. Best Care Practices Regular screening, safe sex practices, complete prescribed treatments, manage stress, boost immune system. Alkaline Diet: Maintain a diet rich in alkaline foods to support the body's natural healing processes. Avoid Trigger Foods: Eliminate foods that can trigger outbreaks, such as chocolate and nuts.

General Tips for Supporting Health and Healing

Detoxification: Regular detoxification is essential for removing toxins from the body. This can be achieved through fasting, consuming herbal teas, and adhering to a clean, alkaline diet. *Hydration:* Drinking ample water is crucial for flushing out toxins and supporting overall health. *Alkaline Foods:* Focus on consuming alkaline-forming foods, such as fruits, vegetables, nuts, and seeds, to help balance the body's pH and support the immune system. *Natural Herbs:* Incorporate herbs with antimicrobial, antiviral, and immune-boosting properties into your daily routine. *Lifestyle Changes:* Avoiding stress, getting enough rest, and maintaining a positive mindset are important for overall health and recovery.

Disclaimer:

It is important to note that with natural healing, it is essential to consult with a healthcare professional for accurate diagnosis and appropriate treatment of sexually transmitted diseases. Natural remedies can complement but should not replace conventional medical treatments.

Sexual Health
Sexually Transmitted Diseases (STDs)

Sexually transmitted diseases (STDs) are infections transmitted through sexual contact. Common STDs include chlamydia, gonorrhea, syphilis, herpes, and human papillomavirus (HPV). Symptoms vary depending on the specific STD but can include unusual vaginal discharge, genital sores or warts, itching, burning during urination, and pelvic pain.

Herbal remedies and best care practices for STDs include: Garlic: Known for its antiviral and antibacterial properties, consuming garlic can help support the immune system in fighting infections. Echinacea: This herb boosts the immune system and can help the body combat viral and bacterial infections. Best care for managing STDs involves regular screening, practicing safe sex, using condoms, and maintaining open communication with sexual partners. It is crucial to follow the prescribed treatments by healthcare providers and complete the full course of medication even if symptoms subside.

QUESTIONS TO ASK HEALTHCARE PROVIDERS
What are the best preventive measures for avoiding STDs?
How often should I get screened for STDs?
What are the most effective treatments and natural remedies for my condition?

Melanin Journey Health and Wellness

Sexually Transmitted Infections (STIs)

Sexually transmitted infections (STIs) often refer to the initial infection phase before symptoms develop into diseases. Common STIs include the same pathogens responsible for STDs. Symptoms might be mild or absent initially, making regular screenings essential for early detection.

Herbal remedies and best care practices for STIs include: Goldenseal: This herb has antimicrobial properties and can be used to support the body in fighting infections. Olive leaf extract: Known for its antiviral properties, olive leaf extract can help manage viral STIs. Preventive care involves safe sex practices, regular STI screenings, and maintaining overall health through a balanced diet and exercise. Early detection and treatment are key to preventing the progression of STIs to more serious STDs.

> **QUESTIONS TO ASK HEALTHCARE PROVIDERS**
> How can I detect STIs early, even if there are no symptoms?
> What lifestyle changes can help prevent STIs?
> Are there specific natural remedies that can support treatment?

Yeast Infections

Yeast infections, caused by the overgrowth of Candida fungus, are common and can cause significant discomfort. Symptoms include thick, white discharge resembling cottage cheese, intense itching, burning, and redness around the vaginal area. Herbal remedies and best care practices for yeast infections include: Probiotics: Taking probiotic supplements or eating yogurt with live cultures can help restore the natural balance of bacteria and yeast in the vagina. Coconut oil: Applying coconut oil externally can help reduce yeast growth due to its antifungal properties.

Maintaining a balanced diet low in sugar and refined carbohydrates can help prevent yeast infections. Wearing breathable cotton underwear and avoiding tight-fitting clothes can also reduce the risk.

QUESTIONS TO ASK HEALTHCARE PROVIDERS
What are the most effective treatments for yeast infections?
How can I prevent recurrent yeast infections?
Are there any dietary changes that can help manage my symptoms?

Bacterial Vaginosis (BV)

Bacterial vaginosis (BV) occurs when there is an imbalance of the natural bacteria in the vagina, leading to an overgrowth of harmful bacteria. Symptoms include a thin, gray discharge with a fishy odor, itching, and burning during urination. Herbal remedies and best care practices for BV include: Tea tree oil: Known for its antimicrobial properties, it can be used in diluted form as a vaginal suppository. Garlic: Consuming garlic can help combat bacterial infections due to its natural antibiotic properties. Maintaining good hygiene, avoiding douching, and using mild, unscented soaps for cleaning the vaginal area can help prevent BV. Probiotics can also support the balance of healthy bacteria.

QUESTIONS TO ASK HEALTHCARE PROVIDERS
How can I prevent bacterial vaginosis from recurring?
What are the best natural treatments for managing BV?
Are there any lifestyle changes that can help maintain a healthy vaginal flora?

General Care for Vaginal Health

Maintaining overall vaginal health involves practicing good hygiene, wearing breathable cotton underwear, avoiding douching, and adhering to a balanced diet rich in nutrients. Drinking plenty of water and limiting sugar intake can also help prevent infections. Regular gynecological check-ups and proactive communication with healthcare providers about any symptoms are crucial for early detection and effective management of vaginal health issues.

Burdock Root: Known for its blood-purifying properties and ability to detoxify the body. Yellow Dock: Used for its detoxifying and anti-inflammatory properties. Sarsaparilla: Known for its blood-purifying and anti-inflammatory benefits. Chaparral: Used for its antimicrobial properties. Elderberry: Boosts the immune system and has antiviral properties. Red Clover: Known for its ability to detoxify the body and support the immune system.

Best Care Practices: Regular Screening: Ensuring regular check-ups and STD screenings to catch and treat infections early. Safe Sex Practices: Using condoms and having open discussions with partners about sexual health. Complete Prescribed Treatments: Following through with all prescribed treatments even if symptoms improve. Maintain Hygiene: Keeping the genital area clean and dry, using mild, unscented soaps. Diet and Lifestyle: Eating a balanced diet rich in nutrients, staying hydrated, managing stress, and avoiding irritants and smoking.

Chlamydia Symptoms Unusual discharge, burning during urination, pain during intercourse **Herbal Remedies** Elderberry: Boosts the immune system and has antiviral properties. Goldenseal: Contains berberine, which has antibacterial properties. Chaparral: Known for its antiviral and antimicrobial effects. **Best Care Practices** Regular screening, safe sex practices, complete prescribed treatments, maintain hygiene, avoid irritants Raw Foods: Incorporate raw fruits and vegetables to enhance nutrient intake and support the immune system. Avoid Mucus-Forming Foods: Eliminate dairy, wheat, and processed foods that can increase mucus production.

Gonorrhea Symptoms Thick discharge, burning during urination, swollen testicles (men), pelvic pain (women) **Herbal Remedies**
Burdock Root: Known for its blood-purifying properties, it helps cleanse the body of toxins. Sarsaparilla: Contains natural compounds that may help reduce inflammation and fight infections. Dandelion Root: Supports liver detoxification and promotes urinary tract health. **Best Care Practices** Regular screening, safe sex practices, complete prescribed treatments, maintain hygiene, stay hydrated. Alkaline Diet: Focus on consuming alkaline foods such as leafy greens, fruits, and vegetables to help restore the body's pH balance. Hydration: Drink plenty of water to help flush out toxins.

Syphilis
Symptoms Sores at infection site, skin rashes, swollen lymph nodes, fever
Herbal Remedies Pau d'Arco: Contains lapachol, which has antimicrobial properties. Red Clover: Helps purify the blood and supports overall detoxification. Burdock Root: Assists in cleansing the blood and removing impurities. **Best Care Practices** Regular screening, safe sex practices, complete prescribed treatments, monitor symptoms, maintain a balanced diet. Fasting: Periodic fasting can help detoxify the body and boost the immune system. Herbal Teas: Drink teas made from recommended herbs to support detoxification and healing.

Human Papillomavirus (HPV)
Symptoms Genital warts, abnormal Pap test results, some strains can lead to cancer **Herbal Remedies**
Cat's Claw: Known for its immune-boosting and antiviral properties. Echinacea: Supports immune function and helps fight infections. Astragalus: Enhances immune response and helps in reducing viral loads. **Best Care Practices** Regular screening (Pap smears), safe sex practices, complete prescribed treatments, HPV vaccination, maintain immune health. Green Leafy Vegetables: Rich in folate and antioxidants which support the immune system. Vitamin C-Rich Foods: Citrus fruits, bell peppers, and strawberries to enhance immune function. Avoid Processed Foods: Focus on whole, nutrient-dense foods to support overall health.

Herpes Symptoms Painful sores or blisters on genitals or mouth, itching, flu-like symptoms **Herbal Remedies**
Lysine-Rich Foods: Consuming foods high in lysine, such as avocados and papayas, may help reduce herpes outbreaks. Sea Moss: Rich in minerals and supports immune function. Hydrangea Root: Traditionally used to treat infections and support urinary tract health. **Best Care Practices** Regular screening, safe sex practices, complete prescribed treatments, manage stress, boost immune system. Alkaline Diet: Maintain a diet rich in alkaline foods to support the body's natural healing processes. Avoid Trigger Foods: Eliminate foods that can trigger outbreaks, such as chocolate and nuts.

General Tips for Supporting Health and Healing

Detoxification: Regular detoxification is essential for removing toxins from the body. This can be achieved through fasting, consuming herbal teas, and adhering to a clean, alkaline diet. Hydration: Drinking ample water is crucial for flushing out toxins and supporting overall health. Alkaline Foods: Focus on consuming alkaline-forming foods, such as fruits, vegetables, nuts, and seeds, to help balance the body's pH and support the immune system. Natural Herbs: Incorporate herbs with antimicrobial, antiviral, and immune-boosting properties into your daily routine. Lifestyle Changes: Avoiding stress, getting enough rest, and maintaining a positive mindset are important for overall health and recovery.

Disclaimer: *It is important to note that with natural healing, it is essential to consult with a healthcare professional for accurate diagnosis and appropriate treatment of sexually transmitted diseases. Natural remedies can complement but should not replace conventional medical treatments*

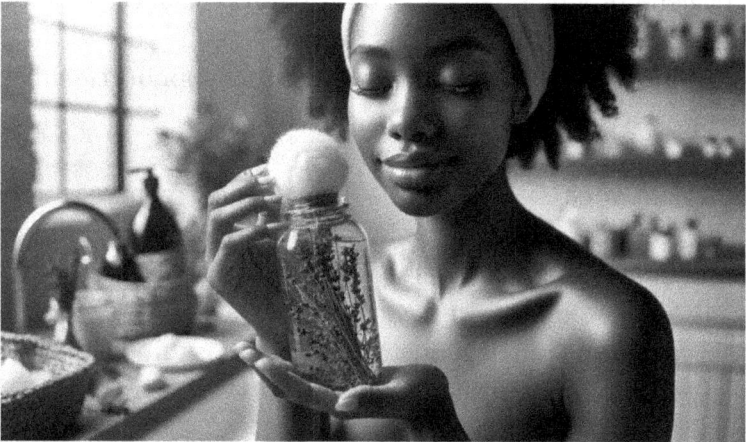

Journey into Feminine Hygiene

This section explores the essential aspects of female hygiene, focusing on the proper care of sensitive body areas like the breasts, vaginal, and anal regions. Understanding the science and appropriate hygiene practices can help prevent or reduce odors, maintain balanced pH levels, and promote overall health. Personal hygiene requires thoughtful daily routines, attention to product ingredients, and mindful dietary choices. Through natural and chemical-free methods, combined with modern products where needed, women can maintain balanced health in their intimate areas. Remember, the journey to optimal hygiene is individual, and listening to your body and collaborating with a healthcare provider will help you make the best choices for your health.

Understanding Female Hygiene

Our bodies have natural mechanisms designed to keep sensitive areas clean, such as beneficial bacteria that maintain the vaginal pH and protect against infections. However, factors like diet, lifestyle, and hygiene products can impact this natural balance. This section addresses the anatomy and hygiene needs of each part, highlighting daily practices and products that support cleanliness.

The Importance of pH Balance

The vaginal area has a unique pH balance, generally ranging between 3.8 and 4.5, which maintains a slightly acidic environment ideal for preventing bacterial infections. Factors that may disrupt this pH balance include menstruation, sexual activity, douching, certain soaps, and medications. When the pH is thrown off, women may experience odor, itching, or discomfort.

pH between 3.8 and 4.5

Why pH Matters for Feminine Health

An unbalanced pH can disrupt the vaginal microbiome, leading to bacterial or yeast overgrowth, which causes symptoms like odor, itching, and discomfort. Common disruptors include douching, scented products, certain medications, hormonal changes, and diet.

Maintaining a Healthy pH

Daily washing with a pH-balanced, gentle cleanser *Avoid harsh soaps, douches, and products with synthetic fragrances* as they can upset this balance. *Instead, use gentle, pH-balanced cleansers specifically designed for sensitive areas.* Stay hydrated, drinking water supports a natural balance by flushing out toxins. Incorporating probiotics in your diet (found in yogurt, kefir, and supplements) can support a balanced pH by introducing good bacteria.

Causes of Vaginal Odor and pH Disruption

Many factors can influence vaginal odor, including diet, hydration, sexual activity, and menstrual cycles. Diets high in sugar or processed foods can encourage bacterial growth, which contributes to odor. Hydrating with water and avoiding sugary drinks can aid in maintaining a healthy balance. Electrolyte drinks can also benefit hydration and reduce sweating, indirectly affecting odor.

Additional Tips for Feminine Hygiene

Diet and Probiotics play a significant role in feminine hygiene. A diet rich in fruits, vegetables, and whole grains promotes good bacteria, helping balance pH and reduce odor. Listen to Your Body. Noticing unusual changes in odor or discomfort could indicate an imbalance or infection. Regular check-ups and lab tests are essential for proactive health management. Consider your birth conditions. Factors such as being born prematurely or experiencing complications at birth can influence overall health, affecting how the body responds to certain products and hygiene practices.

Certain Foods Affect Odor: Foods like garlic, onions, and red meat can impact body odor. Electrolyte Drinks: Drinking electrolyte drinks can help reduce excessive sweating by balancing fluid in the body, which indirectly supports odor control.

Common Concerns in Female Hygiene

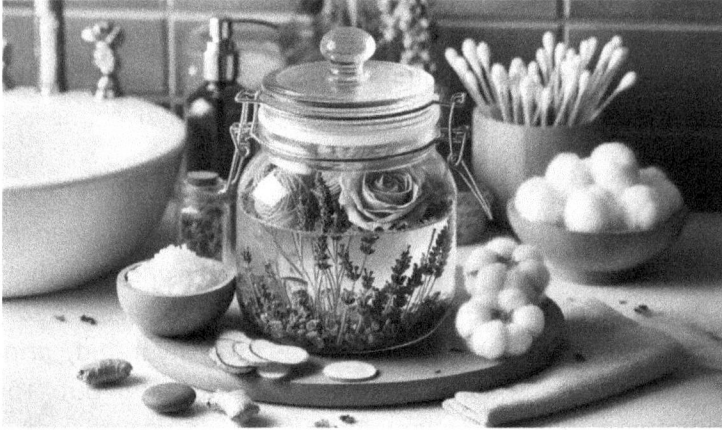

Menstrual Cycle Hygiene

Menstrual cycles can cause a temporary change in odor due to hormonal shifts, and using the right products can help manage this. Change pads and tampons regularly. Change every 4-6 hours (Or more often depending on the menstrual flow and or the heaviness of your cycles) to prevent odor and bacterial buildup. Avoid scented products that may cause irritation. Consider menstrual cups or period underwear, which are less likely to disrupt pH balance.

Post-Sex Hygiene

After sexual activity, the vaginal pH may be temporarily affected. Urinate and Cleanse! Urinating after sex can help prevent urinary tract infections. Gently cleanse with lukewarm water or a mild pH-balanced wash. Using a mild, unscented cleanser or plain water is usually enough. For external cleansing, avoid antibacterial soaps, which can be too harsh. Taking a probiotic supplement can support a healthy balance of bacteria after sexual activity. Certain chemicals in commercial products can irritate sensitive areas and disrupt natural balance. Avoid douches, scented soaps, and antibacterial products. Douching, in particular, can flush out beneficial bacteria and alter pH. making the vagina more susceptible to infections. Studies show that douching may increase the risk of bacterial vaginosis and even reproductive issues.

Avoid Parabens and Phthalates

These synthetic chemicals are commonly found in personal care products and may disrupt hormone function. **Fragrances and Dyes**: Scented products often contain synthetic ingredients that can irritate the skin and cause allergic reactions. **Sulfates**: Found in many soaps and shampoos, sulfates can be too harsh for sensitive areas.

Vaginal Hygiene Cleansing Routines

When cleansing daily, rinse the vulva gently with lukewarm water or a pH-balanced feminine wash. Avoid scrubbing or using strong soaps, as these can strip natural oils and disrupt pH. Using a yoni bar made from natural oils and herbs is a gentle way to cleanse. Consider feminine oil deodorants with essential oils like tea tree or lavender for odor control. A Vinegar Rinse consist of a diluted vinegar solution (1-2 tablespoons of apple cider vinegar in 1 cup of water) can be used occasionally to balance pH. Do not douche, as it can disrupt natural bacteria.

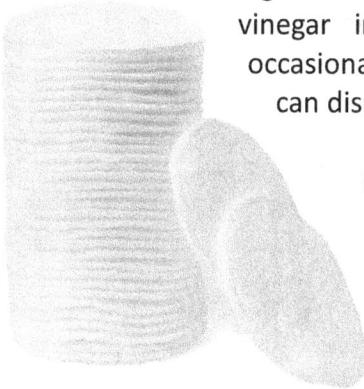

Use cotton rounds and balls to cleanse feminine areas

The Importance of Washcloths

Use a fresh, clean washcloth made of natural material such as cotton, avoid blends. for each wash, as old, damp cloths can harbor bacteria that could disrupt pH. Consider using dye-free washcloths, as dyes may irritate sensitive skin.

Anal Hygiene

Cleanse daily using water or a gentle, fragrance-free soap. Wipe from front to back to prevent bacterial spread to the vaginal area. Proper anal hygiene helps prevent odor and discomfort. The anal area also requires gentle care, as harsh products can irritate the skin. Always clean from front to back to prevent transferring bacteria to the vaginal area.

Natural Hygiene

Witch Hazel Application: Witch hazel is effective for reducing odor and irritation in the anal area. Apply after cleaning with a cotton pad. **Aloe Vera**: Aloe vera can soothe and moisturize the area, reducing the chances of irritation.

The increased pelvic floor pressure during activities like laughing, sneezing, or lifting can cause minor secretions from both the vaginal and anal areas? This is your body's way of managing pressure, but it also underscores the need for regular cleaning to maintain freshness and reduce the risk of infections.

Breast Hygiene and Odor Prevention

Effective hygiene is a combination of gentle cleaning methods, avoiding harsh chemicals, and using safe, pH-balanced products. Sweat and natural oils can accumulate under the breasts, especially in warm weather or during physical activity. This area is prone to bacterial and fungal growth, which can lead to odor or discomfort.

Best Practices for Cleaning and Preventing Odor

Breast Hygiene The breast area, particularly under the breasts, can collect sweat and bacteria that may cause odor or irritation. Good hygiene can help manage this. Cleanse the breast area with a mild, antibacterial soap or natural cleanser. Rinse thoroughly to avoid leaving any residue. Apply a natural feminine deodorant with essential oils like lavender, which has antibacterial properties. Avoid deodorants with aluminum or synthetic fragrances, which may irritate the skin. Drinking plenty of water can help regulate sweat and keep the skin fresh. Including electrolyte-rich drinks supports hydration. Witch hazel is an excellent option for reducing sweat and odor under the breasts. Apply with a cotton pad for a cooling, odor-reducing effect.

Causes of Menstrual Cycle Odor

The odor during the menstrual cycle is normal and usually comes from the combination of blood, tissue, and the natural bacteria that live in the vaginal area. Menstrual blood itself doesn't smell bad, but when it's exposed to air, it can take on a noticeable odor due to bacteria breaking it down. There are several factors, including cleanliness and hygiene, that can influence menstrual odor.

Changing Pads and Tampons Changing pads and tampons every 4-6 hours or more often depending on your flow helps minimize odor by reducing the exposure of blood to air. Avoid scented products, as they can irritate sensitive skin and disrupt the vaginal pH.

Blood and Tissue Breakdown Menstrual blood, composed of blood, uterine tissue, and cervical mucus, can develop an odor when it interacts with air. This natural process often intensifies when pads or tampons are worn for long periods without changing.

Bacteria The vaginal area contains a balance of "good" and "bad" bacteria, primarily Lactobacillus, which helps maintain a slightly acidic environment (pH 3.8-4.5). This acidity naturally minimizes the growth of odor-causing bacteria. However, prolonged exposure of menstrual blood to air can allow bacteria to multiply, causing a stronger smell.

Dietary Factors Foods like garlic, onions, and coffee can sometimes contribute to body odor, which can become more noticeable during menstruation. Staying hydrated and maintaining a balanced diet can reduce this effect.

Hormonal Changes Hormonal fluctuations during menstruation can change the pH of the vagina, which may temporarily alter the smell.

Prevention or Reduction of Menstrual Odor

Opt for Menstrual Cups or Period Underwear Menstrual cups collect, rather than absorb, blood, reducing the odor that can come from blood exposure to air. Period underwear can provide an alternative to pads or tampons and can be easier to change regularly for odor control.

Use Gentle, pH-Balanced Washes Gently cleaning the external vaginal area daily with warm water and a pH-balanced, unscented cleanser can help remove sweat and bacteria, reducing odor. Avoid douching or using scented washes internally, as they disrupt the natural balance of bacteria and can worsen odor issues.

Stay Hydrated Drinking enough water throughout the day helps flush out toxins, keeping the body and vaginal area healthier, which can indirectly reduce odor. Hydration supports overall hygiene and may help reduce any body odors.

Consider a Yoni Wash A homemade yoni wash can help cleanse the external area without disrupting pH. For example, a mild solution of 1 cup warm water and 1 tablespoon apple cider vinegar can gently clean without disturbing natural bacteria.

Wear Breathable Fabrics Try opting for cotton underwear, which allows air circulation and can reduce moisture buildup that could lead to odor. Avoid tight synthetic fabrics that trap heat and sweat, as these can promote bacterial growth.

Dietary Changes Eating a balanced diet with plenty of fruits, vegetables, and water can help keep natural body odors at bay. Reducing caffeine and spicy foods can sometimes help with minimizing body odor, especially during the menstrual cycle.

Does Odor Indicate Poor Hygiene?

A mild odor during menstruation is natural and doesn't indicate poor hygiene. However, a strong or foul smell, especially one that resembles fish or rotten eggs, can indicate an infection like bacterial vaginosis or a forgotten tampon and should be checked by a healthcare provider. Practicing good hygiene, such as regularly changing menstrual products and using mild cleansers, helps manage odor effectively. By understanding the causes and taking a few preventive steps, you can manage menstrual odor while maintaining a healthy and balanced environment in the vaginal area.

Proper Post-Partum Feminine Hygiene

After childbirth, maintaining proper hygiene is critical for healing, preventing infections, and overall comfort. The postpartum period is marked by physical changes, hormonal shifts, and increased vulnerability to infections, especially in the vaginal and perineal areas. The postpartum period is not only about physical healing but also about nurturing your emotional, mental, and spiritual health. This is a critical time for new mothers, and adopting a natural approach can make the journey smoother, healthier, and more empowering.

Reducing Post-Partum Stress and Stabilize Hormones
Meditation and Deep Breathing

Taking a few moments each day to engage in deep breathing exercises can help reduce stress, stabilize hormones, and enhance emotional well-being. Aim for 5-10 minutes of focused breathing, inhaling deeply through your nose and exhaling slowly through your mouth. Visualize healing energy surrounding your womb area. Maintaining a healthy vaginal microbiome is crucial postpartum, as the body's natural balance can be disrupted by hormonal changes, medications, and even stress.

Journaling Your Emotions

Writing down your thoughts and feelings can be a powerful tool for emotional release. Journaling about your postpartum experiences can help you process the changes your body is undergoing and support mental clarity. Your body's hormonal shifts can affect your emotional state significantly postpartum. Oxytocin, known as the "love hormone," is released during breastfeeding and bonding with your baby. This hormone not only aids in milk production but also helps enhance the emotional connection between you and your newborn.

In-Between the Crevices: Regular Cleansing and Wiping

During the postpartum phase, the body undergoes several changes that can increase vaginal and anal secretions. Natural movements like laughing, coughing, and walking can cause subtle leaks of fluid, including lochia (vaginal discharge post-birth), sweat, and natural lubrication. This can result in moisture buildup, especially in the crevices between the labia and around the perineal area.

Crevice Care Tips

Use Unscented Wipes: Opt for **unscented, alcohol-free wipes** throughout the day, especially after using the bathroom. Wiping gently in the crevices can help keep the area dry, reduce odor, and prevent bacterial growth. **Pat, Don't Rub**: The skin around the vaginal area is delicate, particularly after childbirth. Patting rather than rubbing will help prevent irritation and tearing of the sensitive skin. **Change Pads Frequently**: If you are using maternity pads to manage postpartum bleeding, change them every 2-3 hours, even if the pad isn't fully soaked. This will help reduce the risk of bacterial infections and discomfort. **Wear Breathable Underwear**: Choose cotton underwear to allow better airflow and reduce moisture. Avoid synthetic fabrics, as they can trap heat and moisture, creating an environment where bacteria thrive.

Natural Hygiene Practices for Postpartum Care

Use a Peri Bottle: A **peri bottle** (perineal irrigation bottle) is essential for postpartum hygiene. Fill it with lukewarm filtered water and use it to gently cleanse the vaginal and anal area after using the toilet. **Air Dry When Possible**: After cleansing, allow the area to air dry for a few minutes if possible. This helps prevent moisture buildup and reduces the risk of yeast infections. **Opt for Natural, Non-Toxic Products**: Choose **unscented, non-toxic** postpartum care products like pads and ointments. Look for ingredients like **aloe vera, calendula, and coconut oil**, which have natural healing properties and are less likely to irritate the sensitive skin. **Stay Hydrated and Eat Well**: Good hydration and a balanced diet rich in vitamins (especially vitamin C and zinc) can support your body's natural healing process and help maintain healthy vaginal flora. Proper postpartum feminine hygiene is vital for comfort, healing, and infection prevention. Regular cleaning, especially in the crevices, can help manage increased secretions due to natural body movements. Being mindful of water quality and avoiding potential toxins can support vaginal health during this delicate period. Embracing gentle, holistic practices will aid in the body's recovery and help maintain optimal well-being.

Feminine hygiene is the human experience!

Yoni Feminine Hygiene Practices

The Sanskrit word, Yoni is that has been interpreted to literally mean the "womb", the "source", or "vagina", "vulva", and "uterus". and the female organs of generation.

Yoni Steaming

Yoni steaming is a traditional practice where women sit or squat over a bowl of steaming water infused with herbs like mugwort, rosemary, lavender, and calendula. The steam is believed to help increase blood flow, soothe menstrual discomfort, and promote relaxation. *How to Do It:* Boil water and add 1-2 tablespoons of dried herbs. Let it steep for about 5 minutes. Place the bowl in a comfortable position where you can safely sit or squat over it. Wrap a towel around yourself to keep the steam contained and steam for about 20-30 minutes. *Caution:* Avoid steaming if you are pregnant, menstruating, or have any open wounds.

Yoni Bombs

Yoni bombs are like bath bombs but are specifically designed for vaginal health. They are usually made with herbs, natural oils, and sometimes baking soda, and are used to freshen the area and support pH balance. *How to Use:* These can be dissolved in warm water for a soak. Note that it's essential to avoid any harsh chemicals, synthetic fragrances, or dyes in these products, as they can irritate the vaginal area.

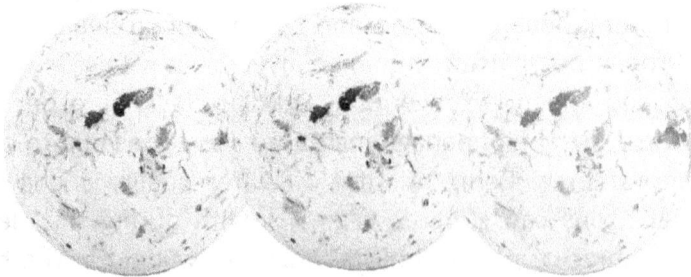

Yoni Oils

Yoni oils are gentle, all-natural oils used to moisturize and soothe the external vaginal area. They may contain ingredients like coconut oil, tea tree oil, lavender oil, and calendula extract. *Benefits*: Yoni oils can help prevent dryness, itching, and odor. They're best used after a shower or bath, and only on the external area.

Herbal Yoni Washes

Yoni washes are gentle cleansers specifically formulated for the vaginal area, often containing pH-balanced and natural ingredients. *How to Use*: Use a small amount to cleanse the external area only. Avoid using these products internally, as the vagina is self-cleaning and internal cleansing can disrupt natural pH.

Impact of Diet and Hydration on Hygiene

Staying hydrated is essential for flushing out toxins and supporting healthy skin. Drinking enough water also helps reduce body odor, including in sensitive areas. A diet high in fruits, vegetables, and whole grains promotes good bacteria and can help maintain pH balance. Reducing sugar and processed foods may prevent yeast overgrowth and body odor.

Preventing Vaginal Toxins from Water Quality

Water quality is a commonly overlooked factor in feminine hygiene. Contaminated water can introduce toxins, bacteria, and chemicals into the vaginal area, disrupting the natural microbiome and potentially leading to infections.

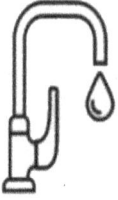

Tap Water Contaminants

Tap water can contain chlorine, fluoride, heavy metals, and even traces of pharmaceuticals. These can irritate the sensitive vaginal tissues, especially after childbirth when the area is more susceptible to infections. In certain areas, water quality may be compromised by bacterial contamination, which can exacerbate issues like bacterial vaginosis (BV) or yeast infections. Hard water contains high levels of minerals like calcium and magnesium. This can affect the natural pH balance of the vagina, increasing the risk of irritation and infection.

Tips to Reduce Vaginal Toxin Exposure from Water

Consider using filtered or boiled and cooled water for feminine area cleansing, especially during sitz baths. This can help minimize exposure to harsh chemicals and contaminants. A sitz bath can be a soothing way to promote healing and reduce discomfort. Fill a basin with filtered warm water and add natural ingredients like Epsom salt or witch hazel to help reduce swelling and support healing.

The Role of Boric Acid in Feminine Health

Boric acid suppositories (a safe form of boric acid specifically made for vaginal use) can help treat infections like bacterial vaginosis. This boric acid differs from the type used for pesticides and should be used only with medical advice. Boric acid is a natural compound with antifungal and antibacterial properties. In low doses, it's safe for treating vaginal infections like bacterial vaginosis and yeast infections. However, *vaginal boric acid is different* from the boric acid used in pest control, which is a highly concentrated form that is toxic for human use. Vaginal boric acid is formulated in safe dosages for internal use. Only use boric acid in the form of a medical-grade suppository recommended by a healthcare provider. This is often used as a last resort when other treatments are ineffective.

Probiotics and Vaginal Health

Probiotics are beneficial bacteria that support a healthy balance in the body. They're often found in foods like yogurt, kefir, and sauerkraut, as well as in supplements. Probiotics help balance the vaginal microbiome by promoting the growth of good bacteria, particularly *Lactobacillus*, which helps maintain a healthy pH. Foods such as yogurt (with live cultures), sauerkraut, and kimchi in addition to supplements with strains like *Lactobacillus acidophilus* and *Lactobacillus reuteri* supports vaginal health.

Common Bacteria and Fungi in the Vaginal Area

In the vaginal area, a balance of "good" and "bad" bacteria is essential for maintaining a healthy environment.

Lactobacillus Bacteria

Lactobacillus is the "good" bacteria that dominates a healthy vaginal environment. It produces lactic acid, which keeps the pH slightly acidic (3.8-4.5), helping prevent harmful bacteria and fungi from thriving. *Why It's Important*: *Lactobacillus* protects against infections like bacterial vaginosis (BV) and yeast infections. This bacteria helps keep other, potentially harmful organisms in check.

Candida Albicans

A yeast (fungus) that lives naturally in the body, including the vaginal area, in small amounts. However, an imbalance (such as from antibiotics, high sugar intake, or hormonal changes) can cause overgrowth, leading to a yeast infection. *Symptoms of Overgrowth*: Itching, thick white discharge, and discomfort.

Gardnerella Vaginalis

A bacterium often associated with bacterial vaginosis (BV), a common infection caused by an imbalance in vaginal bacteria. *Symptoms of Overgrowth*: Thin, gray discharge with a strong fishy odor, itching, and irritation.

Streptococcus agalactiae (Group B Strep)

A bacterium that can exist in the vaginal area without causing symptoms in most cases. However, it's a concern during pregnancy, as it can be passed to the baby during childbirth. *Symptoms of Overgrowth*: Rarely causes symptoms in adults but can pose risks to newborns.

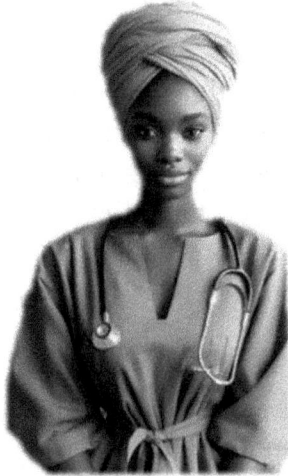

Maintaining the female body can be Complex Do Not Be Embarrassed. Do Your Research! Health Professionals Have Seen It All Seek Help!

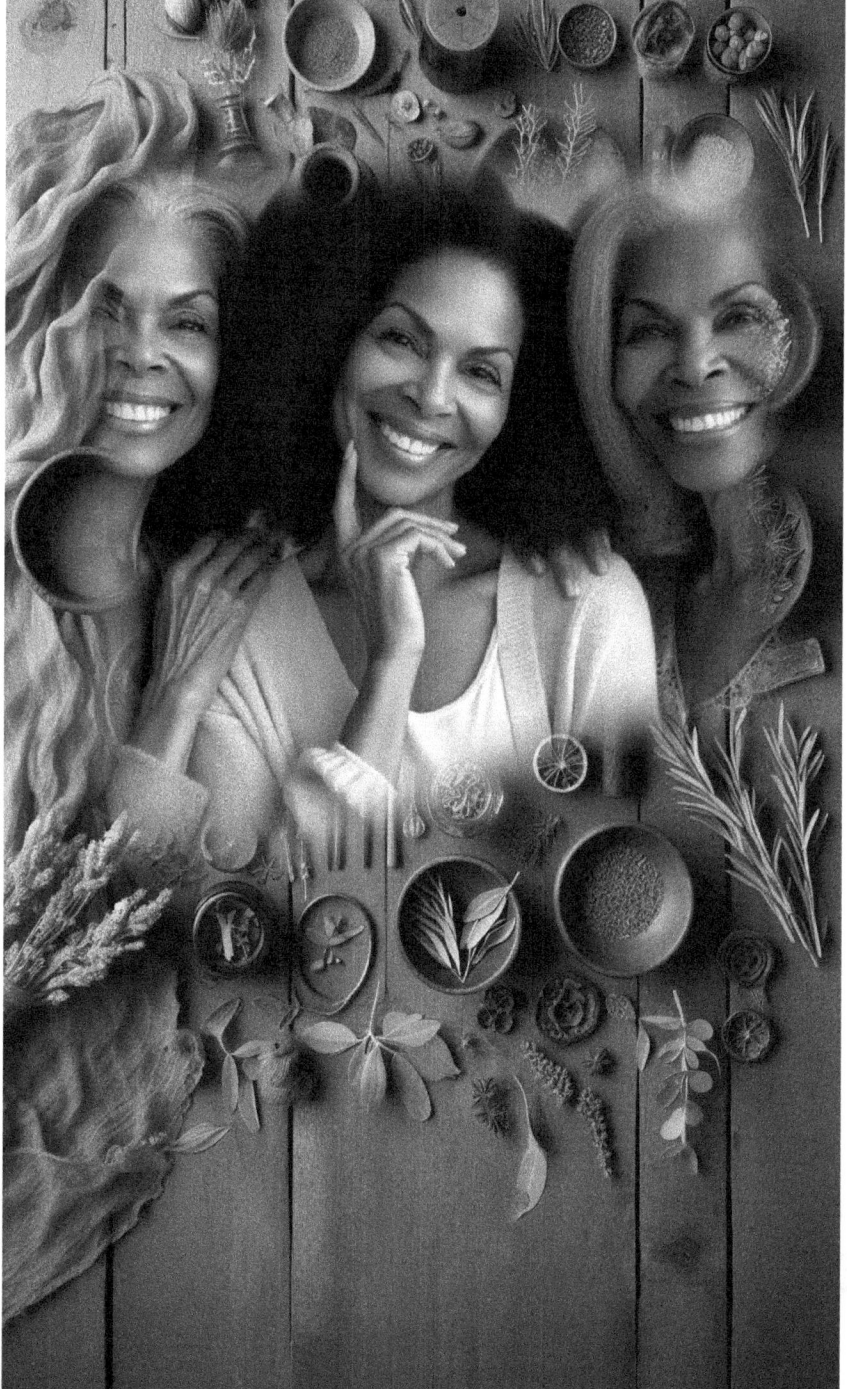

Chapter 16
Journey Into Aging and Longevity

Healthy Aging Tips Active Lifestyle

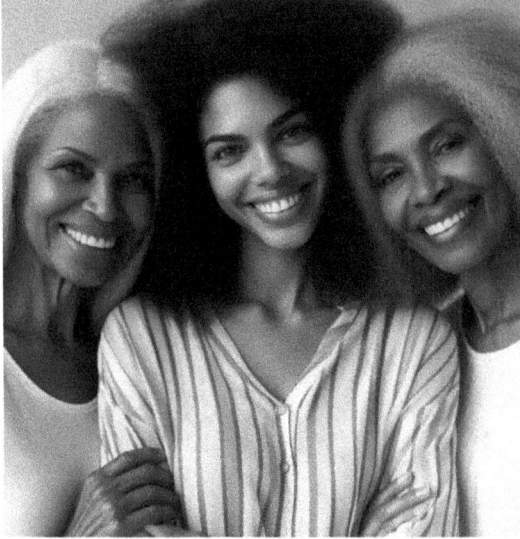

Aging is a natural process that can bring a wealth of wisdom and experience. However, it also requires a proactive approach to maintain health and vitality. This section focuses on essential tips and strategies for Black women to age gracefully and live a long, fulfilling life.

Maintaining an active lifestyle is crucial as you age. Regular physical activity helps to keep your body strong, improve balance, and reduce the risk of chronic diseases. Activities such as walking, swimming, dancing, and yoga can be both enjoyable and beneficial. Aim for at least 150 minutes of moderate exercise per week. Remember, it's never too late to start moving, and every bit of activity counts towards better health.

Healthy Diet

A balanced diet rich in nutrients is vital for healthy aging. Focus on eating a variety of fruits, vegetables, whole grains, lean proteins, and healthy fats. Nutrient-dense foods provide the essential vitamins and minerals your body needs to function optimally. Pay particular attention to calcium and vitamin D for bone health, and antioxidants from fruits and vegetables to combat oxidative stress. Hydration is equally important, so drink plenty of water throughout the day.

Social Engagement

Maintaining social connections is essential for mental and emotional health. Engage in activities that foster social interaction, such as joining clubs, participating in community events, or volunteering. Staying connected with family and friends can provide emotional support and reduce feelings of loneliness and isolation. Social engagement helps keep your mind sharp and your spirits high.

Common Health Concerns in Older Age

Arthritis is a common issue that can cause joint pain and stiffness. Managing arthritis involves regular exercise to maintain joint function and reduce pain. Low-impact activities like swimming and cycling are excellent choices. Additionally, maintaining a healthy weight can reduce stress on the joints. Anti-inflammatory foods, such as fish rich in omega-3 fatty acids, nuts, and green leafy vegetables, can help manage symptoms.

Heart Health is a leading concern as you age. Monitoring blood pressure and cholesterol levels is crucial. Regular exercise, a healthy diet low in saturated fats and high in fiber and avoiding smoking can significantly reduce the risk of heart disease. Consider incorporating heart-healthy foods like berries, nuts, whole grains, and fatty fish into your diet. Regular check-ups with your healthcare provider can help manage and prevent heart-related issues.

Cognitive Health Maintaining cognitive health is important for overall well-being. Engage in activities that challenge your mind, such as reading, puzzles, and learning new skills. Staying mentally active can help preserve cognitive function and delay the onset of dementia. Social engagement and physical activity also play a role in maintaining cognitive health. Consider activities that combine physical and mental challenges, like dancing or gardening.

Maintaining Vitality and Wellness Mental Stimulation
Keeping your mind active is key to staying sharp. Engage in activities that require thinking and problem-solving. This can include reading books, doing crossword puzzles, playing board games, or taking up a new hobby. Lifelong learning is beneficial, so consider enrolling in a class or workshop to learn something new. Staying mentally stimulated helps keep your brain healthy and engaged.

Routine Health Check-ups
Regular visits to your healthcare provider are essential for early detection and management of health issues. Routine check-ups can help monitor blood pressure, cholesterol levels, bone density, and other important health markers. Health screenings and preventive measures can catch potential problems early, making them easier to treat. Build a good relationship with your healthcare provider and keep them informed about any changes in your health.

Balanced Life
Achieving a balanced life involves nurturing your physical, mental, and emotional well-being. Find time for activities that you enjoy and that bring you peace and happiness. Practice stress management techniques such as meditation, deep breathing, or yoga. Ensure you get enough sleep and maintain a regular sleep schedule. A balanced life helps you stay resilient and better equipped to handle the challenges of aging.

Aging gracefully involves a holistic approach to health and wellness. By staying active, eating a balanced diet, engaging socially, and keeping your mind stimulated, you can maintain your vitality and enjoy a fulfilling life. Regular health check-ups and a balanced lifestyle are crucial to managing common health concerns and promoting longevity. Remember, it's never too late to adopt healthy habits that will support you through the aging process. Embrace this journey with confidence and joy, knowing that you are taking steps to live your best life.

THERE IS BEAUTY AND WISDOM
THAT COMES WITH AGE

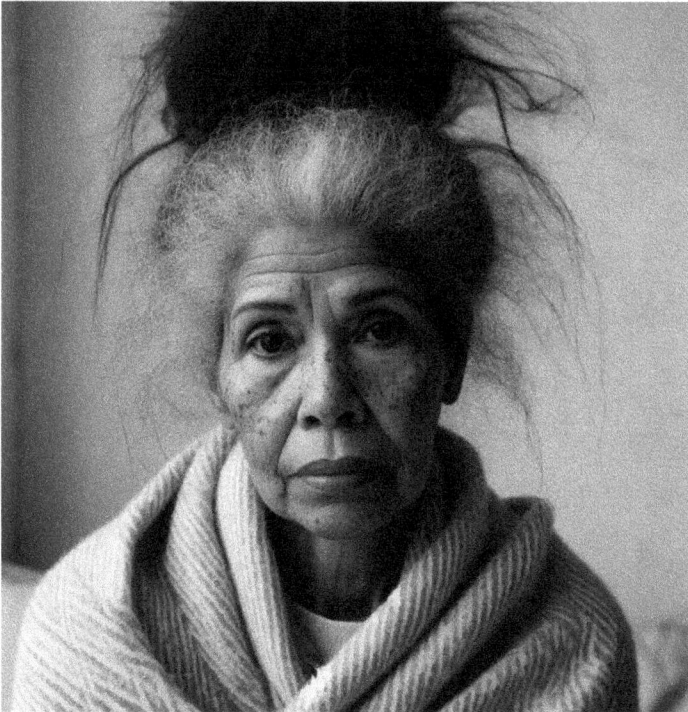

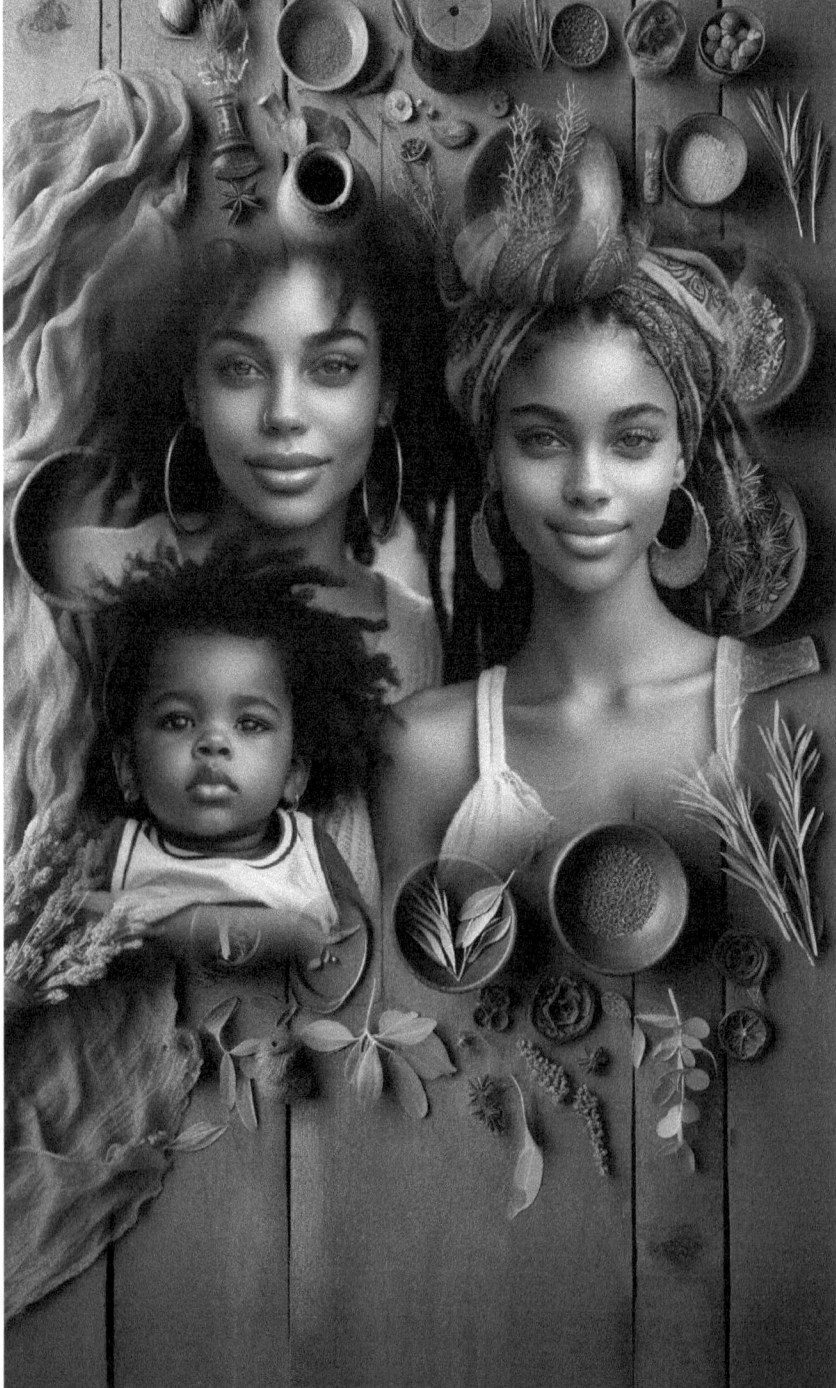

Chapter 17
Journey Into Motherhood

Gut Health and Postnatal Wellness

Maintaining optimal gut health and achieving postnatal wellness, including regaining a flat tummy and addressing stretch marks, are important considerations for the holistic well-being of Black women. This section explores strategies and remedies to support gut health and address postnatal concerns in a holistic manner.

Understanding Gut Health

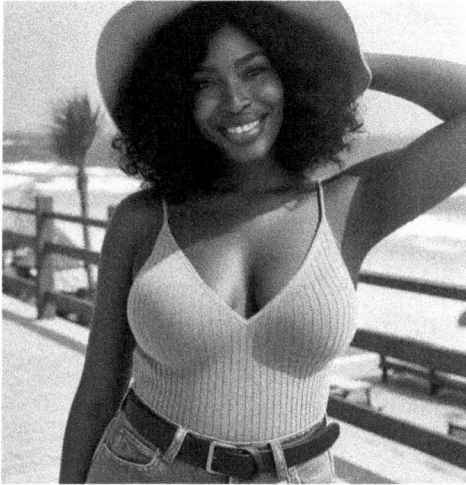

The gut microbiome plays a crucial role in overall health, influencing digestion, immune function, and even mental well-being. For Black women, factors such as diet, stress, and lifestyle can impact gut health, making it essential to prioritize strategies that promote a healthy gut microbiome.

.Strategies for Gut Health

Nutrient-Dense Diet: Consuming a diet rich in fiber, fruits, vegetables, and fermented foods can support a diverse and balanced gut microbiome. *Probiotics and Prebiotics:* Incorporating probiotic-rich foods like yogurt and kefir, as well as prebiotic foods such as garlic and onions, can promote gut health by nourishing beneficial bacteria. *Stress Management:* Practices like mindfulness, meditation, and adequate sleep are crucial for managing stress levels, which can affect gut health. *Hydration:* Drinking plenty of water helps maintain proper digestion and supports a healthy gut environment.

Postnatal Wellness
Flat Tummy After Postnatal

Engaging in postnatal exercises that target the core muscles, such as pelvic tilts, kegels, and gentle abdominal exercises, can help tighten and strengthen the abdominal muscles. **Healthy Eating**: Following a balanced diet that includes lean proteins, whole grains, fruits, and vegetables can aid in postnatal weight loss and contribute to a flatter tummy. **Pelvic Floor Exercises**: Performing pelvic floor exercises, such as Kegels, can help improve muscle tone and support the abdominal region.

Addressing Stubborn Flat Tummy and Stretch Marks

Herbal Remedies: Natural remedies like shea butter, coconut oil, and almond oil can help moisturize the skin and reduce the appearance of stretch marks. Massage Therapy: Gentle massage with essential oils like lavender or rosehip oil can improve blood circulation and promote skin elasticity, aiding in the reduction of stretch marks. Hydration: Drinking plenty of water hydrates the skin from within, improving elasticity and reducing the appearance of stretch marks. Healthy Diet: Consuming foods rich in vitamins C and E, such as citrus fruits, berries, and nuts, can support skin health and reduce the appearance of stretch marks.

Prioritizing gut health and postnatal wellness is essential for the holistic well-being of Black women. By incorporating strategies such as a nutrient-dense diet, stress management techniques, and targeted exercises, Black women can support their gut health and address postnatal concerns like regaining a flat tummy and reducing stretch marks in a holistic manner. Additionally, utilizing natural remedies and lifestyle modifications can promote overall health and confidence during the postnatal period.

The Cultural Role of Traditional Practices in Motherhood

Historically, African American women have relied on traditional practices rooted in African heritage to support their journey into motherhood. These practices not only focus on physical health but also honor the spiritual and communal aspects of raising a child.

Key Traditional Practices

African American mothers have long used herbal infusions like red raspberry leaf tea for uterine health and ginger tea for postpartum nausea. Incorporating herbs like fenugreek and blessed thistle can support milk production. **Postpartum Belly Binding** is a practice that involves wrapping the abdomen with a cloth to help the uterus contract and support core muscles. It's a comforting way to honor the changes the body has undergone and promote physical recovery. A **moon bath** or herbal sitz bath can help with healing tears, reducing swelling, and promoting relaxation. Use a combination of calendula, comfrey, and lavender for their anti-inflammatory and soothing properties.

The Role of Community Support

The concept of "it takes a village" is deeply rooted in African American culture. Leaning on the support of elders and extended family members can provide emotional relief, guidance, and a connection to ancestral knowledge. Adopt and grandparent elderly people in assisted living will enjoy the company and sense of family. Accept help from trusted friends and family for tasks like meal preparation, childcare, and emotional support.

Navigating Racism and Medical Bias in Maternal Healthcare

African American women face disproportionate risks in maternal healthcare, including higher rates of maternal mortality, preeclampsia, and postpartum complications. These disparities are often linked to systemic racism and implicit biases within the medical system.

Tips for Self-Advocacy in Healthcare

Create a birth plan. Outline your preferences for labor, delivery, and postpartum care. Include specifics about pain management, interventions, and breastfeeding. Share this plan with your healthcare provider early on. Bring a doula or advocate. Having a **doula** or trusted advocate present during medical appointments and delivery can help ensure that your concerns are heard. Doulas provide emotional and physical support, and studies have shown they can reduce the likelihood of interventions. Know your rights! Educate yourself on patient rights, including the right to informed consent and the ability to refuse procedures you do not feel comfortable with. Do not be afraid to ask for a second opinion if you feel unheard.

Resources for Support

Groups like *Black Mamas Matter Alliance* offers advocacy and educational resources to help address the needs of Black mothers. *The National Birth Equity Collaborative* works to eliminate racial disparities in maternal and infant health through research, training, and advocacy.

Hormonal and Skin Health for Melanin-Rich Women

Hormonal changes during and after pregnancy can have a unique impact on women with melanin-rich skin, leading to issues like hyperpigmentation, hormonal acne, and melasma. Postpartum hair loss is also a common concern due to fluctuations in estrogen levels.

Tips for Balancing Hormones

Herbs like ashwagandha and maca root can help stabilize cortisol levels and support adrenal health, reducing stress-related hormonal imbalances. Incorporate foods high in omega-3 fatty acids, such as salmon, chia seeds, and flaxseeds, to support hormonal balance and reduce inflammation. Also, consider vitamin D supplementation, as melanin-rich skin may require more exposure to produce adequate levels of vitamin D.

Natural Skin Care for Melanin-Rich Skin

For hyperpigmentation use natural treatments like aloe vera, turmeric masks, and serums with vitamin C to brighten dark spots and even out skin tone. For stretch marks use shea butter, cocoa butter, and rosehip oil are excellent choices for reducing the appearance of stretch marks and supporting skin elasticity. For postpartum hair loss massage the scalp with castor oil or jojoba oil can stimulate hair growth and improve circulation.

Support for Breastfeeding Challenges and Mental Health Care

Breastfeeding can present unique challenges for African American women, including lower rates of initiation and continuation due to cultural, socioeconomic, and historical factors. Mental health is also a critical concern, as postpartum depression (PPD) often goes underdiagnosed in Black women.

Tips for Successful Breastfeeding

Seek the help of a lactation consultant, especially if you encounter issues like latching difficulties. Many community health centers offer free lactation support. Incorporate galactagogue foods like oats, almonds, and fenugreek tea to increase milk production. Stay hydrated with herbal teas like fennel tea.

Natural Tips for Enhancing Milk Production

For breastfeeding mothers, maintaining milk supply can be a concern. Here are some natural ways to boost lactation. Eat Galactagogue Foods. Foods like oats, fennel seeds, fenugreek, and almonds are known to increase milk production. Dehydration can affect your milk supply. Aim for at least 10-12 cups of water per day and consider drinking herbal teas like fennel tea or milk thistle tea. Gently massaging your breasts can help stimulate milk flow and reduce the risk of clogged ducts.

Addressing Postpartum Depression

Seek therapy early. Find a culturally competent therapist who understands the unique stressors faced by African American mothers. Online platforms like *Therapy for Black Girls* offer directories for finding mental health professionals. Omega-3 supplements, magnesium, and B vitamins can help alleviate mood swings and support mental well-being.

Addressing Postnatal Anemia and Sickle Cell Trait

African American women are at higher risk for postnatal anemia and may carry the sickle cell trait, which can affect overall health during the postpartum period.

Managing Postnatal Anemia

Iron-rich foods like dark leafy greens, beans, lentils, and molasses in your diet. Pair them with vitamin C-rich foods (e.g., citrus fruits, bell peppers) to enhance iron absorption. Nettle tea and dandelion root are effective herbal remedies for increasing iron levels naturally.

Sickle Cell Trait Awareness

It is important to know your status, if you carry the sickle cell trait, it's essential to discuss it with your healthcare provider, as it can impact your pregnancy and postpartum recovery. Staying well-hydrated and getting adequate rest are key for preventing complications related to sickle cell trait.

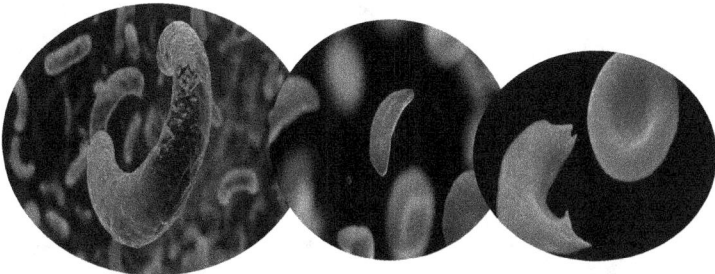

Coping, Balancing, and Managing Overwhelm as an African American Mother and Single Mother

The intersection of race, motherhood, and single parenthood can lead to unique stressors for African American women. Here are strategies for managing the emotional and physical demands:

Strategies for Balance

Time Management: Establish a daily routine that includes time for self-care, even if it's just 10-15 minutes of meditation or a relaxing bath. **Set Boundaries**: Learn to say "no" to non-essential tasks and prioritize your well-being. Delegate responsibilities when possible. Join **support groups** for single mothers or connect with community organizations that offer resources tailored to African American women.

Self-Care Tips for Overwhelm

Grounding Practices: Engage in grounding activities like **yoga, deep breathing, or walking in nature** to calm your mind and body. **Affirmations**: Use daily affirmations to boost your confidence and remind yourself of your strength. Examples include: "I am enough," "I am capable," and "I am deserving of rest and care." **Therapeutic Outlets**: Consider **journaling**, creative arts, or **talk therapy** as tools for processing emotions and relieving stress.

Being a Mother is The Hardest Frightening Job Ever!
There Is No Proper Handbook or Guide.
You Are Doing Great!

The Importance of Being Your Child's First Teacher

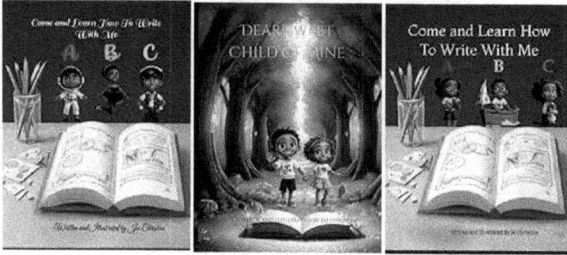

As parents, we are our children's first and most influential teachers. Long before they set foot in a classroom, children learn from observing, listening, and engaging with the world around them, guided primarily by their parents or caregivers. Reading to your child, sharing images, and telling stories that reflect their identity not only strengthens literacy but also instills pride, confidence, and cultural awareness. For African American children, seeing themselves represented in books can be transformative, helping them to connect deeply with their heritage and develop a sense of belonging.

Relying solely on the educational system is not enough; our children's self-image and understanding of the world are largely shaped at home. That's why Black authors like **Jai Christine** are so important. Jai Christine, a passionate advocate for culturally reflective storytelling, writes children's books that celebrate Black culture and uplift young readers. Her works, such as *Dear Sweet Child of Mine* and *Come and Learn How to Write with Me*, offer stories and images that resonate with African American children, providing them with characters and narratives that reflect their experiences and aspirations. Available on Amazon, these books serve as valuable tools for parents who want to actively engage in their children's education, helping them to see themselves in literature and, ultimately, in the broader world.

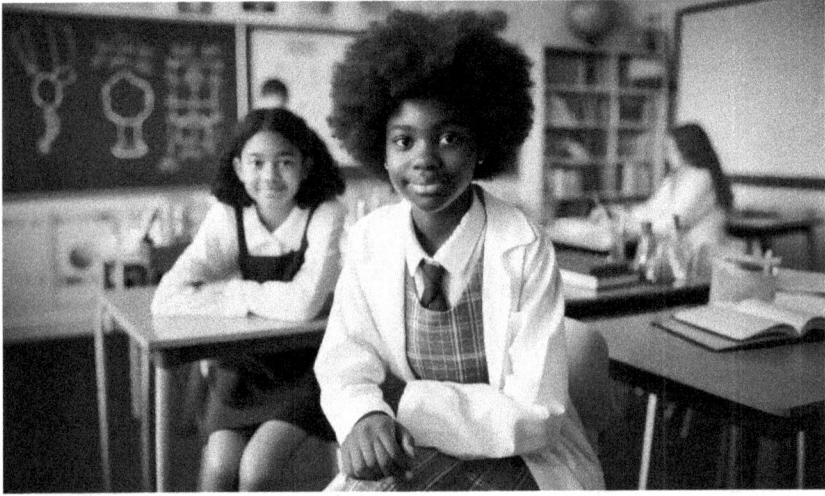

Dealing with Learning Disabilities

Learning disabilities are neurological disorders that can interfere with a person's ability to learn, read, write, speak, or process information. In African American communities, early diagnosis and intervention are essential, as these conditions can often be misunderstood, overlooked, or improperly addressed due to lack of access to resources or misdiagnosis. Learning disabilities affect each child differently, but with timely, tailored support, children can thrive in both academic and social environments.

Common Learning Disabilities Among African American Children

Some of the most prevalent learning disabilities that affect children across all populations, including African American children.

Dyslexia: Dyslexia is a reading disorder that makes it challenging for children to identify speech sounds and how they relate to letters and words. It's one of the most commonly diagnosed learning disabilities and can lead to struggles with reading fluency, spelling, and comprehension.

Dyscalculia: This learning disorder affects mathematical ability. Children with dyscalculia may have difficulty grasping number-related concepts, memorizing math facts, or performing calculations accurately and confidently.

Dysgraphia: Dysgraphia affects a child's handwriting skills and can interfere with the ability to express themselves in writing. Children may have trouble with spelling, organizing thoughts on paper, or maintaining legible handwriting.

Auditory Processing Disorder (APD): Children with APD have trouble processing sounds, including spoken words, making it challenging to follow verbal instructions, distinguish similar-sounding words, or remember details from conversations.

Attention-Deficit/Hyperactivity Disorder (ADHD): Although not technically classified as a learning disability, ADHD often coexists with learning disabilities and can significantly affect a child's learning experience. African American children are sometimes underdiagnosed or misdiagnosed with ADHD, leading to challenges in getting appropriate support.

Oppositional Defiant Disorder (ODD): Often associated with learning challenges, ODD is characterized by a pattern of angry, irritable, argumentative, or defiant behavior towards authority figures. African American children with ODD often face additional stigma and may be more likely to be punished rather than treated, underscoring the need for understanding and appropriate care.

Importance of Early Diagnosis and Intervention

Early identification of learning disabilities can profoundly impact a child's development, enabling tailored support and reducing negative emotional effects such as frustration, low self-esteem, or behavioral issues. Parents should advocate for comprehensive evaluations from professionals trained in assessing learning disabilities. Schools often provide evaluations, but it's also possible to seek private evaluations from psychologists and educational specialists.

Individualized Education Plans (IEPs) and Specialized Support

An **Individualized Education Plan (IEP)** is a critical tool that outlines specialized goals and accommodations designed to meet a child's unique educational needs. Collaborating with teachers, school counselors, and other professionals ensures a well-rounded support network. IEPs may include extra time on tests, access to specialized teaching methods, or the use of technology to assist with reading or writing.

Support from specialists can also play a crucial role. For instance: **Speech therapists** assist children with language-based learning disabilities by helping them improve language comprehension and verbal communication. **Occupational therapists** focus on developing fine motor skills, especially helpful for children with dysgraphia or other motor-skill-related challenges. **Psychologists** work on emotional and cognitive assessments and can provide behavioral therapies to help children adapt and succeed.

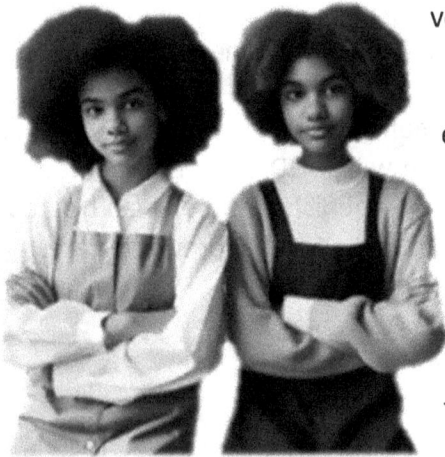

Oppositional Defiant Disorder (ODD)

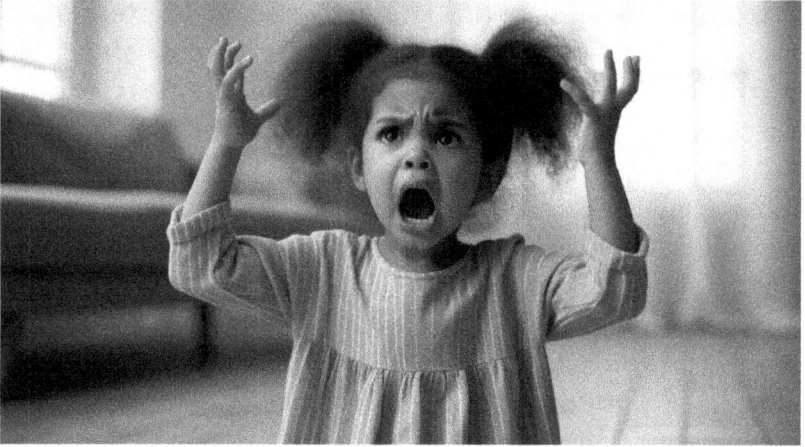

Oppositional Defiant Disorder (ODD) is often misunderstood, especially within communities where behavioral symptoms may be mistaken for general defiance or personality traits. ODD is a pattern of uncooperative, defiant, and hostile behavior towards authority figures, which significantly impacts family dynamics, school performance, and social relationships.

Symptoms of ODD
Frequent temper tantrums or outbursts
Arguing with adults or refusing to comply with rules
Blaming others for personal mistakes or difficulties
Being easily annoyed or touchy
Frequent displays of anger and resentment
Deliberate actions to annoy or upset others

Getting Help for ODD
If a child exhibits signs of ODD, a professional evaluation is essential. A mental health professional, such as a psychologist or psychiatrist, can provide a comprehensive assessment. Treatment options may include behavioral therapy, which focuses on teaching children how to handle frustration and anger constructively, and family therapy, which supports parents in managing challenging behaviors.

Managing ODD at Home

While professional support is crucial, there are also steps parents can take at home to help manage ODD symptoms: **Set Clear Boundaries**: Establish and consistently enforce clear rules and expectations. A structured environment can help children with ODD understand limits and predict outcomes. **Positive Reinforcement**: Acknowledge and reward positive behaviors. Focus on small, specific actions to build up the child's self-esteem and reinforce desired behaviors. **Practice Patience and Understanding**: Children with ODD benefit from calm, composed responses. Avoid engaging in power struggles, which can escalate situations. **Seek to Understand the Root of Behaviors**: Children with ODD may be reacting to underlying frustrations, misunderstandings, or insecurities. Compassion and open dialogue can help uncover the source of negative behaviors.

Dietary and Natural Approaches for Learning Disabilities and ODD

Diet plays an influential role in mood, behavior, and cognitive performance. Many families have observed that dietary adjustments can benefit children with learning disabilities and behavioral challenges like ODD.

Reduce Sugar and Processed Foods: Excessive sugar and processed foods can lead to fluctuations in blood sugar levels, affecting mood, energy, and focus. Reducing these foods may help children maintain a more stable emotional and mental state. **Incorporate Omega-3 Fatty Acids**: Omega-3s, found in fish, flaxseed, and walnuts, support brain health and have been linked to improved focus and mood. **Focus on Whole Foods**: A diet rich in fruits, vegetables, lean proteins, and whole grains supports balanced nutrition and can reduce behavioral issues. **Avoid Food Dyes and Additives**: Artificial colors and preservatives, particularly those found in processed snacks, have been linked to hyperactivity and irritability in some children.

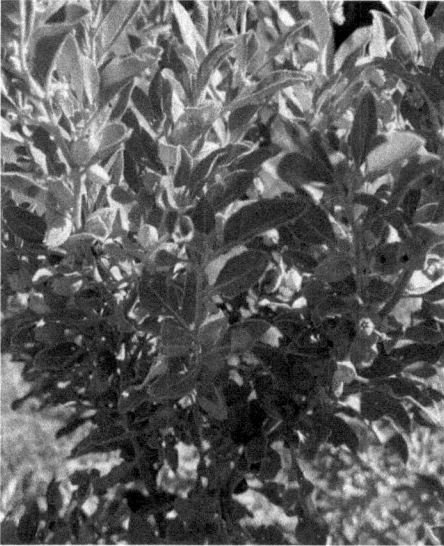

Certain natural remedies can also support behavioral and cognitive health, though they should be used with caution and under a professional's supervision: **Ashwagandha**: This adaptogenic herb has been known to help reduce stress and promote calm, which can be beneficial for children with ODD. **Bacopa Monnieri**: Often used to enhance memory and learning, bacopa may assist children with learning disabilities in managing cognitive functions. **Magnesium**: Many children are deficient in magnesium, which plays a critical role in mood regulation and relaxation. Magnesium supplements can support emotional balance and reduce irritability. **Chamomile Tea**: Known for its calming effects, chamomile tea may help with anxiety and sleep disturbances, especially for children experiencing frustration or anger due to ODD.

Learning disabilities and behavioral disorders like ODD present unique challenges, particularly for African American children, who may encounter additional social and systemic barriers. Through early diagnosis, structured support systems, dietary adjustments, and, if appropriate, natural remedies, parents can offer their children the best chances of overcoming these obstacles and thriving. Resilience, patience, and a focus on individual strengths can empower both parents and children to navigate these challenges with confidence and hope for a bright future.

Immunizations Effects on our Bodies

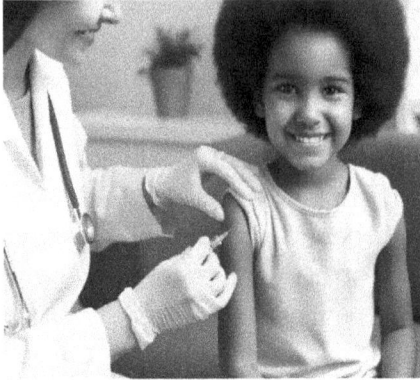

The topic of potential correlations between immunization shots and adverse health effects, especially among African American populations, is an area of active debate. While scientific consensus broadly supports immunization as a critical public health measure to prevent contagious diseases, discussions and studies about potential side effects and health outcomes have raised questions. These concerns include possible correlations between immunization and conditions like autism, although mainstream scientific research has consistently found no causal link between vaccines and autism. Below is a structured exploration of required immunization shots in the U.S., their mechanisms of action, noted adverse effects, and alternative considerations.

Required Immunizations in the United States

The most common immunization shots required in the U.S.

MMR (Measles, Mumps, Rubella)
DTaP (Diphtheria, Tetanus, Pertussis)
Polio (IPV)
Hepatitis B
Varicella (Chickenpox)
Pneumococcal (PCV13)
Haemophilus influenzae type b (Hib)
Rotavirus
Influenza

Mechanisms of Action for Each Vaccine

MMR (Measles, Mumps, Rubella)

MMR is a live attenuated vaccine, which means it uses a weakened form of the virus to prompt immune response. *Potential Effects:* The MMR vaccine is associated with mild side effects like fever or rash. A concern arose in the late 1990s regarding the MMR vaccine and autism, primarily from a now-retracted study by Andrew Wakefield. However, subsequent research has consistently shown no causal link between the MMR vaccine and autism, though some community skepticism remains.

DTaP (Diphtheria, Tetanus, Pertussis)

This inactivated vaccine combines protection against three diseases by stimulating immunity against the toxins produced by these bacteria. *Potential Effects:* Common side effects include fever, fatigue, and swelling at the injection site. Rarely, neurological events and seizures have been reported, though these are extremely rare.

Polio (IPV)

IPV contains inactivated poliovirus, which cannot cause disease but triggers an immune response. **Potential Effects:** Minimal side effects are reported, such as soreness at the injection site. Past issues were associated with live vaccines, which are no longer used in the U.S.

Hepatitis B

This vaccine contains parts of the Hepatitis B virus protein, which prompts an immune response without causing disease. *Potential Effects:* Mild side effects include pain at the injection site and low-grade fever. Concerns have been raised about potential links to autoimmune conditions, though evidence is limited.

Varicella (Chickenpox)

A live attenuated vaccine that provides immunity against chickenpox. *Potential Effects:* Potential side effects include rash and fever. There's no established evidence of long-term harm or chronic adverse conditions directly associated with this vaccine.

Pneumococcal (PCV13)
This conjugate vaccine targets several strains of Streptococcus pneumoniae by using proteins to prompt a strong immune response. *Potential Effects:* Common side effects include drowsiness, irritability, and swelling at the injection site. Severe reactions are rare.

Haemophilus influenzae type b (Hib)
A conjugate vaccine that protects against Hib bacteria, which can cause severe infections in children. *Potential Effects:* Minor reactions like redness or swelling at the injection site. There is limited evidence of long-term effects.

Rotavirus
A live attenuated vaccine taken orally, which stimulates immunity against rotavirus. *Potential Effects:* Some risk of mild gastrointestinal upset. There has been a rare association with intussusception (a bowel obstruction) in infants.

Influenza
Available as both inactivated and live attenuated vaccines, designed to prompt an immune response to flu viruses. *Potential Effects:* Typical side effects include fever, muscle aches, and soreness at the injection site. Neurological concerns, such as Guillain-Barré Syndrome, have been reported but are extremely rare.

Autism and Immunizations

Despite strong scientific consensus, public concerns about vaccines potentially increasing autism risk, particularly among African American males, persist. A 2014 study by Dr. William Thompson at the CDC raised concerns that MMR might be correlated with autism in African American boys if administered before age three. However, the findings were controversial, and the CDC maintains that comprehensive evidence refutes any causal relationship between vaccines and autism. Research continues to explore genetic and environmental risk factors for autism, though no definitive link to vaccines has been established in peer-reviewed studies.

Natural Approaches

In some communities, herbal and natural remedies are explored as alternatives or complements to immunization.

Elderberry (Sambucus nigra): Used for its antiviral and immune-boosting properties, elderberry is a common alternative to bolster immunity.

Echinacea: Often used to reduce the severity and duration of respiratory infections.

Vitamin D: Linked to immune health, especially important for those with darker skin due to lower synthesis from sunlight.

Turmeric (Curcuma longa): Known for its anti-inflammatory properties, turmeric is used to promote general wellness.

While these natural remedies can support general immune health, they are not a replacement for vaccines when it comes to protecting against highly contagious or severe diseases.

Systemic Factors and Health Inequities

African American populations face unique health challenges due to systemic issues such as socioeconomic barriers, access to healthcare, and historical distrust due to unethical research practices, such as the Tuskegee Syphilis Study. This distrust impacts immunization rates, leading to disparities in health outcomes.

Limited representation in clinical trials also makes it difficult to evaluate potential adverse effects on Black individuals, leading to advocacy for more inclusive research.

Vaccination remains a cornerstone of modern public health, but questions around its effects on diverse populations emphasize the need for comprehensive, transparent, and inclusive research. Until more data is available, those considering alternative approaches should work closely with healthcare providers.

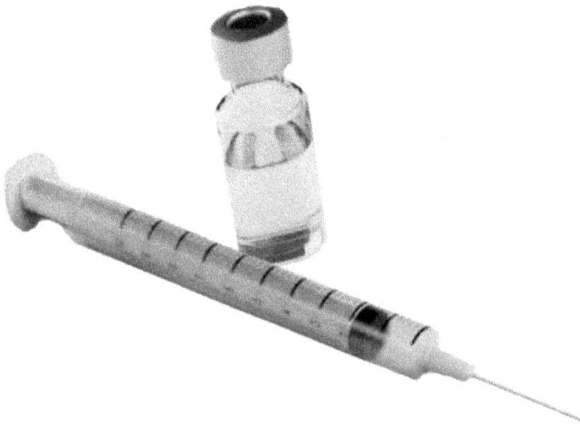

Motherhood as Caretakers for Children with Special Needs

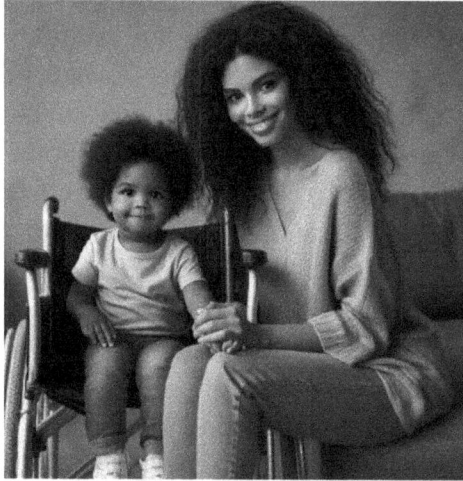

Understanding the Role of a Caretaker

Black mothers who are caretakers for children with special needs embody resilience and dedication, often providing around-the-clock care that demands both physical and emotional strength. This role requires a deep understanding of their child's unique needs and the ability to adapt to an ever-changing routine. Being a caretaker can be incredibly rewarding, but it also comes with significant challenges, including mental endurance, finding support, and maintaining one's well-being.

Early Detection and Diagnosis

Early detection of special needs is crucial for ensuring that a child receives the appropriate care and interventions. Black mothers should be vigilant about developmental milestones and seek professional evaluations if they have concerns. Pediatricians, developmental specialists, and genetic counselors can offer diagnoses and suggest early intervention programs. These programs often include physical, occupational, and speech therapy, which are essential for supporting the child's development.

Where to Get Help

Navigating the healthcare and support systems can be daunting. It's important for mothers to connect with local and national organizations that provide resources for children with special needs. Organizations such as the National Down Syndrome Society (NDSS) and local support groups can offer valuable information, financial assistance, and community connections. Additionally, state and federal programs, like Medicaid and Social Security Disability Insurance (SSDI), can help cover the costs of care.

Mental Endurance

The mental endurance required to care for a child with special needs is immense. Black mothers often face additional stressors, including systemic racism and economic challenges, which can compound the emotional toll of caregiving. It's essential to prioritize mental health through self-care practices such as meditation, therapy, and stress-relief activities. Building a strong support network of family, friends, and professionals can provide emotional sustenance and practical assistance.

Support Groups and Finding Help

Joining support groups can offer emotional and practical support to Black mothers. These groups provide a space to share experiences, gain insights, and receive encouragement from others who understand the challenges of raising a child with special needs. Online communities and local groups can be valuable resources for finding respite care, accessing educational resources, and navigating the complexities of special needs parenting.

Establishing Routines

Routines are vital for both the child and the caregiver. A structured daily schedule helps children with special needs feel secure and can reduce anxiety. For mothers, routines create a sense of order and predictability, making the caregiving responsibilities more manageable. It's important to include time for the child's therapies, recreational activities, and personal care, as well as time for the mother to rest and recharge.

Creating routines for caregivers, whether they are mothers, family members, or professionals, is essential for managing the daily needs of children, individuals with disabilities, and the elderly.

Morning Routine

Gentle Wake-Up & Personal Care (7 AM - 8 AM):

Begin with a calming wake-up, using natural light if possible.

Assist with personal hygiene: brushing teeth, washing face, and dressing.

For individuals with special needs, use visual or verbal cues to guide each step.

Nutritious Breakfast (8 AM - 8:30 AM):

Prepare a balanced breakfast rich in fiber and protein to support energy levels.

Incorporate choices to promote independence (e.g., selecting their cereal).

For elderly individuals, ensure food is easy to chew and swallow.

Mid-Morning Activities

Exercise or Movement (9 AM - 10 AM):

Engage in gentle physical activities like stretching, walking, or seated exercises.

For children, incorporate fun activities like dancing or yoga to improve mood and focus.

Learning or Cognitive Activities (10 AM - 11 AM):

Set aside time for reading, puzzles, or interactive games.

Adapt activities to match the individual's developmental level or cognitive ability.

Afternoon Routine

Lunch & Quiet Time (12 PM - 1 PM):

Serve a healthy lunch with plenty of hydration.

Encourage a rest period or quiet time, which may include reading or listening to soothing music.

Skill-Building or Sensory Activities (2 PM - 3 PM):

Use this time for activities that promote sensory engagement, like arts and crafts, tactile play, or gardening.

Incorporate therapy exercises if applicable (e.g., speech therapy or occupational therapy).

Evening Routine

Family Time & Social Connection (5 PM - 6 PM):
Engage in family activities such as board games, storytelling, or watching a favorite TV show.
For elderly individuals, encourage conversation and reminiscence to foster connection.

Dinner & Wind-Down (6 PM - 7 PM):
Serve a nutritious dinner that is easy to digest. For those with special dietary needs, ensure food is prepared accordingly.
Begin the wind-down process with calming activities like listening to soft music or a short meditation session.

Bedtime Routine

Hygiene & Relaxation (7 PM - 8 PM):
Assist with nightly hygiene, such as bathing, brushing teeth, and changing into comfortable sleepwear.
Incorporate a relaxation technique like reading a bedtime story, deep breathing, or guided imagery.

Consistent Sleep Schedule (8 PM - 9 PM):
Establish a consistent bedtime to promote better sleep quality.

Create a calming environment by dimming lights and minimizing noise. These routines help structure the day, providing stability and predictability, which is especially beneficial for individuals with special needs or cognitive impairments. Flexibility is key, and routines can be adjusted based on energy levels, preferences, or unexpected changes in circumstances.

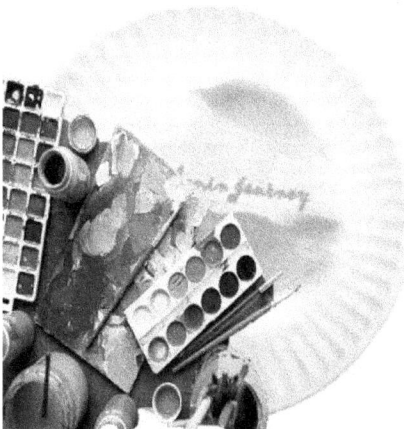

Taking Breaks and Time Away

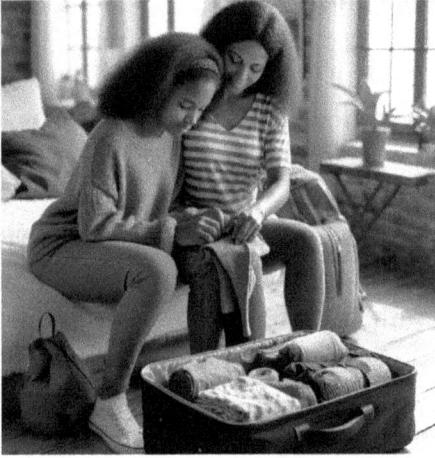

Taking breaks is essential for preventing caregiver burnout. Black mothers should not feel guilty about needing time away from their caregiving duties. Respite care services can provide temporary relief, allowing mothers to address their own needs, whether it's for rest, social activities, or personal hobbies. Family members, friends, and professional caregivers can step in to provide care, ensuring that the child is well looked after while the mother takes a necessary break.

Dealing with Guilt and Feeling Overwhelmed

Feelings of guilt and being overwhelmed are common among caregivers. Black mothers may feel immense pressure to do everything perfectly, often neglecting their own needs. It's important to acknowledge these feelings and seek support through therapy, support groups, or counseling. Remembering that doing one's best is enough, and that taking care of oneself is crucial for being able to care for the child effectively, can help alleviate some of these pressures.

Early Detection and Diagnosis

Monitoring developmental milestones and seeking evaluations.	Pediatricians, developmental specialists, genetic counselors, early intervention programs

Where to Get Help

Accessing local and national organizations, financial assistance, and community connections.	NDSS, local support groups, Medicaid, SSDI

Mental Endurance

Prioritizing mental health through self-care and building a support network.	Meditation, therapy, support from family and friends

Support Groups

Joining groups for emotional and practical support.	Online communities, local support groups

Establishing Routines

Creating structured daily schedules for predictability and security.	Include therapy sessions, recreational activities, and personal care time

Taking Breaks and Time Away

Using respite care services to prevent burnout and address personal needs.	Family members, friends, professional caregivers

Dealing with Guilt and Overwhelm

Acknowledging feelings and seeking support to manage them.	Therapy, counseling, support groups

Spotting and Tracking Early Signs of Autism and Progress

Symptoms	Early Signs	Interventions	Progress Indicators
Communication Difficulties	Limited speech or non-verbal communication, difficulty responding to name, lack of eye contact	Speech therapy, social skills training, dietary changes, probiotics	Improved eye contact, increased verbal communication, social engagement
Repetitive Behaviors	Repetitive movements (e.g., hand-flapping), strict adherence to routines	Behavioral therapy, stress-reduction techniques, dietary modifications	Reduced frequency of repetitive behaviors, flexibility in routines
Sensory Sensitivities	Extreme reactions to sounds, lights, or textures	Sensory integration therapy, mindfulness practices, environmental adjustments	Increased tolerance to sensory stimuli, reduced distress
Gastrointestinal Issues	Chronic constipation, diarrhea, bloating, or abdominal pain	Probiotics, GFCF diet, anti-inflammatory supplements	Improved bowel movements, reduced abdominal discomfort
Sleep Disturbances	Difficulty falling or staying asleep, irregular sleep patterns	Sleep hygiene practices, melatonin supplements, gut-healing diets	More consistent sleep patterns, increased duration of restful sleep

Autism as a Gut/Brain Disorder: Exploring the Connection

Autism Spectrum Disorder (ASD) is a complex neurodevelopmental condition characterized by challenges with social skills, repetitive behaviors, and communication difficulties. In recent years, emerging research has shed light on the potential link between the gut and the brain, often referred to as the "gut-brain axis," in influencing autism. This section explores the role of the gut-brain axis in ASD, the symptoms associated with this connection, mechanisms involved, holistic approaches that may offer new avenues for treatment, and the role of detoxification in gut health.

The Gut-Brain Axis

The gut-brain axis is a bidirectional communication network that connects the gastrointestinal (GI) tract and the brain. This axis involves various systems, including the central nervous system (CNS), the enteric nervous system (ENS), the immune system, and the gut microbiome (the community of microorganisms living in the digestive tract). The gut-brain axis allows for the exchange of information between the brain and the gut, influencing digestion, mood, behavior, and overall health.

Mechanisms of the Gut-Brain Axis in Autism

Several mechanisms illustrate how the gut-brain axis may impact autism: *Microbiome Imbalance (Dysbiosis):* The gut microbiome plays a crucial role in maintaining health, including producing neurotransmitters like serotonin, which affects mood and behavior. Dysbiosis, or an imbalance in gut bacteria, has been linked to autism symptoms such as irritability, anxiety, and gastrointestinal distress. *Gut Inflammation:* Inflammation in the gut can trigger systemic inflammation that impacts the brain. Chronic inflammation is common in individuals with ASD and may contribute to the neurological and behavioral symptoms of the disorder. *Leaky Gut Syndrome:* This condition occurs when the lining of the gut becomes more permeable than normal, allowing toxins and harmful substances to enter the bloodstream.

These substances can cross the blood-brain barrier, potentially affecting brain function and exacerbating autism symptoms. *Vagus Nerve Communication:* The vagus nerve, which runs from the brain to the abdomen, plays a key role in the gut-brain connection. Dysfunction in vagus nerve signaling may lead to disruptions in mood regulation, stress responses, and social behavior, all of which are relevant to autism.

Symptoms of Gut-Brain Dysfunction in Autism

Individuals with autism often experience a range of symptoms that may be linked to gut-brain axis dysfunction: *Gastrointestinal Issues:* Many individuals with ASD suffer from chronic GI problems such as constipation, diarrhea, bloating, and abdominal pain. These issues may be signs of gut-brain axis disruption. *Behavioral Symptoms:* Irritability, anxiety, and aggression are common in autism and may be exacerbated by gut-related issues. For instance, discomfort from GI problems can lead to increased behavioral challenges. *Sensory Sensitivities:* Alterations in the gut-brain axis may influence sensory processing, leading to heightened sensitivity to stimuli like noise, light, and textures. *Sleep Disturbances:* Sleep problems are prevalent in individuals with autism and may be related to gut-brain interactions. Disruptions in the microbiome or vagus nerve signaling can interfere with sleep patterns.

Detoxification of the Gut

Detoxification is an important aspect of restoring gut health and enhancing the function of the gut-brain axis. The buildup of toxins in the body, such as heavy metals, can exacerbate autism symptoms and impact overall well-being. Here are some effective methods for gut detoxification: ***Bentonite Clay:*** Bentonite clay is a natural detoxifier that binds to toxins, including heavy metals, in the digestive tract and removes them from the body. Regular consumption of bentonite clay, under the guidance of a healthcare provider, may support gut health by reducing the toxic load in the body. ***Zeolite:*** Zeolite is a naturally occurring mineral with a unique cage-like structure that traps toxins and heavy metals, facilitating their elimination from the body. Zeolite supplements are often used as part of a detox regimen to support gut and brain health by reducing the burden of harmful substances.

Detox Baths for Autism

Detox baths are a simple yet effective way to support the body's natural detoxification processes, calm the nervous system, and alleviate symptoms associated with autism. The following ingredients can be used in a detox bath regimen: ***Baking Soda:*** Baking soda helps neutralize water and has detoxifying properties that can aid in removing toxins from the skin. It also helps balance the body's pH levels, which is important for maintaining optimal health. ***Epsom Salt:*** Epsom salt is rich in magnesium, a mineral that calms the nervous system, relaxes muscles, and reduces stress. Epsom salt baths can help alleviate irritability and anxiety, which are common in individuals with autism. ***Bentonite Clay:*** Bentonite clay can also be added to bathwater to help pull out heavy metals and other toxins from the skin, further supporting the body's detoxification process.

Healing Approaches

Holistic approaches to managing autism often involve addressing gut health alongside traditional therapies. Some strategies include: **Dietary Interventions:** Many families and practitioners explore gluten-free, casein-free (GFCF) diets, or diets rich in probiotics and prebiotics, to improve gut health. These dietary changes may reduce inflammation and promote a healthier gut microbiome. **Nutritional Supplements:** Supplements such as omega-3 fatty acids, vitamins (e.g., vitamin D, B vitamins), and minerals (e.g., magnesium, zinc) may support brain and gut health. **Probiotics and Prebiotics:** Probiotics (beneficial bacteria) and prebiotics (food for probiotics) can help restore balance in the gut microbiome, potentially improving GI function and reducing autism-related symptoms. **Mind-Body Therapies:** Techniques such as yoga, meditation, and deep-breathing exercises can stimulate the vagus nerve, promoting relaxation and enhancing gut-brain communication. **Environmental and Lifestyle Modifications:** Reducing exposure to toxins, managing stress, and ensuring adequate sleep are essential for supporting overall health and well-being.

? QUESTIONS TO ASK YOUR DOCTOR ?

Are there any gastrointestinal issues that could be contributing to my child's symptoms? *Exploring GI health is crucial in understanding the potential impact of gut dysfunction on autism.*

Can we test for gut dysbiosis or leaky gut syndrome? *These tests can help identify imbalances in the gut that may need addressing.*

Are there specific dietary or supplement recommendations you suggest? *Tailoring dietary changes or supplements to the individual's needs can optimize treatment outcomes.*

What tests can evaluate the integrity of the gut-brain axis? *Tests measuring inflammation markers, vagus nerve function, or neurotransmitter levels may provide insights into gut-brain health.*

How can we incorporate holistic approaches alongside traditional therapies? *Discussing a balanced approach that combines medical treatments with holistic strategies ensures comprehensive care.*

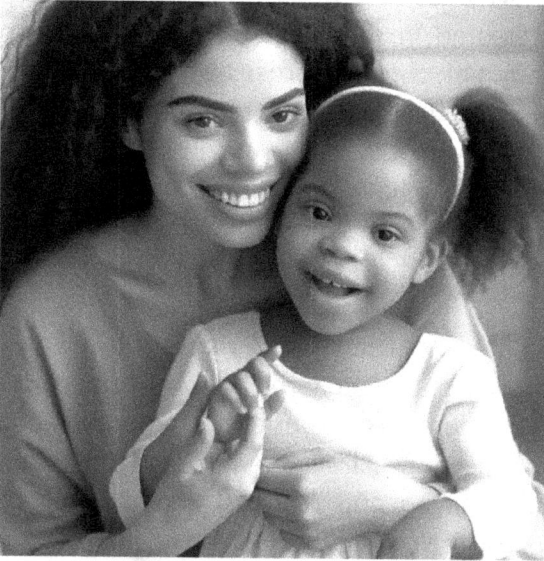

Autism and Methylated Folate Supplements

Autism spectrum disorder (ASD) is a developmental condition that affects communication, behavior, and social interaction. Researchers have been exploring various treatments to help improve symptoms of autism. One area of interest is the use of methylated folate supplements.

Folate is a type of B vitamin that is important for many bodily functions, including DNA production and repair. Methylated folate is a form of folate that the body can easily use. Methylated folate, also known as 5-MTHF or L-methylfolate, is a form of folate that is already in its active form, ready for the body to use. Unlike regular folate, which needs to be converted into its active form by the body, methylated folate can be directly absorbed and utilized. Some people, including those with autism, may have difficulty converting regular folate into its usable form. Methylated folate bypasses this conversion step.

Why Methylated Folate?

Researchers are interested in methylated folate because it can directly enter the body's biochemical processes. This is particularly important for people who have a genetic mutation called MTHFR, which affects their ability to convert folate into its active form. Many individuals with autism have this genetic mutation.

Several studies have looked into whether methylated folate can help improve symptoms of autism.

Improvement in Behavior and Communication

Some studies have shown that children with autism who took methylated folate supplements experienced improvements in behavior and communication skills. Parents reported that their children were more engaged and responsive after starting the supplement. *Reduction in Irritability:* Research also found that methylated folate helped reduce irritability and hyperactivity in some children with autism. This made it easier for them to participate in social activities and learning. *Enhanced Cognitive Function:* There is evidence suggesting that methylated folate might support cognitive functions such as attention, memory, and learning. This is particularly beneficial for children with autism who often face challenges in these areas.

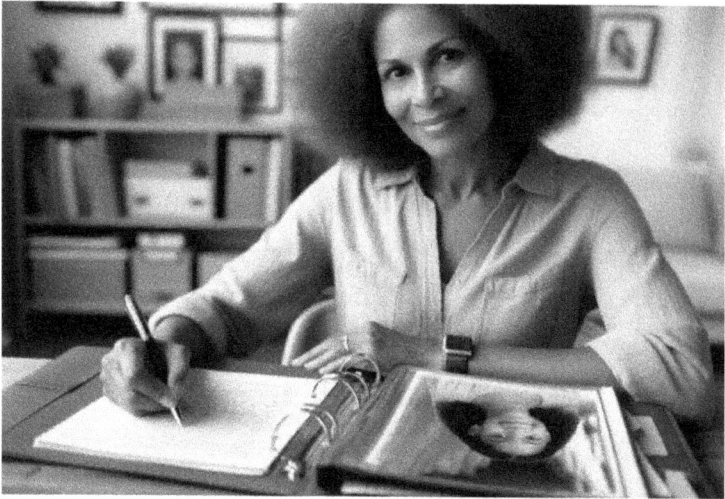

Taking Care of Yourself and Planning for the Future

When you feel overwhelmed, don't hesitate to reach out to family and friends for support. It's important to take breaks to mentally and physically recharge—you are doing an amazing job! Remember, caring for someone with special needs is a significant responsibility, and it's essential to have a plan in place for the future, should anything happen to you.

Create a comprehensive binder that outlines everything about the person's care. Include their daily routines, food preferences, and any specific dietary needs. Document their medical history, including a list of doctors, past treatments, and medications. Note any behavioral patterns, such as what triggers aggressive behavior or what soothes them. Include detailed information on their allergies, sensitivities, and any other health concerns.

In the binder, you should also answer important questions.

What calms them down when they're upset?
How do they communicate discomfort?
What activities do they enjoy?
What are their favorite and least favorite foods?
Do they have specific bedtime routines that help them sleep?
Pertinent medical information

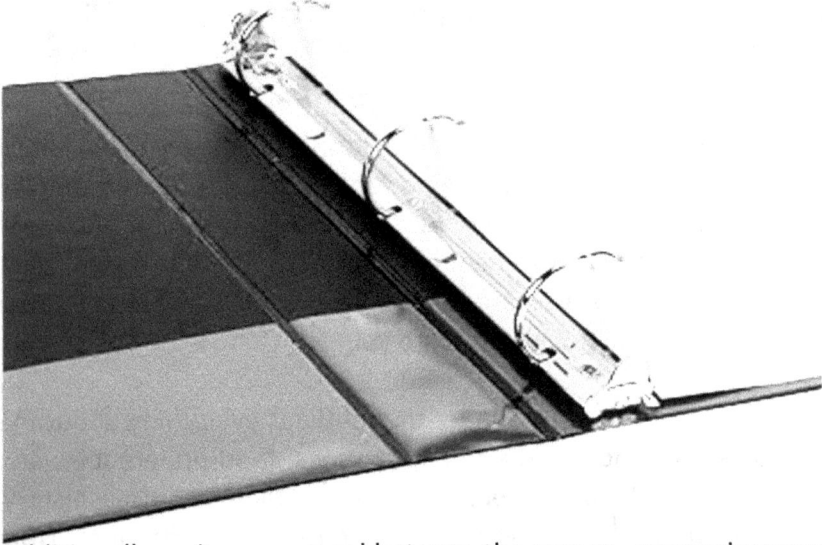

Additionally, write a personal letter to the person, expressing your love and hopes for them. This can be a comforting message for them in your absence. Finally, designate a trusted individual to be their caretaker if you're no longer able to care for them, and ensure that person is aware of and prepared for this responsibility. This binder will be invaluable in ensuring continuity of care and providing peace of mind, knowing that their needs will continue to be met, even in your absence.

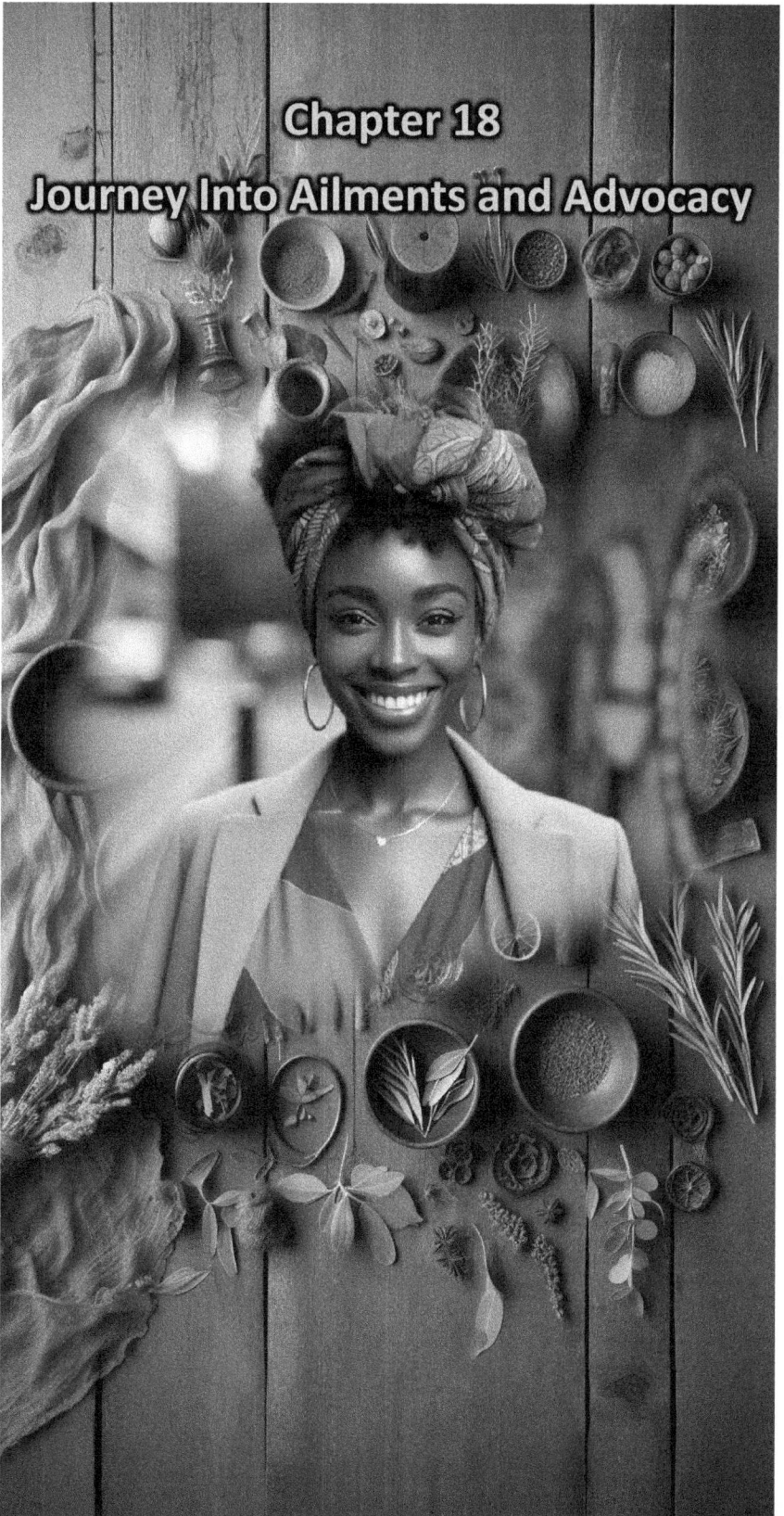

Chapter 18
Journey Into Ailments and Advocacy

Candida Overgrowth in the Body

Candida is a type of yeast that naturally lives in small amounts in the human body, particularly in the mouth, gut, and on the skin. However, when the balance of healthy bacteria in the body is disrupted, Candida can grow out of control, leading to a condition known as candidiasis or Candida overgrowth. This overgrowth can cause various health issues, particularly affecting the digestive system, skin, and mucous membranes.

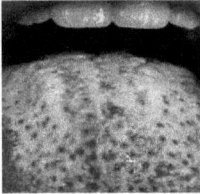

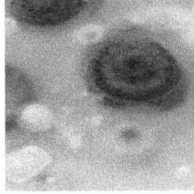

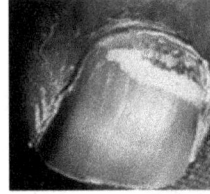

Causes of Candida Overgrowth

Antibiotic Use: Antibiotics can kill off beneficial bacteria in the gut, allowing Candida to multiply unchecked. *High Sugar Diet:* Candida thrives on sugar, so a diet high in refined sugars and carbohydrates can promote its growth. *Weakened Immune System:* A compromised immune system, due to stress, illness, or chronic conditions, can make it easier for Candida to overgrow. *Hormonal Imbalances:* Hormonal changes, such as those during pregnancy, menstruation, or menopause, can disrupt the body's natural balance and encourage Candida growth. *Chronic Stress:* Stress can affect gut health and weaken the immune system, both of which can contribute to Candida overgrowth.

Symptoms of Candida Overgrowth

Digestive Issues: Bloating, gas, constipation, or diarrhea. ***Fatigue:*** Persistent tiredness or brain fog. ***Skin and Nail Fungal Infections:*** Athlete's foot, ringworm, or nail fungus. ***Oral Thrush:*** White patches on the tongue or inside the mouth. ***Recurrent Yeast Infections:*** Frequent vaginal yeast infections, especially with itching, discharge, and discomfort. ***Sugar Cravings:*** Intense cravings for sweets and carbohydrates. ***Mood Swings:*** Irritability, anxiety, or depression. ***Joint Pain:*** Unexplained joint pain or stiffness. ***Sinus Infections:*** Candida fungal infections have been linked to a high percentage of sinus infections. Symptoms include a runny nose, nasal congestion, loss of smell, and headaches.

How Candida Overgrowth Affects African American Women

Candida overgrowth can be particularly challenging for African American women due to potential factors like higher rates of diabetes, which can make the body more susceptible to fungal infections, and the unique microbiome influenced by genetics and diet. Additionally, traditional diets high in refined carbohydrates and sugars can exacerbate Candida growth.

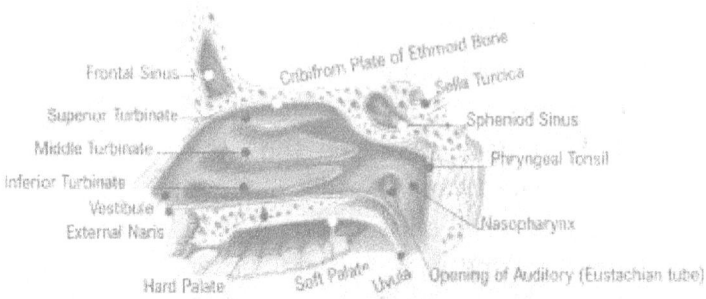

Frontal Sinus — Cribriform Plate of Ethmoid Bone
Sella Turcica
Superior Turbinate — Spheniod Sinus
Middle Turbinate —
Pharyngeal Tonsil
Inferior Turbinate
Vestibule
External Naris — Nasopharynx
Hard Palate — Soft Palate Uvula Opening of Auditory (Eustachian tube)

Candida-Related Sinus Infections

Saline Nasal Rinse with Apple Cider Vinegar A saline rinse helps clear out mucus, allergens, and pathogens from the nasal passages. Adding raw, unfiltered apple cider vinegar (ACV) can help restore the pH balance and provide antifungal properties. *How to Use:* Mix 1/4 teaspoon of sea salt with 1/4 teaspoon of baking soda in a cup of warm distilled water. Add 1 tablespoon of raw ACV. Use a neti pot or nasal syringe to rinse your nasal passages twice daily.

Oregano oil has strong antifungal, antibacterial, and antiviral properties, making it effective against sinus infections caused by Candida. *How to Use:* Mix a few drops of oregano oil with a carrier oil (like coconut oil) and apply it externally to the sinuses (forehead, nose, and cheekbones). Alternatively, you can take oregano oil capsules or add a drop to a glass of water and drink it.

Steam Inhalation with Essential Oils Inhaling steam infused with antifungal essential oils can help open up nasal passages and reduce Candida growth. *How to Use:* Boil water and pour it into a large bowl. Add a few drops of essential oils like eucalyptus, tea tree, or peppermint. Place a towel over your head and lean over the bowl to inhale the steam for 5-10 minutes.

Garlic has potent antifungal and antibacterial properties that can help fight Candida overgrowth and reduce sinus infection symptoms. *How to Use:* Incorporate raw garlic into your diet by adding it to salads, or soups, or taking garlic supplements. You can also create a garlic-infused oil by soaking crushed garlic in olive oil and applying it externally to the sinus areas.

Probiotics can help restore the balance of good bacteria in your gut and sinuses, reducing the chances of Candida overgrowth and subsequent sinus infections. *How to Use:* Take a high-quality probiotic supplement or include fermented foods like yogurt, kefir, sauerkraut, and kimchi in your diet.

Dietary Changes Reducing sugar and refined carbohydrates can help starve Candida and reduce the likelihood of sinus infections. *How to Do It:* Focus on a diet rich in vegetables, lean proteins, healthy fats, and low-sugar fruits. Avoid foods that feed Candida, such as sugars, refined carbs, alcohol, and yeasted bread.

Staying hydrated helps thin mucus, making it easier to clear out from the sinuses, and supports overall immune function. *How to Do It:* Drink plenty of water, herbal teas, and broths throughout the day.

Both **vitamin C and Echinacea** support the immune system and help fight off infections, including those caused by Candida overgrowth. *How to Use:* Take a vitamin C supplement (1000 mg daily) and Echinacea tincture or capsules as directed, particularly during sinus infection flare-ups.

Additional Tips:
Avoid Environmental Triggers: Minimize exposure to mold, dust, and other environmental allergens that can exacerbate sinus infections. *Sleep with a Humidifier:* A humidifier can keep the air moist, reducing irritation in your sinuses and helping mucus drain more easily. *Practice Good Oral Hygiene:* Candida can also thrive in the mouth, so maintaining good oral hygiene can help prevent its spread to the sinuses.

Natural Remedies for Candida Overgrowth

Probiotic Foods: Incorporate fermented foods like sauerkraut, kimchi, kefir, and yogurt into your diet to help restore the balance of good bacteria in the gut. *Apple Cider Vinegar:* Raw, unfiltered apple cider vinegar can help restore the body's pH balance and has antifungal properties. Mix a tablespoon in water and drink before meals. *Garlic:* Garlic is a powerful antifungal agent. Include raw garlic in your diet or take garlic supplements to combat Candida. *Coconut Oil:* Coconut oil contains caprylic acid, which has antifungal properties. Use it in cooking or take a spoonful daily. *Reduce Sugar Intake:* Eliminate refined sugars, alcohol, and processed foods from your diet to starve the Candida. *Herbal Teas:* Drink teas made from antifungal herbs like pau d'arco, oregano, and calendula.

Prevention

Adopt an Anti-Candida Diet: Focus on a diet rich in non-starchy vegetables, lean proteins, and healthy fats while avoiding sugars, refined carbs, and yeast-containing foods. *Boost Immune Health:* Support your immune system with a balanced diet, regular exercise, adequate sleep, and stress management techniques. *Consult a Healthcare Provider:* If symptoms persist, consult a healthcare provider, preferably one familiar with holistic and integrative approaches, to ensure proper diagnosis and treatment.

Common and Little-Known Diseases and Conditions

Black women face unique health challenges due to genetic, socioeconomic, and cultural factors. Understanding these conditions, advocating for proper care, and knowing the right tests to request from healthcare providers can improve health outcomes. Additionally, incorporating herbal remedies can offer complementary support.

Sickle Cell Disease

Sickle cell disease (SCD) is a genetic disorder prevalent among Black women, characterized by abnormally shaped red blood cells that can cause blockages in blood flow. Sickle cell disease (SCD) affects hemoglobin in red blood cells, causing them to take on a sickle shape. These cells can get stuck in small blood vessels, leading to pain, organ damage, and increased risk of infection. Symptoms include severe pain (often referred to as sickle cell crises), fatigue, and frequent infections.

Sickle Cell Disease Advocacy and Testing Advocate for yourself by asking your physician for a hemoglobin electrophoresis test to confirm the diagnosis. Regular blood tests, such as complete blood counts (CBCs), are essential for monitoring health. Discuss pain management options and infection prevention strategies with your healthcare provider.

Sickle Cell Disease Herbalist Information
Herbs such as *nettle leaf* and *red clover* can help improve blood quality. *Burdock root* is known for its detoxifying properties, which can support overall health. Always consult with a healthcare provider before starting any herbal treatments.

Heart Problems

Black women are at higher risk for cardiovascular diseases, including hypertension, heart disease, and stroke. Symptoms can include chest pain, shortness of breath, palpitations, and fatigue. **Heart Problems Advocacy and Testing** Request regular screenings for blood pressure, cholesterol levels, and blood glucose levels. An electrocardiogram (ECG) and echocardiogram can help detect heart abnormalities. Discuss family history and risk factors with your physician. **Heart Problems Herbalist Information** Herbs like hawthorn berry and garlic can support heart health by improving circulation and reducing blood pressure. *Ginger* is also beneficial for its anti-inflammatory properties.

Scoliosis

Scoliosis a condition characterized by an abnormal curvature of the spine, can affect Black women, causing back pain, uneven shoulders, and noticeable spinal curvature. **Scoliosis Advocacy and Testing** Ask your physician for a physical examination and X-rays to diagnose scoliosis. For severe cases, an MRI may be needed. Physical therapy and regular monitoring are crucial for managing this condition. **Scoliosis Herbalist Information** Turmeric and willow bark are known for their anti-inflammatory properties, which can help manage pain. *Boswellia* may also provide relief from inflammation and pain.

Diabetes

Black women are disproportionately affected by Type 2 diabetes. Symptoms include increased thirst, frequent urination, extreme fatigue, and slow-healing sores. **Diabetes Advocacy and Testing** Request regular blood glucose tests, including fasting blood sugar and HbA1c tests, to monitor and manage diabetes. Discuss lifestyle changes and medication options with your healthcare provider. **Diabetes Herbalist Information** *Bitter melon, fenugreek*, and *cinnamon* can help regulate blood sugar levels. Always consult with a healthcare provider before incorporating these into your regimen.

Breast Cancer

Black women are at higher risk for aggressive forms of breast cancer. Symptoms can include lumps, changes in breast shape, and nipple discharge. **Breast Cancer Advocacy and Testing** Request regular mammograms and breast exams, especially if you have a family history of breast cancer. Genetic testing for BRCA1 and BRCA2 mutations can also be discussed. **Breast Cancer Herbalist Information** *Green tea, flaxseed,* and *curcumin* (from turmeric) have been studied for their potential anti-cancer properties.

Anemia

Anemia is a common condition among Black women, often exacerbated by heavy menstrual bleeding. Symptoms include fatigue, dizziness, and pale skin. One peculiar symptom associated with anemia is the craving for ice, known as pagophagia. This craving can be a sign of iron deficiency, which requires medical attention. **Anemia Advocacy and Testing** Request a complete blood count (CBC) and ferritin test to check for iron levels. If anemia is detected, discuss treatment options with your healthcare provider, including iron supplements and dietary changes. **Anemia Herbalist Information** Herbs such as nettles and *yellow dock root* are rich in iron and can help improve anemia. *Dandelion root* can also support iron absorption.

Sickle Cell Disease
Symptoms Severe pain, anemia, infections
Common Tests Hemoglobin electrophoresis, CBC
Natural Rememdies Nettle leaf, red clover, burdock root

Heart Disease
Symptoms Chest pain, shortness of breath
Common Tests Blood pressure, cholesterol, ECG, echo
Natural Rememdies Hawthorn berry, garlic, ginger

Diabetes
Symptoms Increased thirst, frequent urination
Common Tests Fasting blood sugar, HbA1c
Natural Rememdies Bitter melon, fenugreek, cinnamon

Breast Cancer
Symptoms Lumps, breast shape changes
Common Tests Mammogram, BRCA1/BRCA2 genetic tests
Natural Rememdies Green tea, flaxseed, curcumin

Scoliosis
Symptoms Back pain, uneven shoulders
Common Tests Physical exam, X-ray, MRIn
Natural Rememdies Turmeric, willow bark, Boswellia

Genetic Diseases and Conditions

Autoimmune diseases are conditions in which the body's immune system mistakenly attacks its own tissues. While these diseases can affect anyone, Black women are at a higher risk for certain autoimmune disorders that are often rare, underdiagnosed, or misdiagnosed. Understanding these diseases, their symptoms, and the appropriate tests to request is crucial for accurate diagnosis and effective treatment. Additionally, a holistic approach that includes natural remedies can be beneficial in managing these conditions.

Constant Unexplained Pain: Fibromyalgia and Related Conditions
One of the most challenging autoimmune-related conditions that Black women may face is fibromyalgia, a disorder characterized by widespread, constant, and unexplained pain throughout the body. This condition is often misunderstood and misdiagnosed because its symptoms overlap with other disorders such as chronic fatigue syndrome and rheumatoid arthritis.

Symptoms
Persistent pain in muscles, ligaments, and tendons, Fatigue and sleep disturbances, Cognitive difficulties (often referred to as "fibro fog"), Sensitivity to touch, light, and sound

!TESTS TO REQUEST!
Tender Point Exam: A physical exam where the doctor checks for specific tender points on the body. Thyroid Function Tests: To rule out hypothyroidism, which can cause similar symptoms. Complete Blood Count (CBC): To check for anemia or other blood-related issues. Vitamin D Levels: Low levels can contribute to muscle pain and fatigue.

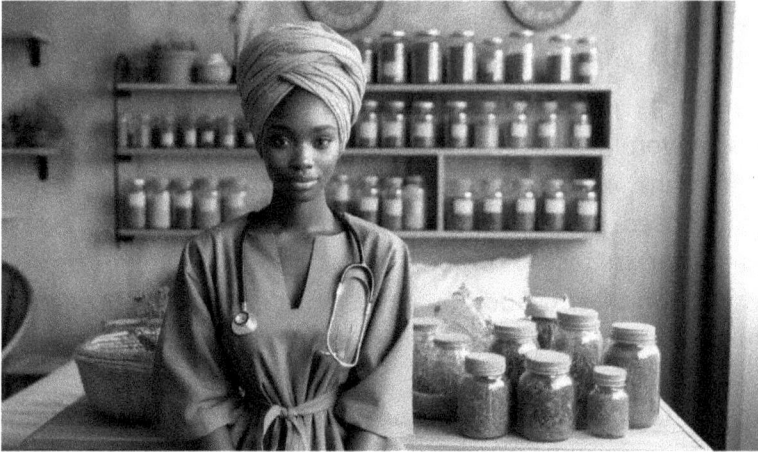

Natural Treatments

Anti-inflammatory Diet Incorporate foods rich in omega-3 fatty acids, such as flaxseeds and walnuts, as well as plenty of fruits and vegetables. Avoid processed foods and sugars that can increase inflammation. *Herbal Remedies:* Turmeric and ginger have anti-inflammatory properties that can help reduce pain. *Mind-Body Practices:* Yoga, tai chi, and meditation can help manage pain and improve sleep quality. *Acupuncture:* This traditional Chinese medicine technique may relieve pain by balancing the body's energy flow.

Unexplained Fainting: Vasovagal Syncope and Dysautonomia

Vasovagal syncope and dysautonomia are conditions that can cause sudden fainting spells, which are often misdiagnosed as anxiety or other psychological disorders. These conditions affect the autonomic nervous system, which controls involuntary body functions such as heart rate and blood pressure.

Symptoms

Sudden fainting, often triggered by stress, pain, or standing for long periods, Dizziness and lightheadedness, Nausea and sweating before fainting, Rapid or irregular heartbeat.

!TESTS TO REQUEST!

Tilt Table Test: To assess how your body responds to changes in position, which can trigger fainting. Electrocardiogram (EKG): To check for heart-related issues that could cause fainting. Holter Monitor: A portable device worn for 24-48 hours to monitor heart activity and detect irregularities. Blood Tests: To check for electrolyte imbalances or other metabolic issues.

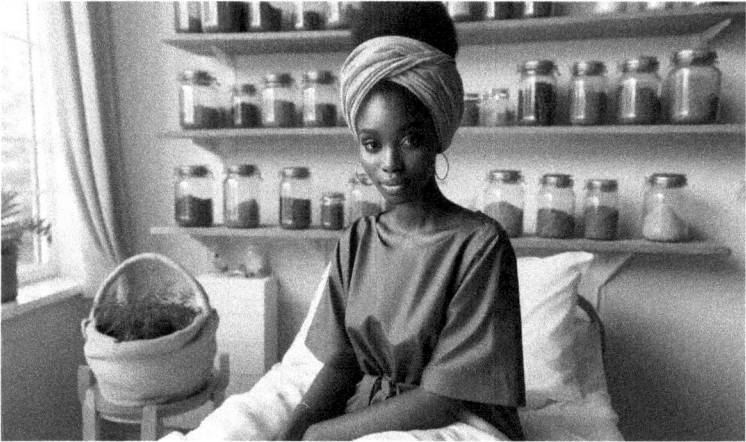

Holistic Natural Treatments

Hydration and Salt Intake: Increase water and salt intake to maintain blood pressure and prevent fainting spells. *Herbal Teas:* Ginseng tea can support the nervous system and improve circulation, reducing the likelihood of fainting. *Compression Stockings:* Wearing compression stockings can help improve blood flow and prevent blood from pooling in the legs, reducing the risk of fainting. *Breathing Exercises:* Practicing deep breathing can help manage stress and prevent the onset of a vasovagal response.

Advocating for a Diagnosis

Due to the rarity and complexity of these conditions, Black women are often misdiagnosed or dismissed when they report symptoms. Advocacy is crucial in navigating the healthcare system to obtain a proper diagnosis. Here's how to effectively advocate for yourself.

Document Your Symptoms Keep a detailed record of your symptoms, including when they occur, their intensity, and any potential triggers. This documentation can provide your healthcare provider with a clearer picture of what you are experiencing.

Research and Educate Yourself Learn about the possible conditions that could be causing your symptoms. Familiarize yourself with the tests that are available and appropriate for your situation.

Ask Specific Questions When meeting with your doctor, ask direct questions about the possibility of rare autoimmune diseases. Inquire about specific tests like the Tilt Table Test for fainting or the Tender Point Exam for fibromyalgia.

Seek a Second Opinion If you feel that your symptoms are not being taken seriously or that your concerns are being dismissed, don't hesitate to seek a second opinion. Consulting with a specialist who has experience with autoimmune diseases might lead to more accurate diagnosis and treatment.

Be Persistent It's essential to be persistent in your pursuit of answers. If initial tests come back normal, but your symptoms persist, request further testing or alternative approaches. Your health is too important to be left to guesswork.

Consider Holistic and Natural Therapies While seeking a medical diagnosis, also explore holistic and natural therapies that can support your health. These therapies may not only alleviate symptoms but also contribute to overall well-being while you continue to seek a definitive diagnosis.

? QUESTIONS TO ASK YOUR DOCTOR ?

Could my symptoms be related to an autoimmune disorder?
What tests can we run to rule out conditions like fibromyalgia, dysautonomia, or thyroid dysfunction?
Are there any lifestyle changes or natural treatments that can support my treatment plan?
How can we monitor my condition over time to adjust my care as needed?

Fibromyalgia

Symptoms Persistent body pain, fatigue, sleep disturbances, cognitive difficulties, sensitivity to touch
Common Tender Point Exam, Thyroid Function Tests, Complete Blood Count (CBC), Vitamin D Levels
Herbal Turmeric, Ginger, Omega-3-rich foods (flaxseeds, walnuts), Yoga, Acupuncture

Vasovagal Syncope

Symptoms Sudden fainting, dizziness, lightheadedness, nausea, sweating, irregular heartbeat
Common Tests Tilt Table Test, Electrocardiogram (EKG), Holter Monitor, Blood Tests
Herbal Remedies Ginseng tea, Increased hydration, Salt intake, Compression stockings, Deep breathing exercises.

Dysautonomia
Symptoms Similar to Vasovagal Syncope, with added symptoms of heart palpitations, digestive issues, fatigue
Common Tests Tilt Table Test, Electrocardiogram (EKG), Autonomic Testing, Blood Tests
Herbal Remedies Adaptogenic herbs (Ashwagandha, Rhodiola), Hydration, Breathing exercises, Ginger

Thyroid Dysfunction
Symptoms Fatigue, weight changes, muscle weakness, sensitivity to cold, depression
Common Tests Thyroid Function Tests (TSH, T3, T4), CBC, Ultrasound of the Thyroid
Herbal Remedies Bladderwrack, Selenium-rich foods (Brazil nuts), Omega-3 fatty acids, Ashwagandha, Iodine-rich foods (seaweed)

Dysautonomia Types
(POTS) Postural Orthostatic Tachycardia Syndrome
(FD) Familial dysautonomia
(IST) Inappropriate Sinus Tachycardia
(AAG) Autoimmune Autonomic Ganglionopathy
Reflex Syndromes
(PAF) Pure Autonomic Failure
(OI) Orthostatic Intolerance
(DBHD) Dopamine Beta-Hydroxylase Deficiency
(MSA) Multiple System Atrophy
(NCS) Neurocardiogenic Syncope
(NMH) Neurally Mediated Hypotension
(VS) Vasovagal Syncope
Chronic Fatigue Syndrome
(nOH) Neurogenic Orthostatic Hypotension
Carotid Sinus Hypersensitivity Syndrome
Orthostatic hypotension | Vasovagal syncope
Pure autonomic failure | Multiple system atrophy

The Health Benefits of Lysine

Lysine, an essential amino acid, plays a pivotal role in numerous bodily functions and health practices. Unlike non-essential amino acids, lysine cannot be synthesized by the human body and must be obtained through diet or supplementation. This section delves into the multifaceted benefits of lysine, its role in maintaining overall health, the symptoms and consequences of deficiencies, natural dietary sources presented in a detailed chart, and its significant impact on managing genital herpes. Additionally, we explore lesser-known aspects of lysine that highlight its importance in holistic healing.

What is Lysine?

Lysine, scientifically known as ε-lysine, is one of the nine essential amino acids required for human health. Amino acids are the building blocks of proteins, which are crucial for the structure, function, and regulation of the body's tissues and organs. Lysine is particularly important for growth, tissue repair, and the production of enzymes and hormones.

Biochemically, lysine is involved in the synthesis of collagen, which is vital for skin, bone, and connective tissue health. It also aids in calcium absorption, plays a role in energy production, and supports immune function. Given its essential status, ensuring adequate lysine intake is fundamental for maintaining optimal health and preventing various deficiency-related conditions.

Health Benefits of Lysine

Lysine offers a wide array of health benefits that contribute to both physical and mental well-being.

Protein Synthesis and Muscle Growth Lysine is integral to the synthesis of proteins, facilitating muscle repair and growth. This makes it particularly beneficial for athletes and individuals engaged in regular physical activity.

Bone Health By enhancing calcium absorption, lysine supports bone density and strength, reducing the risk of osteoporosis and fractures.

Collagen Formation Lysine is essential for collagen production, which maintains the integrity of skin, hair, nails, and connective tissues. This contributes to youthful skin and overall structural health.

Immune System Support Lysine boosts the immune system by promoting the production of antibodies and enzymes that defend against infections and illnesses.

Hormone and Enzyme Production Lysine is involved in the synthesis of hormones such as insulin, which regulates blood sugar levels, and various enzymes that facilitate biochemical reactions in the body.

Energy Production Lysine plays a role in converting fatty acids into energy, thereby supporting metabolic processes and maintaining energy levels throughout the day.

Anxiety and Stress Reduction Emerging research suggests that lysine may help reduce anxiety and stress by modulating the body's stress response systems, including cortisol levels.

Cardiovascular Health Lysine may contribute to cardiovascular health by preventing the buildup of certain fats in the arteries, thus reducing the risk of atherosclerosis and heart disease.

Symptoms and Deficiencies of Lysine

A deficiency in lysine can lead to a range of health issues, given its involvement in critical bodily functions. Common symptoms and consequences of lysine deficiency include:

Fatigue and Weakness Insufficient lysine can result in reduced energy levels, leading to persistent fatigue and muscle weakness.

Anemia Lysine deficiency may impair the production of hemoglobin, the protein in red blood cells that carries oxygen, potentially leading to anemia.

Hair Loss Collagen synthesis is essential for hair health. A lack of lysine can contribute to thinning hair and increased hair loss.

Delayed Growth in Children Adequate lysine intake is crucial for proper growth and development in children. Deficiency can hinder height and overall physical development.

Reproductive Issues Lysine plays a role in reproductive health. Deficiency may lead to menstrual irregularities and fertility issues.

Poor Calcium Absorption Without sufficient lysine, the body struggles to absorb calcium effectively, increasing the risk of bone-related conditions.

Weakened Immune Function A deficient lysine level can compromise the immune system, making the body more susceptible to infections and illnesses.

Mental Health Concerns Low lysine levels have been linked to increased anxiety and stress, as lysine influences neurotransmitter regulation and stress response mechanisms.

Natural Food Sources of Lysine

Incorporating lysine-rich foods into the diet is essential for preventing deficiencies and harnessing its health benefits. The following chart details natural food sources high in lysine, along with their lysine content and additional health benefits.

Food Source	Lysine Content (mg per 100g)	Additional Health Benefits
Lean Beef	2,500	High in iron, zinc, and vitamin B12
Chicken Breast	2,300	Rich in protein, niacin, and selenium
Salmon	2,100	High in omega-3 fatty acids, vitamin D
Eggs	880	Contains vitamins B2, B12, and choline
Quinoa	1,100	Complete protein, high in fiber and magnesium
Lentils	1,300	Rich in fiber, folate, and iron
Cheese (Parmesan)	2,700	High in calcium, phosphorus, and vitamin A
Pumpkin Seeds	900	Good source of magnesium, iron, and antioxidants
Tofu	900	Plant-based protein, contains calcium and iron
Greek Yogurt	1,000	High in probiotics, calcium, and potassium
Soybeans	2,100	High in protein, fiber, and essential vitamins
Spirulina	2,700	Rich in vitamins, minerals, and antioxidants
Black Beans	1,200	High in fiber, folate, and antioxidants
Turkey Breast	2,400	Lean protein, rich in selenium and vitamin B6
Edamame	1,800	High in protein, fiber, and essential vitamins

Lysine and Genital Herpes

One of the most well-documented benefits of lysine is its role in managing and preventing genital herpes outbreaks. Genital herpes, caused by the herpes simplex virus (HSV), is a common viral infection characterized by recurrent sores and blisters.

Mechanism of Action

Lysine interferes with the replication of the herpes simplex virus by inhibiting the enzyme arginase, which is necessary for the virus to multiply. By competing with arginine (another amino acid that promotes viral replication), lysine effectively reduces the frequency and severity of herpes outbreaks.

Clinical Evidence

Numerous studies have demonstrated that lysine supplementation can decrease the number of herpes episodes and shorten their duration. Regular intake of lysine has been associated with fewer and less severe outbreaks, making it a valuable adjunct in herpes management.

Dosage and Usage

For individuals with frequent herpes outbreaks, a daily dosage of 1,000 mg to 3,000 mg of lysine is commonly recommended. It is advisable to consult with a healthcare professional before starting any supplementation regimen to determine the appropriate dosage based on individual health needs.

Additional Benefits for Herpes Patients

Beyond reducing outbreaks, lysine may help alleviate associated symptoms such as pain and inflammation, improving the overall quality of life for those affected by genital herpes. Additionally, lysine supports immune function, which is crucial for the body's ability to fight off viral infections.

Benefits of Lysine

Lysine's impact extends beyond its immediate physiological roles, contributing to health in various ways:

Enhanced Mental Well-being Lysine supports the production of serotonin, a neurotransmitter that regulates mood. By promoting serotonin synthesis, lysine can help alleviate symptoms of depression and anxiety, fostering emotional balance.

Skin Health Through its role in collagen production, lysine contributes to skin elasticity and wound healing. It aids in the repair of damaged skin tissues, reducing scarring and promoting a healthy complexion.

Bone Strength Lysine's facilitation of calcium absorption is crucial for maintaining strong bones and preventing osteoporosis, especially in aging populations.

Athletic Performance For athletes and active individuals, lysine supports muscle recovery and growth, enhancing physical performance and reducing the risk of injuries.

Cardiovascular Health Lysine may help lower cholesterol levels and reduce the risk of heart disease by preventing the buildup of plaque in the arteries.

Immune Enhancement By boosting immune function, lysine helps the body defend against infections and illnesses, contributing to overall resilience and health.

Anti-Inflammatory Properties Lysine exhibits anti-inflammatory effects, which can help manage chronic inflammatory conditions and promote overall well-being.

Little-Known Information About Lysine

While lysine is widely recognized for its role in protein synthesis and herpes management, several lesser-known aspects highlight its comprehensive benefits:

Lysine and Anxiety Emerging research suggests that lysine may play a role in reducing anxiety by modulating serotonin and cortisol levels, offering a natural approach to managing stress.

Lysine for Collagen Synthesis Beyond general skin health, lysine is essential for the formation of collagen fibers, which are critical for the structural integrity of tendons, ligaments, and cartilage.

Lysine in Fertility Lysine has been linked to improved fertility in both men and women by supporting reproductive health and hormone balance.

Lysine and Iron Absorption Lysine enhances the absorption of iron from plant-based foods, helping to prevent iron-deficiency anemia, particularly in vegetarians and vegans.

Lysine's Role in Metabolism Lysine is involved in the synthesis of carnitine, a nutrient responsible for converting fatty acids into energy, thus supporting metabolic health and energy levels.

High-Fructose Corn Syrup (HFCS) vs. Lysine

While lysine supports various aspects of health, high-fructose corn syrup (HFCS) poses significant risks. Understanding the contrast between these two substances highlights the importance of mindful dietary choices: HFCS is an additive commonly found in processed foods and beverages. Unlike lysine, HFCS is associated with numerous health issues, including obesity, diabetes, and heart disease. Its high sugar content leads to rapid blood sugar spikes and crashes, fostering addiction-like cravings and contributing to metabolic imbalances.

In contrast, lysine is an essential nutrient that supports metabolic processes, muscle growth, and immune function. It promotes overall health without the detrimental effects associated with excessive sugar consumption.

Sugar, HFCS, and Links to Chronic Disease

Excessive consumption of sugar and HFCS has been linked to various physical and mental health disorders, particularly affecting the Black community in America:

Obesity and Metabolic Syndrome High intake of HFCS contributes to excessive calorie consumption, leading to weight gain and metabolic syndrome, a cluster of conditions that increase the risk of heart disease, stroke, and diabetes.

Type 2 Diabetes HFCS consumption is closely linked to the development of insulin resistance, a precursor to type 2 diabetes. This condition is prevalent in the Black community, exacerbating existing health disparities.

Cardiovascular Diseases High sugar intake, especially from HFCS, elevates triglyceride levels and blood pressure, increasing the risk of cardiovascular diseases, including hypertension and heart attacks.

Liver Disease Excessive fructose from HFCS overloads the liver, leading to non-alcoholic fatty liver disease (NAFLD), which can progress to more severe liver conditions.

Mental Health Disorders There is growing evidence that high sugar consumption can affect brain health, contributing to mood disorders such as depression and anxiety. Sugar-induced inflammation may impair cognitive function and emotional regulation.

Addiction and Behavioral Issues The addictive nature of sugar can lead to compulsive eating behaviors, mood swings, and decreased self-control, impacting overall mental well-being and quality of life.

Lysine

Essential amino acids
It is necessary for a healthy body
Get lysine from foods
The body cannot make Lysine

L-lysine

Little-Known Information About Lysine

While lysine is widely recognized for its role in protein synthesis and herpes management, several lesser-known aspects highlight its comprehensive benefits:

Lysine and Anxiety Emerging research suggests that lysine may play a role in reducing anxiety by modulating serotonin and cortisol levels, offering a natural approach to managing stress.

Lysine for Collagen Synthesis Beyond general skin health, lysine is essential for the formation of collagen fibers, which are critical for the structural integrity of tendons, ligaments, and cartilage.

Lysine in Fertility Lysine has been linked to improved fertility in both men and women by supporting reproductive health and hormone balance.

Lysine and Iron Absorption Lysine enhances the absorption of iron from plant-based foods, helping to prevent iron-deficiency anemia, particularly in vegetarians and vegans.

Lysine's Role in Metabolism Lysine is involved in the synthesis of carnitine, a nutrient responsible for converting fatty acids into energy, thus supporting metabolic health and energy levels.

Lysine stands out as a vital amino acid with profound health benefits, from supporting muscle growth and bone health to enhancing immune function and managing genital herpes. Its role in overall well-being underscores the importance of adequate lysine intake through diet or supplementation. Conversely, the pervasive consumption of sugar and high-fructose corn syrup poses significant health risks, particularly within the Black community, contributing to chronic diseases and mental health challenges.

Understanding the stark contrast between the essential benefits of lysine and the detrimental effects of excessive sugar intake highlights the need for mindful dietary choices. By embracing natural alternatives, incorporating lysine-rich foods, and utilizing natural remedies to counteract the effects of sugar and HFCS, individuals can promote health and mitigate the adverse impacts of modern dietary practices.

Lysine-Rich Foods and Their Health Benefits

Food Source	Lysine (mg per100g)	Additional Health Benefits
Lean Beef	2,500	High in iron, zinc, and vitamin B12
Chicken Breast	2,300	Rich in protein, niacin, and selenium
Salmon	2,100	High in omega-3 fatty acids, vitamin D
Eggs	880	Contains vitamins B2, B12, and choline
Quinoa	1,100	Complete protein, high in fiber and magnesium
Lentils	1,300	Rich in fiber, folate, and iron
Cheese (Parmesan)	2,700	High in calcium, phosphorus, and vitamin A
Pumpkin Seeds	900	Good source of magnesium, iron, and antioxidants
Tofu	900	Plant-based protein, contains calcium and iron
Greek Yogurt	1,000	High in probiotics, calcium, and potassium
Soybeans	2,100	High in protein, fiber, and essential vitamins
Spirulina	2,700	Rich in vitamins, minerals, and antioxidants
Black Beans	1,200	High in fiber, folate, and antioxidants
Turkey Breast	2,400	Lean protein, rich in selenium and vitamin B6
Edamame	1,800	High in protein, fiber, and essential vitamins

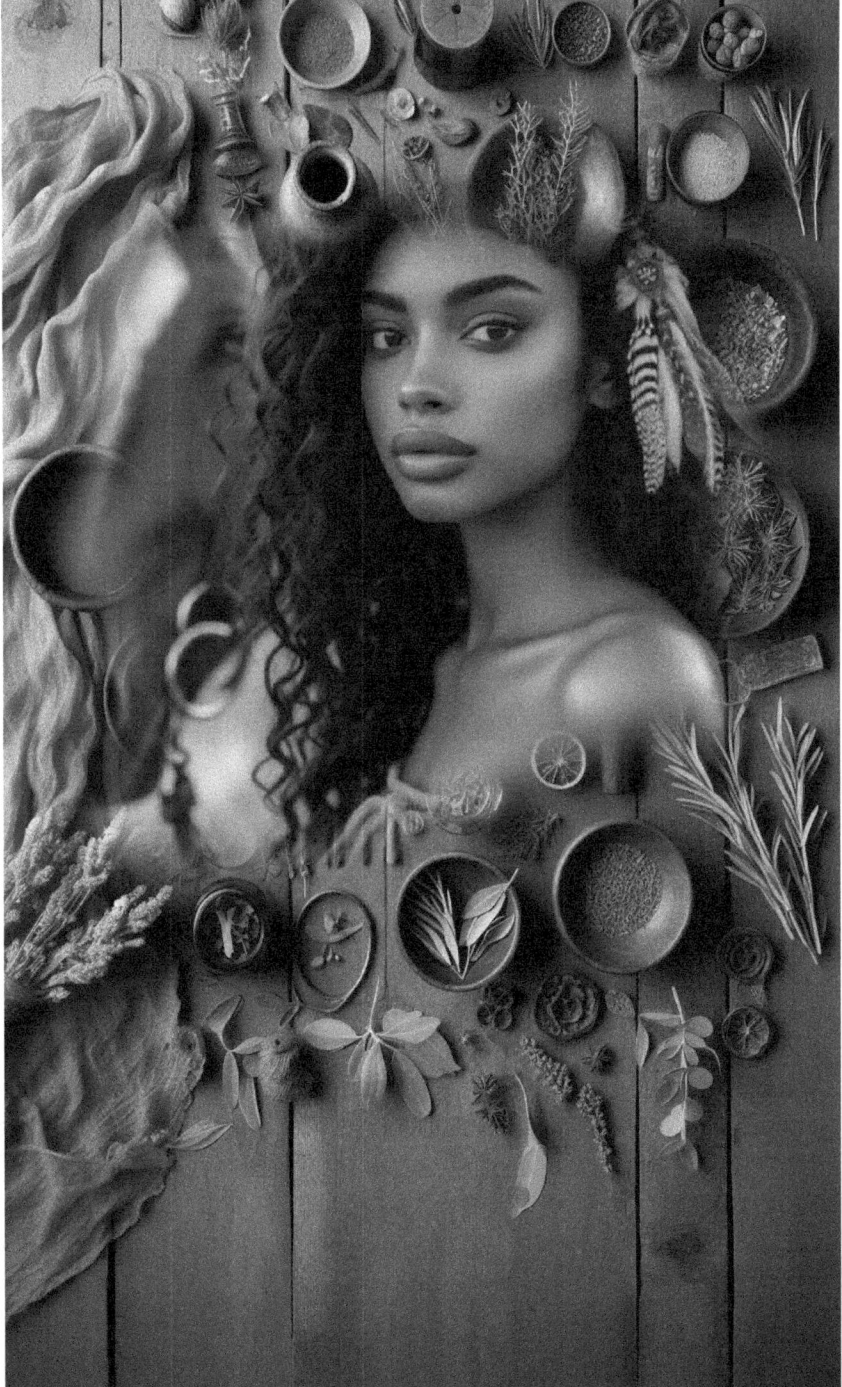

Chapter 19
Journey Into Understanding Diabetes

Prevalence and Impact of Diabetes

African Americans are disproportionately affected by diabetes. According to the Centers for Disease Control and Prevention (CDC), African Americans are 60% more likely than non-Hispanic whites to be diagnosed with diabetes. Additionally, they are more likely to suffer from complications such as kidney failure, amputations, and blindness. *Socioeconomic and Genetic Factors* Several factors contribute to this disparity, including socioeconomic status, access to healthcare, and genetic predispositions. High rates of obesity and hypertension, which are prevalent in the African American community, also increase the risk of developing diabetes.

Types of Diabetes

Type 1 Diabetes Type 1 diabetes is an autoimmune condition where the body attacks insulin-producing cells in the pancreas. It is less common but can occur at any age. *Type 2 Diabetes* Type 2 diabetes is the most common form and occurs when the body becomes resistant to insulin or when the pancreas cannot produce enough insulin. Lifestyle factors, such as diet and physical activity, play a significant role in its development. **Gestational Diabetes** Gestational diabetes occurs during pregnancy and can increase the risk of developing type 2 diabetes later in life. African American women have a higher incidence of gestational diabetes compared to other groups.

Symptoms and Complications

Common symptoms of diabetes include frequent urination, excessive thirst, extreme fatigue, blurry vision, and slow-healing wounds. Recognizing these symptoms early can lead to timely diagnosis and treatment. **Complications** Diabetes can lead to severe complications, including cardiovascular disease, nerve damage (neuropathy), kidney disease (nephropathy), eye damage (retinopathy), and increased risk of infections. These complications highlight the importance of effective management and control of the condition.

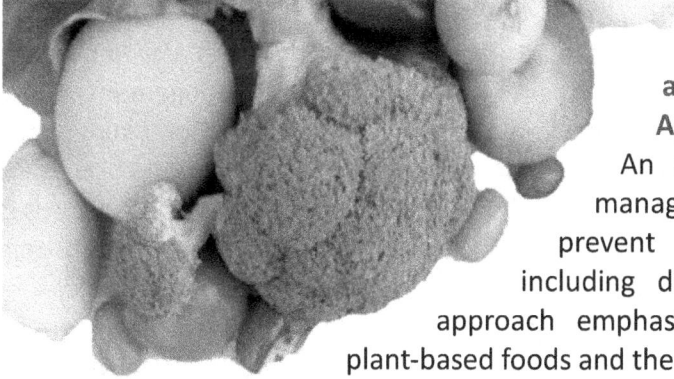

Holistic and Herbal Approaches An alkaline diet manages and prevent diseases, including diabetes. The approach emphasizes natural, plant-based foods and the avoidance of processed foods and animal products. **Alkaline Diet** The alkaline diet includes a variety of fruits, vegetables, nuts, seeds, and grains that are believed to reduce acidity in the body and promote overall health.

Key components to an Alkaline Diet

Vegetables: Leafy greens, cucumbers, and squash.

Fruits: Berries, apples, and bananas.

Grains: Amaranth, quinoa, and wild rice.

Herbs: Burdock root, dandelion root, and sarsaparilla.

Recommended Specific Herbs For Managing Diabetes

Burdock Root: Known for its blood-purifying properties and ability to lower blood sugar levels.

Dandelion Root: Supports liver health and detoxification.

Sarsaparilla: Rich in iron, which is crucial for those with diabetes-related anemia.

Role of Blood Type in Diabetes Management

Blood Type and Diet There is an ongoing debate about the influence of blood type on diet and disease management. Some theories suggest that individuals with different blood types may benefit from specific dietary plans.

For individuals with blood type A, a diet rich in plant-based foods is recommended which emphasizes vegetables, fruits, and whole grains. Foods such as tofu, legumes, and green vegetables are beneficial for blood type A individuals and can help manage diabetes by improving insulin sensitivity and reducing inflammation.

Prevention and Management Strategies Lifestyle

Adopting a balanced, nutrient-rich diet that focuses on whole foods, such as fruits, vegetables, lean proteins, and whole grains, is crucial. Avoiding processed foods and sugars can help control blood sugar levels. **Physical Activity:** Regular exercise helps maintain a healthy weight, improve insulin sensitivity, and reduce the risk of complications. **Weight Management:** Maintaining a healthy weight through diet and exercise is key to preventing and managing diabetes.

Medical Treatments

Oral medications and insulin therapy are commonly prescribed to manage blood sugar levels. It's important to follow the treatment plan recommended by healthcare professionals. **Regular Monitoring:** Frequent monitoring of blood sugar levels helps track progress and adjust treatment plans as necessary.

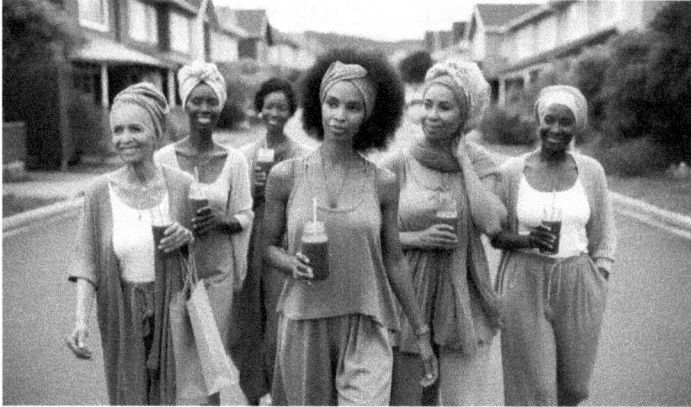

Testing for Diabetes and Advocating for Your Health

Detecting and managing diabetes requires proper testing, effective communication with healthcare providers, and informed self-care practices. This section outlines the tests for diagnosing diabetes, questions to ask your doctor, understanding normal ranges, and essential at-home care tips.

Fasting Plasma Glucose (FPG) Test

Measures blood sugar levels after an overnight fast. This test is commonly used to diagnose diabetes and prediabetes.

Procedure	No food or drink (except water) for at least 8 hours before the test
Normal Range	Less than 100 mg/dL
Prediabetes Range	100 to 125 mg/dL
Diabetes Range	126 mg/dL or higher on two separate tests

Oral Glucose Tolerance Test (OGTT)

Measures blood sugar levels before and after consuming a glucose-rich drink. It is particularly used to diagnose gestational diabetes.

Procedure	Fasting overnight, followed by drinking a glucose solution, with blood sugar levels measured at intervals.
Normal Range	Less than 140 mg/dL after 2 hours
Prediabetes Range	140 to 199 mg/dL after 2 hours
Diabetes Range	200 mg/dL or higher after 2 hours

Hemoglobin A1c (HbA1c) Test

Measures the average blood sugar levels over the past two to three months, providing a long-term indication of blood sugar control.

Procedure	A blood sample is taken at any time of the day; no fasting required.
Normal Range	Less than 5.7%
Prediabetes Range	5.7% to 6.4%
Diabetes Range	6.5% or higher

Random Plasma Glucose Test

Measures blood sugar levels at any time, regardless of when you last ate. This test is used when diabetes symptoms are present.

Diabetes Range 200 mg/dL or higher

QUESTIONS TO ASK HEALTHCARE PROVIDERS
Initial Diagnosis
What type of diabetes do I have?
What are the differences between type 1, type 2, and gestational diabetes?
What are the potential complications of diabetes?
Monitoring and Management
How often should I test my blood sugar levels?
What are my target blood sugar ranges?
What symptoms should I watch for that might indicate my blood sugar is too high or too low?
Treatment and Medication
What medications do I need to take, and how do they work?
What are the potential side effects of my medications?
How can I manage my condition through diet and exercise?
Lifestyle and Diet
What dietary changes should I make to help manage my diabetes?
What types of physical activity are recommended?
How can I effectively manage stress, which can affect my blood sugar levels?
Long-Term Health
How often should I have check-ups and tests to monitor my diabetes?
What other health conditions am I at risk for, and how can I prevent them?
Are there any new treatments or research that I should be aware of?

Understanding Normal Ranges
Blood Sugar Levels
Fasting Blood Sugar 70 to 99 mg/dL (normal)
2hrs Post-Meal Blood Sugar Less than 140 mg/dL (normal)
HbA1c   Less than 5.7% (normal)

Blood Pressure and Cholesterol
Blood Pressure   Less than 120/80 mmHg
LDL Cholesterol Less than 100 mg/dL
HDL Cholesterol
40 mg/dL or higher (men), 50 mg/dL or higher (women)
Triglycerides Less than 150 mg/dL

At-Home Care - Blood Sugar Monitoring

Regularly checking your blood sugar levels at home helps you understand how your body responds to food, exercise, and medications. *Use a Glucometer:* Follow the manufacturer's instructions for accurate readings. *Keep a Log*: Record your blood sugar levels, noting the time of day and any factors that might have influenced the reading (e.g., meals, exercise). *Adjust as Needed:* Use your readings to adjust your diet, exercise, and medications with your doctor's guidance.

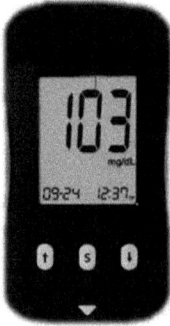

Healthy Eating - Balanced Diet

Focus on a diet rich in fruits, vegetables, whole grains, lean proteins, and healthy fats. *Carbohydrate Counting:* Monitor carbohydrate intake to manage blood sugar levels effectively. *Portion Control:* Eat smaller, more frequent meals to prevent blood sugar spikes.

Physical Activity - Regular Exercise

Aim for at least 150 minutes of moderate aerobic activity (e.g., walking, cycling) per week. *Strength Training*: Include muscle-strengthening activities at least twice a week. *Stay Active:* Incorporate physical activity into your daily routine, such as taking the stairs or walking during breaks.

Stress Management - Relaxation Techniques

Practice deep breathing, meditation, or yoga to reduce stress. *Sleep:* Aim for 7-9 hours of quality sleep each night to help regulate blood sugar levels. *Support Networks:* Engage with friends, family, or support groups to share experiences and advice.

Routine Check-Ups - Regular Appointments

Schedule regular visits with your healthcare provider to monitor your diabetes and adjust treatment plans as needed. *Eye Exams:* Have annual eye exams to check for diabetes-related eye problems. **Foot** *Care*: Inspect your feet daily for any cuts, sores, or changes, and see a podiatrist regularly.

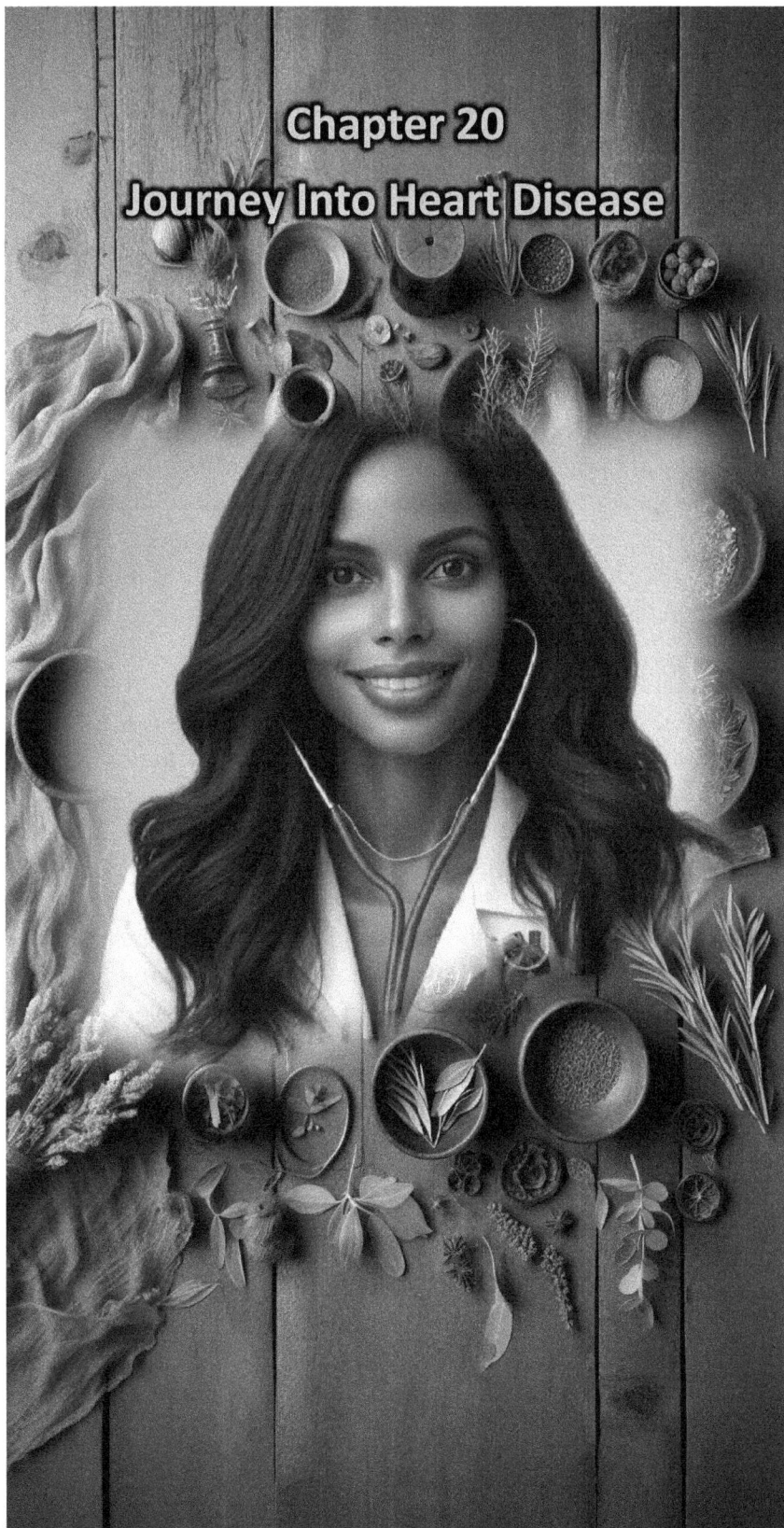
Chapter 20
Journey Into Heart Disease

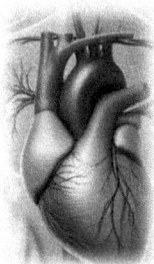

Cardiovascular System
BLOOD VESSLES HEART BLOOD

The cardiovascular system, also known as the circulatory system, is made up of the heart, blood, and blood vessels. The heart is a muscular pump that moves blood through the blood vessels in a closed circuit. The blood vessels include arteries, veins, and capillaries. The cardiovascular system's main function is to transport oxygen and nutrients to the body's cells, tissues, and organs, while also removing waste products. The heart pumps oxygen-rich blood from the left side of the heart into the aorta, which then travels through smaller arteries and capillaries to deliver oxygen and nutrients. As the blood passes through the capillaries, it drops off oxygen and nutrients and picks up carbon dioxide and waste products.

The oxygen-poor blood then returns to the right side of the heart, where it's pumped to the lungs to pick up oxygen and release carbon dioxide. This part of the system is called the pulmonary circuit. The blood vessels are made up of layers of connective tissue, muscle, and elastic fibers. Many problems with the cardiovascular system are related to slowdowns or blockages in the blood vessels. Some conditions and disorders that can affect the cardiovascular system include: **Heart disease:** Caused by narrowed arteries that limit blood supply to the heart. **High blood pressure:** Can be caused by obesity and other factors **Varicose veins:** Caused by problems with the valves that prevent blood from flowing backwards.

The cardiovascular system, also known as the circulatory system, is a vital network consisting of the heart, blood, and blood vessels. This system is essential for sustaining life, as it transports oxygen and nutrients to the body's cells, tissues, and organs while removing waste products. The heart serves as a muscular pump that propels blood through the blood vessels in a closed circuit. Blood vessels include arteries, veins, and capillaries, each playing a critical role in maintaining circulatory efficiency.

The primary function of the cardiovascular system is to deliver oxygen and nutrients to the body's cells and tissues and to remove carbon dioxide and metabolic waste products. The heart pumps oxygen-rich blood from the left side into the aorta, the body's largest artery. From the aorta, blood travels through progressively smaller arteries and capillaries, delivering oxygen and nutrients to cells. As blood passes through the capillaries, it exchanges oxygen and nutrients for carbon dioxide and waste products, which are carried back to the heart via veins. This oxygen-poor blood returns to the right side of the heart and is then pumped to the lungs through the pulmonary circuit to pick up oxygen and release carbon dioxide.

The structure of blood vessels is complex, consisting of layers of connective tissue, muscle, and elastic fibers. This composition allows blood vessels to maintain their shape and function under various pressures. However, many cardiovascular problems arise from slowdowns or blockages in these blood vessels. Common cardiovascular conditions include heart disease, high blood pressure, and varicose veins. Heart disease often results from narrowed arteries that restrict blood flow to the heart, while high blood pressure can be caused by factors such as obesity, stress, and dietary habits. Varicose veins occur when the valves that prevent blood from flowing backward fail, leading to enlarged and twisted veins.

Heart Disease
Narrowed arteries limiting blood supply to the heart
> **Health Tips** Diet rich in leafy greens, berries, omega-3 fatty acids regular exercise

High Blood Pressure
Elevated blood pressure due to various factors
> **Health Tips** Reduce sodium intake, stress management, regular physical activity

Varicose Veins
Enlarged, twisted veins due to valve issues
> **Health Tips** Elevate legs, regular movement, avoid prolonged standing or sitting

Natural Approaches to Cardiovascular Health

Maintaining cardiovascular health is particularly important for Black women, who may face higher risks for certain cardiovascular conditions. A natural approach to cardiovascular health involves a combination of diet, lifestyle modifications, and natural remedies. Incorporating heart-healthy foods into the diet, such as leafy green vegetables, berries, nuts, and seeds, can help manage blood pressure and reduce the risk of heart disease. Omega-3 fatty acids found in flaxseeds and walnuts are beneficial for reducing inflammation and promoting heart health.

Regular physical activity is crucial for maintaining a healthy cardiovascular system. Activities like brisk walking, cycling, and swimming can improve heart function, lower blood pressure, and enhance overall cardiovascular fitness. Additionally, practices that reduce stress, such as yoga and meditation, can have a positive impact on heart health by reducing stress hormones that can strain the heart.

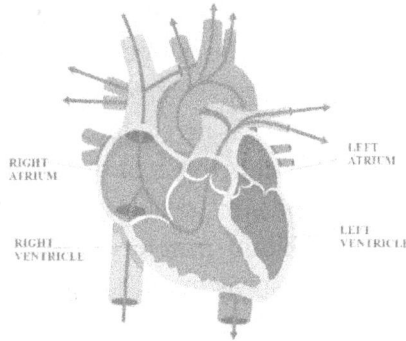

Understanding Common Heart Diseases

The heart is a powerful muscle that pumps blood throughout the body in a continuous cycle. It has four chambers: two atria on the top and two ventricles on the bottom. The right atrium receives oxygen-poor blood from the body, while the right ventricle pumps this oxygen-poor blood to the lungs through the pulmonary valve to get oxygen. The left atrium receives oxygen-rich blood from the lungs, and the left ventricle pumps oxygen-rich blood to the rest of the body through the aortic valve.

The heart's electrical system controls the heartbeat, with the sinoatrial (SA) node, known as the heart's natural pacemaker, generating electrical signals that travel to the atrioventricular (AV) node. The AV node sends these signals to the ventricles, causing them to contract and pump blood. The heart is divided by muscular walls called septa, which prevent the mixing of oxygen-rich and oxygen-poor blood. The circulatory system, made up of arteries and veins, carries blood away from and back to the heart, delivering oxygen and nutrients to cells and removing waste products.

Hypertension (High Blood Pressure)

Hypertension occurs when the blood pressure in the arteries is consistently too high, forcing the heart to work harder to pump blood. Often, hypertension has no symptoms, but it can sometimes present with headaches, shortness of breath, or nosebleeds. It is more common and tends to occur at younger ages in Black populations. A normal blood pressure reading is below 120/80 mmHg. Preventative measures include regular exercise, a healthy diet, reducing salt intake, maintaining a healthy weight, and avoiding tobacco and excessive alcohol. Management involves medications and lifestyle changes; while it cannot be cured, it can be controlled. Holistic approaches include a diet rich in fruits, vegetables, and whole grains and practices like meditation and yoga.

Coronary Artery Disease (CAD)

CAD occurs when the arteries supplying blood to the heart muscle become hardened and narrowed due to plaque buildup. Symptoms include chest pain (angina), shortness of breath, and heart attacks. It is more prevalent in Black populations due to risk factors like hypertension and diabetes. Normal cholesterol levels are an LDL below 100 mg/dL and an HDL above 40 mg/dL for men and above 50 mg/dL for women. Preventative measures include a healthy diet, regular exercise, maintaining a healthy weight, and avoiding smoking. Management involves medications, lifestyle changes, and surgical procedures if necessary. While it cannot be reversed, it can be managed. Holistic approaches include following a Mediterranean diet, engaging in regular physical activity, and utilizing stress management techniques.

Heart Failure

Heart failure is a condition where the heart cannot pump enough blood to meet the body's needs. Symptoms include shortness of breath, fatigue, swollen legs, and a rapid heartbeat. It is more common in Black populations, often due to hypertension. A normal ejection fraction (EF) is between 55-70%. Preventative measures involve managing blood pressure, diabetes, and cholesterol, along with a healthy lifestyle. Management includes medications, lifestyle changes, devices, or surgery. While it cannot be cured, it can be managed. Holistic approaches include a low-sodium diet, regular exercise, and stress reduction techniques.

Stroke

A stroke occurs when the blood supply to part of the brain is interrupted, causing brain cells to die. Symptoms include sudden numbness, confusion, trouble speaking, loss of balance, and severe headache. It is more prevalent in Black populations due to factors like hypertension and diabetes. A normal blood pressure reading is below 120/80 mmHg. Preventative measures involve controlling blood pressure, maintaining a healthy diet, regular exercise, and not smoking. Management includes emergency treatment, medications, and rehabilitation. The effects can be mitigated if treated promptly. Holistic approaches include a diet rich in antioxidants and regular physical activity.

Peripheral Artery Disease (PAD)

PAD is a condition where the blood vessels outside the heart become narrowed, reducing blood flow to the limbs. Symptoms include leg pain when walking, numbness, and coldness in the lower leg or foot. It is more common in Black populations, increasing the risk of heart disease and stroke. A normal ankle-brachial index (ABI) is between 1.0 to 1.4. Preventative measures include a healthy lifestyle and controlling blood pressure, diabetes, and cholesterol. Management involves lifestyle changes, medications, and surgical procedures if necessary. Holistic approaches include a plant-based diet, regular exercise, and quitting smoking.

Left Ventricular Hypertrophy (LVH)

LVH is the thickening of the heart's left ventricle muscle, often due to high blood pressure. Symptoms include shortness of breath, chest pain, dizziness, and palpitations. It is more common in Black populations due to higher rates of hypertension. Preventative measures involve managing blood pressure and maintaining a healthy lifestyle. Management includes controlling blood pressure, medications, and lifestyle changes. Holistic approaches include a low-sodium diet, regular exercise, and stress management.

Diabetes-Related Heart Disease

Diabetes increases the risk of developing heart disease. Symptoms include chest pain, shortness of breath, and fatigue. Black populations have a higher prevalence of diabetes, which increases the risk of heart disease. A normal HbA1c level for diabetes management is below 7%. Preventative measures include controlling blood sugar, maintaining a healthy diet, and regular exercise. Management involves blood sugar control, medications, and lifestyle changes. Holistic approaches include a plant-based diet and regular physical activity.

Cardiomyopathy

Cardiomyopathy encompasses diseases that affect the heart muscle, leading to heart failure. Symptoms include shortness of breath, swelling, fatigue, and an irregular heartbeat. Black populations are at higher risk for certain types of cardiomyopathy. Preventative measures involve a healthy lifestyle and managing blood pressure and other risk factors. Management includes medications, devices, surgery, and lifestyle changes. Holistic approaches include a balanced diet, regular exercise, and stress management.

Sudden Cardiac Arrest (SCA)

SCA occurs when the heart suddenly stops beating, leading to a loss of blood flow to the brain and other organs. Symptoms include sudden collapse, no pulse, and no breathing. It has a higher incidence in Black populations. Preventative measures involve managing heart disease risk factors and regular health check-ups. Management includes emergency treatment with CPR and defibrillation, along with ongoing management of heart health. Holistic approaches include a heart-healthy diet, regular exercise, and avoiding smoking.

Mitral Valve Prolapse/Regurgitation

Mitral valve prolapse occurs when the valve between the heart's left atrium and left ventricle does not close properly, while mitral regurgitation involves the leaking of blood backward through the mitral valve. Symptoms are often absent but can include palpitations, shortness of breath, and chest pain. It is less common in Black populations than other heart conditions. Preventative measures include regular monitoring and maintaining a healthy lifestyle. Management involves medications, lifestyle changes, and surgery if severe. Holistic approaches include a healthy diet, regular exercise, and stress management.

? QUESTIONS TO ASK YOUR DOCTOR ?

What is my risk of developing heart disease based on my current health and family history?

What lifestyle changes can I make to lower my risk of heart disease?

Are there specific screenings or tests I should have regularly?

How do my current medications affect my heart health?

Can you explain my blood pressure, cholesterol, and blood sugar readings?

What are the warning signs of heart disease that I should watch for?

Key tests to request include blood pressure measurement, cholesterol and lipid panel, blood glucose test (for diabetes), electrocardiogram (ECG or EKG), echocardiogram, stress test, and ankle-brachial index (ABI) for PAD.

Genetic and Socioeconomic Factors

Certain genetic traits prevalent in Black populations can increase susceptibility to heart conditions. Socioeconomic factors such as access to healthcare, socioeconomic status, and lifestyle choices also influence the prevalence and management of heart diseases. Preventive measures like regular screening, lifestyle modifications (such as diet and exercise), and managing risk factors like hypertension and diabetes are crucial in reducing the risk of heart diseases.

Hypertension (High Blood Pressure) A condition where the force of the blood against the artery walls is too high, often leading to heart disease and stroke. Black individuals are more likely to develop hypertension at a younger age compared to other races.

Coronary Artery Disease (CAD) A condition characterized by narrowed or blocked coronary arteries due to plaque buildup, leading to reduced blood flow to the heart. It can result in chest pain, heart attacks, and other complications.

Heart Failure A chronic condition where the heart doesn't pump blood as well as it should, leading to fatigue, shortness of breath, and fluid buildup. Black individuals have a higher risk of developing heart failure.

Stroke Occurs when the blood supply to part of the brain is interrupted or reduced, preventing brain tissue from getting oxygen and nutrients. Black individuals are at higher risk due to factors like hypertension and diabetes.

Peripheral Artery Disease (PAD) A circulatory condition in which narrowed blood vessels reduce blood flow to the limbs, particularly the legs. It is more common in Black populations, increasing the risk of heart disease and stroke.

Left Ventricular Hypertrophy (LVH) A condition where the muscle wall of the heart's left ventricle thickens, which can lead to heart disease. This is often a result of hypertension, which is prevalent in Black populations.

Diabetes-Related Heart Disease Diabetes increases the risk of heart disease, and Black individuals are disproportionately affected by diabetes, leading to a higher prevalence of diabetes-related heart complications.

Cardiomyopathy A group of diseases that affect the heart muscle, leading to heart failure. Black individuals are at higher risk for certain types of cardiomyopathy, such as hypertrophic and dilated cardiomyopathy.

Sudden Cardiac Arrest (SCA) A condition in which the heart suddenly and unexpectedly stops beating, leading to a loss of blood flow to the brain and other organs. Black populations have a higher incidence of SCA.

Cardiovascular Health

Black women have higher rates of hypertension and cardiovascular diseases. Prevention and management of cardiovascular health issues involve maintaining a balanced diet that is low in sodium and saturated fats and focuses on whole, plant-based foods. Regular physical activity, such as walking, cycling, swimming, and yoga, is essential. Monitoring blood pressure regularly and maintaining a healthy weight are also crucial steps. Herbal remedies like hibiscus tea, known for its blood pressure-lowering properties, can be beneficial. By focusing on these holistic practices, Black women can better manage their cardiovascular health and reduce the risk of related diseases.

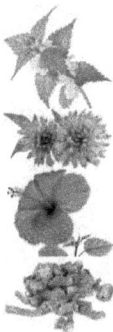

Nettle Leaf High in vitamins and minerals, helps with iron deficiency.

Red Clover Supports bone health due to its isoflavone content.

Hibiscus Tea Helps manage blood pressure.

Sarsaparilla Rich in iron, beneficial for anemia.

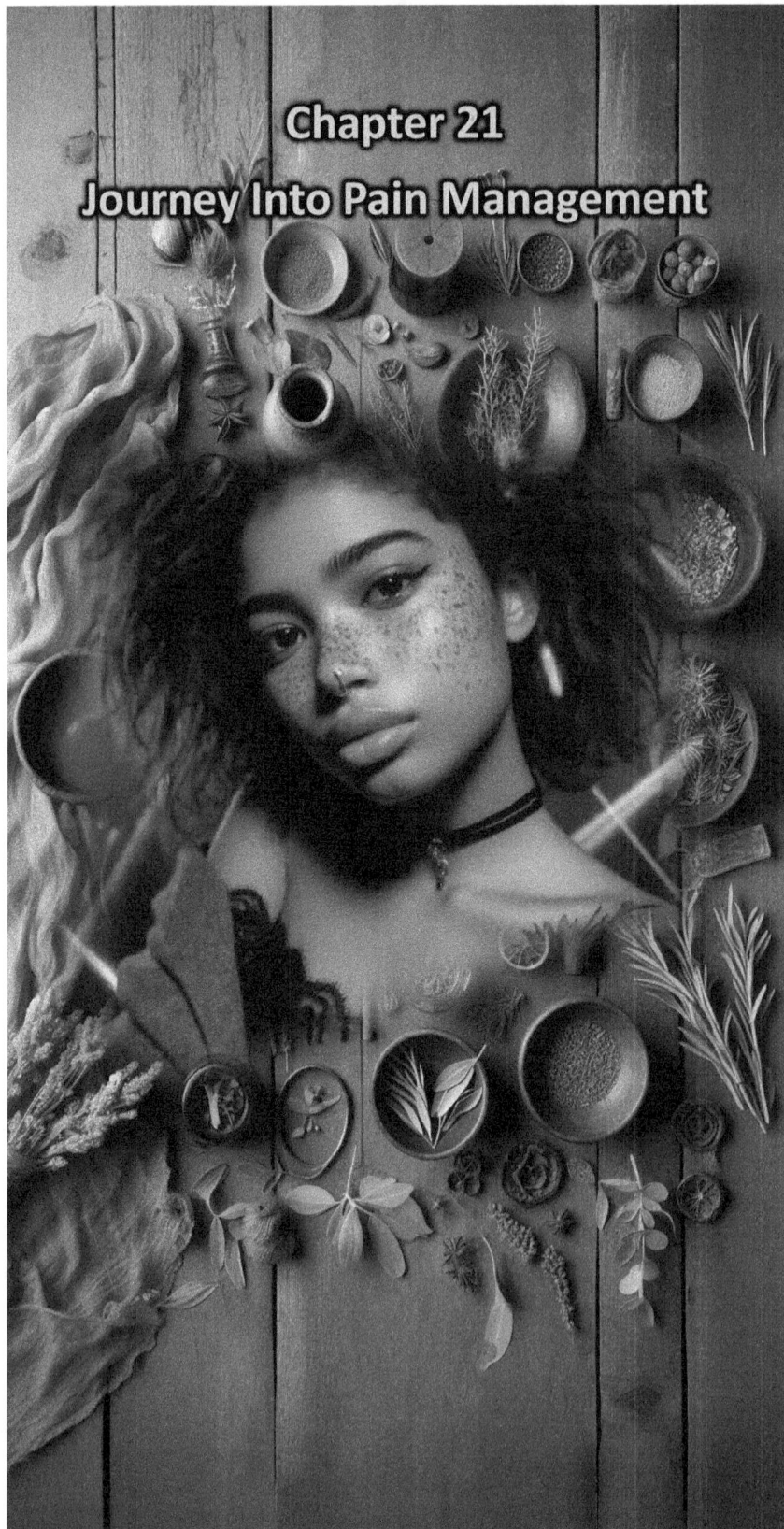

Chapter 21
Journey Into Pain Management

Introduction to Pain Management

Pain management involves various methods and practices used to reduce or alleviate pain. It encompasses pharmacological, physical, and psychological techniques to manage pain in acute, chronic, and palliative care settings. This guide will provide insights into effective pain management practices, focusing on both prescription and over-the-counter (OTC) solutions, homemade remedies, and the importance of safety in preventing substance abuse. Pain management involves a variety of approaches to prevent, reduce, or alleviate pain. It encompasses medication, physical therapy, psychological support, and lifestyle changes. The goal is to improve function and enhance the overall quality of life.

Morphine and Codeine

Morphine and Codeine are commonly used in prescription medications for pain management. These opioids are derived from the opium poppy plant (Papaver somniferum) and are known for their potent analgesic effects. **Morphine**: Used for severe pain, especially after surgeries or for cancer-related pain. **Codeine**: Typically used for milder pain and often combined with other pain relievers like acetaminophen.

Morphine

Source: Derived from the opium poppy (Papaver somniferum). *Usage:* Commonly used for severe pain relief, especially in postoperative settings, cancer pain management, and palliative care. *Mechanism:* Binds to opioid receptors in the brain and spinal cord, blocking pain signals. *Benefits:* Highly effective for severe pain; rapid onset of action. *Risks*: High potential for abuse, addiction, and side effects like respiratory depression and constipation.

Codeine

Source*: Also derived from the opium poppy. ***Usage***: Used for mild to moderate pain relief, often combined with other analgesics like acetaminophen. ***Mechanism***: Similar to morphine but with less potency; also works by binding to opioid receptors. ***Benefits***: Effective for less severe pain; has antitussive (cough suppressant) properties. ***Risks***: Potential for abuse and addiction, though lower than morphine; side effects include drowsiness, constipation, and nausea.

Natural Sources of Codeine
Papaver somniferum (Opium Poppy)

Opium Poppy (Papaver somniferum) is the primary natural source of codeine. It produces several alkaloids, including morphine, thebaine, and codeine, which are used for their analgesic properties. **Description**: The opium poppy plant produces alkaloids extracted from the plant's latex. ***Alkaloids***: The plant contains morphine, codeine, and thebaine. ***Codeine Content***: Codeine makes up about 1-3% of the opium extracted from the poppy plant.

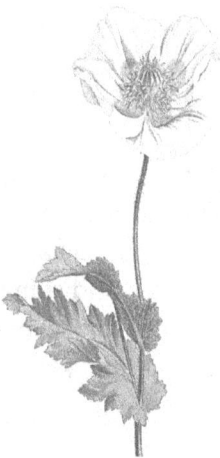

Important Considerations

Legal Restrictions: The cultivation of opium poppy plants and the extraction of opium alkaloids are highly regulated and controlled by law in most countries due to their potential for abuse and addiction. ***Health Risks***: Self-extraction or processing of codeine from natural sources can be dangerous and is illegal without proper licensing and oversight. The potency and dosage of natural opiates can vary significantly, leading to a high risk of overdose and severe side effects. Papaver somniferum (the opium poppy) is used more extensively than other plants for several key reasons.

Potency of Active Compounds

High Concentration of Alkaloids: The opium poppy produces a high concentration of potent alkaloids, such as morphine, codeine, and thebaine. These compounds are highly effective at relieving severe pain and have well-documented pharmacological effects. **Direct Derivatives:** Morphine and codeine, derived directly from the opium poppy, are powerful analgesics that are critical in medical settings for managing acute and chronic pain.

Historical and Medical Use

Long History of Use: The use of the opium poppy dates back thousands of years, with documented use in ancient civilizations for its analgesic and sedative properties. This long history has led to extensive knowledge and documentation of its effects, making it a reliable source for pain management. *Established Medical Applications:* Morphine and codeine have been well-studied and are widely used in modern medicine. They are included in the World Health Organization's list of essential medicines, underscoring their importance in medical treatment.

Predictability and Consistency

Standardized Extraction: The extraction and purification processes for morphine and codeine from the opium poppy are well-established, allowing for consistent and standardized dosages. This predictability is crucial for medical use. *Reliable Effects:* The pharmacokinetics (absorption, distribution, metabolism, and excretion) and pharmacodynamics (mechanism of action) of these alkaloids are well understood, providing predictable and reliable effects for pain relief.

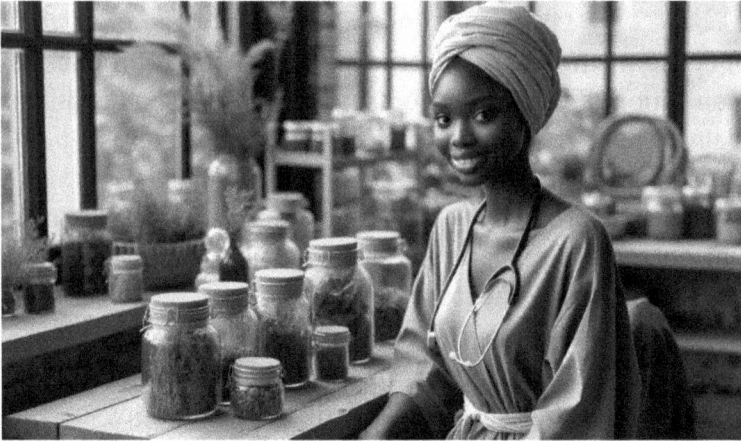
Pharmaceutical Development

Basis for Synthetic Derivatives: Many synthetic opioids (like oxycodone, hydrocodone, and heroin) are chemically derived from thebaine, another alkaloid in the opium poppy. This makes the plant a critical resource for developing various opioid medications.
Regulation and Control: The cultivation and processing of opium poppies are tightly regulated, ensuring that the production of opiates meets medical standards and legal requirements.

Efficacy in Severe Pain Management

Effective for Severe Pain: The analgesic properties of morphine and codeine are particularly effective for managing severe pain, such as postoperative pain, cancer pain, and pain from serious injuries. Other plants, while beneficial for milder pain or as adjunct therapies, generally do not match the potency of opium-derived alkaloids.

Legal and Medical Infrastructure

Integrated into Healthcare Systems: The infrastructure for prescribing, distributing, and monitoring the use of opioids derived from the opium poppy is well-established in many healthcare systems. This integration supports their widespread use and availability for patients in need.

Safe Alternatives for Pain Relief

Instead of attempting to extract codeine or other opiates from natural sources, it is safer to use legal and over-the-counter medications and natural remedies for pain relief. By combining safe medications with effective natural remedies, individuals can manage pain without resorting to potentially dangerous or illegal methods. Always consult with healthcare professionals before starting any new treatment for pain management. While Papaver somniferum (the opium poppy) is the primary natural source of opiates like morphine and codeine, there are other plants that contain compounds with similar analgesic (pain-relieving) effects. However, these plants and their compounds can vary significantly in terms of potency, legal status, and safety. Below are some plants that have similar effects:

Kratom (Mitragyna speciosa) Mitragynine and 7-hydroxymitragynine. *Effects*: Kratom leaves have been used traditionally in Southeast Asia for their stimulant and analgesic properties. In higher doses, they can have sedative and pain-relieving effects similar to opioids. **Legal Status:** Kratom is legal in some countries and states, but it is banned or regulated in others due to concerns about safety and potential for abuse.

Wild Lettuce (Lactuca virosa) Lactucin and lactucopicrin. *Effects:* Often referred to as "opium lettuce," wild lettuce has mild sedative and pain-relieving properties. It has been used in traditional medicine to alleviate pain and promote relaxation. **Legal Status:** Generally legal and available in most places, though its effects are much milder compared to opium-derived substances.

California Poppy (Eschscholzia californica) Alkaloids such as californidine and eschscholtzine. *Effects:* This plant has sedative and mild analgesic effects. It is used in herbal medicine to treat anxiety, insomnia, and mild pain. *Legal Status:* Legal and commonly used in herbal remedies.

Corydalis (Corydalis yanhusuo) Alkaloids such as tetrahydropalmatine (THP). *Effects:* Corydalis has been used in traditional Chinese medicine for its analgesic and sedative properties. It is often used to treat pain, including menstrual pain and headaches. *Legal Status:* Generally legal and available in most places as a supplement.

Turmeric (Curcuma longa) Curcumin. *Effects:* While not an opioid or directly comparable in potency to codeine or morphine, curcumin in turmeric has strong anti-inflammatory and mild pain-relieving effects. It is widely used in both traditional medicine and modern supplements. *Legal Status:* Legal and widely available.

Considerations and Warnings

Potency and Safety: The potency and safety of these plants can vary significantly. While some have been traditionally used for their medicinal properties, others may pose risks if not used correctly. *Legal Status:* The legal status of these plants can vary by country and region. Always check local regulations before using or obtaining these plants. *Consultation:* It is important to consult with a healthcare professional before using any herbal remedies, especially if you have underlying health conditions or are taking other medications. While there are plants with similar effects to Papaver somniferum, they do not contain the same opiate alkaloids and generally have milder effects. Always prioritize safety and legality when considering natural alternatives for pain relief.

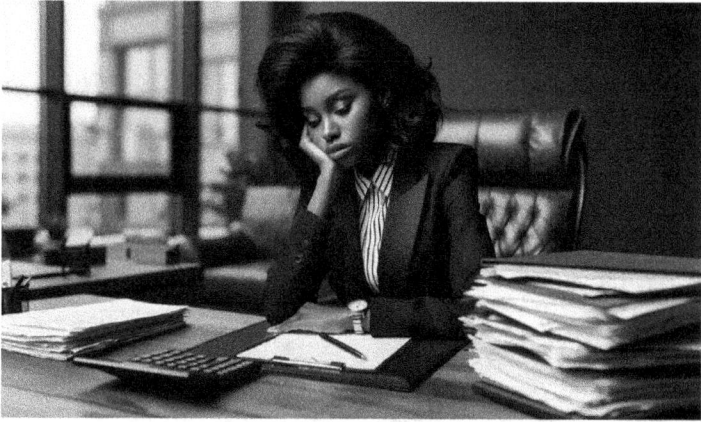

Substance Abuse and Pain Medication

Using pain medications, especially opioids, carries a risk of substance abuse and addiction. It is crucial to follow prescribed dosages and consult healthcare professionals to manage these risks effectively. *Safety Practices: Consult Healthcare Providers:* Always consult with a healthcare professional before starting any pain management regimen. **Monitor Dosages**: Follow the prescribed dosages strictly to avoid the risk of overdose and addiction. *Duration* **of Use**: Do not use pain medications for prolonged periods without medical supervision. *Check for Allergies:* Be aware of potential allergic reactions to pain medications.

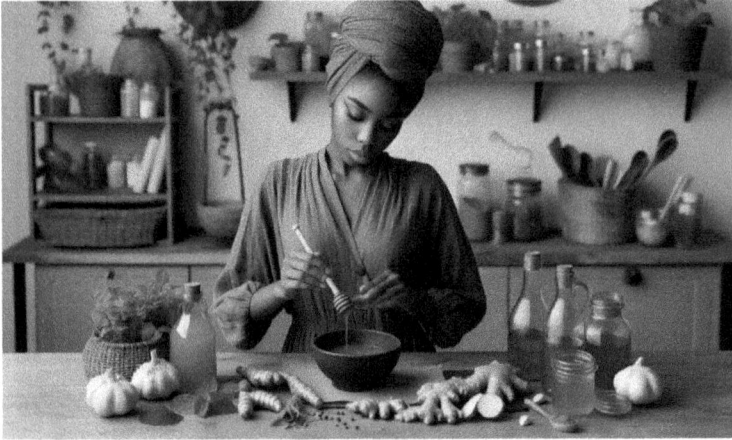

HOMEMADE GENERAL PAIN, FEVER REDUCTION, AND ANTI-INFLAMMATION SYRUP

Ingredients *Turmeric: Effect*: Natural anti-inflammatory and antibacterial properties. **Dose**: 1 teaspoon of turmeric powder. *Clove Oil: Effect*: Natural analgesic (pain relief) and antiseptic properties. **Dose**: 1 teaspoon of clove oil. *Garlic: Effect:* Natural antibiotic and anti-inflammatory properties. **Dose**: 2 cloves of fresh garlic. *Raw Honey: Effect:* Natural antibacterial and soothing properties. **Dose**: 2 tablespoons of raw honey. *Ginger: Effect*: Natural anti-inflammatory and pain relief properties. **Dose**: 1 teaspoon of fresh grated ginger. *Cayenne Pepper: Effect*: Natural pain reliever by reducing substance P, a chemical that transmits pain signals. **Dose**: 1/4 teaspoon of cayenne pepper. *Apple Cider Vinegar: Effect:* Antibacterial properties and helps balance pH levels. **Dose**: 1 tablespoon of apple cider vinegar. *Peppermint Oil: Effect*: Natural pain reliever and soothing properties. **Dose**: 10 drops of peppermint oil.

Preparation Instructions: Turmeric Paste Mix 1 teaspoon of turmeric powder with a few drops of water to form a paste.
Garlic Preparation Crush 2 cloves of fresh garlic and let it sit for 10 minutes to activate its beneficial compounds.

Combining Ingredients: In a small saucepan, combine the turmeric paste, crushed garlic, 1 teaspoon of clove oil, 2 tablespoons of raw honey, 1 teaspoon of grated ginger, 1/4 teaspoon of cayenne pepper, 1 tablespoon of apple cider vinegar, and 10 drops of peppermint oil.
Heat the mixture on low heat for 5 minutes, stirring continuously to ensure all ingredients are well mixed.
Remove from heat and let it cool.
Strain the mixture to remove any solid particles.
Store the syrup in a clean, airtight glass jar.

Dosage Instructions: Adults: Take 1 tablespoon of the syrup up to 3 times a day, as needed for pain and inflammation relief. **Children (over 12 years)**: Take 1 teaspoon of the syrup up to 3 times a day, as needed.

Warnings and Precautions *Consultation: Always consult with a healthcare professional before using any homemade remedies, especially if you have any underlying health conditions or are taking other medications.*
Allergic Reactions: Check for possible allergic reactions to any ingredients. Discontinue use if any adverse reactions occur.
Pregnancy and Breastfeeding: Pregnant or breastfeeding women should consult a healthcare provider before using this syrup.
Diabetes: Raw honey and apple cider vinegar may affect blood sugar levels. Diabetic individuals should monitor their blood sugar levels closely.
Blood Thinners: Ingredients like garlic and turmeric may have blood-thinning effects. Individuals on blood-thinning medications should use this syrup with caution.
Duration: Do not use this remedy for more than 7 days without consulting a healthcare provider, as persistent symptoms may require professional medical intervention.

Natural Remedies

Turmeric and Ginger Tea: **Effect**: Natural anti-inflammatory and pain relief properties. **Preparation**: Mix 1 teaspoon of turmeric powder and 1 teaspoon of grated ginger in hot water. Add honey to taste. Drink 2-3 times a day.

Clove Oil: **Effect**: Natural analgesic and antiseptic properties. **Usage**: Apply a few drops of clove oil directly to the affected area for pain relief.

Peppermint Tea: **Effect**: Natural pain relief and soothing properties. **Preparation**: Brew fresh or dried peppermint leaves in hot water. Drink 2-3 times a day.

Effective pain management requires a comprehensive approach, combining prescription medications, over-the-counter alternatives, natural remedies, and safety practices to prevent substance abuse and ensure overall well-being. Understanding the sources, effects, and appropriate usage of these pain management strategies can help individuals manage pain effectively while minimizing risks. Always seek guidance from healthcare professionals to tailor pain management strategies to individual needs.

Warnings and Precautions

*Consultation: Always consult with a healthcare professional before using any medication or natural remedy, especially if you have any underlying health conditions or are taking other medications. **Allergic Reactions**: Check for possible allergic reactions to any ingredients. Discontinue use if any adverse reactions occur. **Pregnancy and Breastfeeding**: Pregnant or breastfeeding women should consult a healthcare provider before using these medications or remedies. **Dosage Limits**: Do not exceed the recommended dosages for acetaminophen, ibuprofen, or naproxen to avoid potential liver and kidney damage or gastrointestinal issues. **Duration**: Do not use these medications or remedies for more than 7 days without consulting a healthcare provider, as persistent symptoms may require professional medical intervention.*

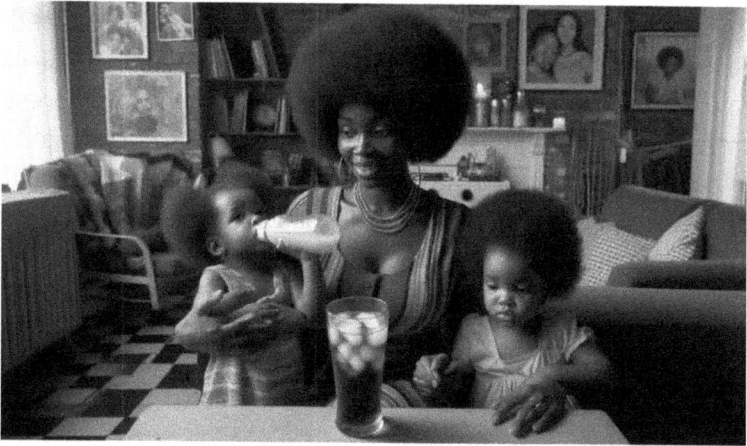

The Silent Drug: Sugar and Its Impact on Health

Sugar, particularly in its refined form, has been likened to a drug in modern health discourse due to its highly addictive nature. Though not often discussed in the same vein as substances like alcohol or opioids, sugar has a similarly powerful grip on the brain's reward system. The body craves it, people overconsume it, and withdrawal symptoms occur when intake is reduced. This epidemic is particularly devastating in the Black community in America, where sugar consumption—particularly in the form of refined sugar and high-fructose corn syrup (HFCS)—has reached alarming levels, leading to chronic health conditions and exacerbating existing socioeconomic health disparities.

The Historical Context of Sugar and High-Fructose Corn Syrup

The history of sugar in the Black community is a long and complex one, intertwined with economic exploitation. From the sugarcane plantations where enslaved Africans toiled to the present-day food deserts that disproportionately affect Black communities, sugar has always been a tool of oppression.

In the 1970s, high-fructose corn syrup (HFCS) was introduced as a cheaper alternative to sugar. Unlike natural sugars, HFCS was a chemically manufactured sweetener that quickly became prevalent in processed foods, sodas, and snacks. Its rise was not accidental. It was heavily promoted by corporate interests, which prioritized profits over the public's health. This malicious intent manifested in the strategic targeting of poor and minority communities, where processed foods containing HFCS were the most affordable and accessible. The result has been devastating for Black bodies, leading to a dramatic rise in obesity, diabetes, heart disease, and even mental health issues.

What is High-Fructose Corn Syrup?

High-fructose corn syrup is a highly processed sweetener derived from corn starch. Through a complex chemical process, the glucose in corn is converted into fructose. This creates a syrup that is much sweeter than regular sugar (sucrose) and cheaper to produce. Because it is inexpensive and enhances flavor, it has been added to countless foods, even in products you wouldn't expect, such as bread, salad dressings, and canned goods.

HFCS is made up of varying ratios of glucose and fructose, with the most common form being a mixture of 55% fructose and 45% glucose. This imbalance is crucial because fructose is processed by the liver, and in large quantities, it can overwhelm the liver, causing fat to accumulate.

How Sugar and HFCS Affect the Body

The consumption of sugar and HFCS triggers a cascade of effects in the body, many of which mirror the effects of addictive substances:

Blood Sugar Spikes and Crashes: Both sugar and HFCS cause blood sugar levels to spike, leading to an immediate burst of energy. However, this is followed by a rapid crash, which can leave a person feeling lethargic and craving more sugar to maintain energy levels.

Insulin Resistance and Diabetes

Excessive sugar consumption, particularly HFCS, increases the risk of insulin resistance. Over time, this can lead to type 2 diabetes—a condition disproportionately affecting the Black community.

Liver Damage

High levels of fructose are metabolized by the liver, which can result in non-alcoholic fatty liver disease (NAFLD). When the liver is overloaded with fructose, it turns it into fat, some of which is stored in the liver itself. This can lead to liver inflammation and long-term damage.

Obesity

The addictive nature of sugar and HFCS leads to overconsumption, which contributes to weight gain and obesity. HFCS has been shown to bypass the body's natural appetite regulation, meaning you can consume large amounts without feeling full.

Mental Health and Cognitive Decline

Recent studies suggest that excessive sugar consumption may affect brain function, leading to memory problems, cognitive decline, and mood disorders such as depression and anxiety. There's evidence that sugar contributes to the inflammation in the brain, impairing cognitive processes and contributing to mental health disorders.

Symptoms of Sugar and HFCS Overconsumption

Constant sugar cravings
Fatigue and lethargy
Mood swings and irritability
Increased abdominal fat
Frequent headaches
Insomnia or poor-quality sleep
Frequent urination or increased thirst
Difficulty focusing and memory problems

Sugar, HFCS, and Links to Chronic Disease

There is a growing body of evidence linking excessive consumption of sugar and HFCS to various chronic diseases that plague the Black community.

Diabetes Sugar consumption has been shown to contribute directly to the development of insulin resistance, a precursor to diabetes.

Heart Disease

Studies show that high sugar intake increases the risk of heart disease. HFCS, in particular, raises triglyceride levels, which can lead to cardiovascular complications.

Obesity High sugar intake leads to weight gain, particularly abdominal fat, which is a significant risk factor for metabolic syndrome and cardiovascular diseases.

Mental Health Disorders Excessive sugar has been linked to depression and anxiety. It's believed that sugar causes chronic inflammation, which may play a role in the development of these mental health issues.

Cancer There is evidence to suggest that sugar can fuel cancer cells. Cancer cells are known to feed on glucose, and high sugar consumption has been linked to certain types of cancer, including breast and colon cancer.

Natural Alternatives to Sugar and HFCS

There are several natural alternatives to sugar and HFCS that can satisfy your sweet tooth without the harmful effects.

Raw Honey Unlike processed sugar, raw honey contains vitamins, minerals, and antioxidants. It is a great option to sweeten food naturally while boosting the immune system.

Stevia A plant-derived sweetener, stevia is much sweeter than sugar but has no calories and doesn't affect blood sugar levels, making it a great option for diabetics.

Dates are naturally sweet and loaded with fiber, which helps regulate the body's sugar absorption. Date syrup or whole dates can be used in smoothies, desserts, or even baking.

Maple Syrup Pure maple syrup contains antioxidants and a variety of minerals such as zinc and manganese. While still a source of sugar, it is much less processed than HFCS.

Counteracting the Effects of Sugar and HFCS with Natural Remedies

Fiber-Rich Foods Increase your intake of fiber from vegetables, fruits, and whole grains. Fiber helps slow down the absorption of sugar in the body and can improve digestion.

Herbal Detox Herbal teas such as dandelion, milk thistle, and burdock root can support liver detoxification and help the body process excess sugars.

Haritaki This powerful Ayurvedic herb is known for detoxifying the body and decalcifying the pineal gland. It can help cleanse the system of the toxic buildup caused by HFCS consumption.

Chlorophyll Found in leafy greens and algae like spirulina and chlorella, chlorophyll helps detoxify the body at a cellular level, improving digestion, balancing blood sugar, and supporting overall health.

Magnesium A mineral often depleted by sugar consumption, magnesium is crucial for regulating blood sugar levels, supporting the nervous system, and reducing cravings.

While sugar and high-fructose corn syrup have become ubiquitous in the modern diet, their impact on health—particularly in the Black community—cannot be overstated. The addictive nature of these substances, combined with their links to chronic diseases, calls for a conscious shift toward natural alternatives and a focus on health. Awareness is the first step toward healing, and by adopting natural sweeteners, detoxifying the body, and making mindful dietary choices, we can begin to reverse the damage caused by sugar addiction. The road to better health starts with knowledge and the empowerment to make better choices.

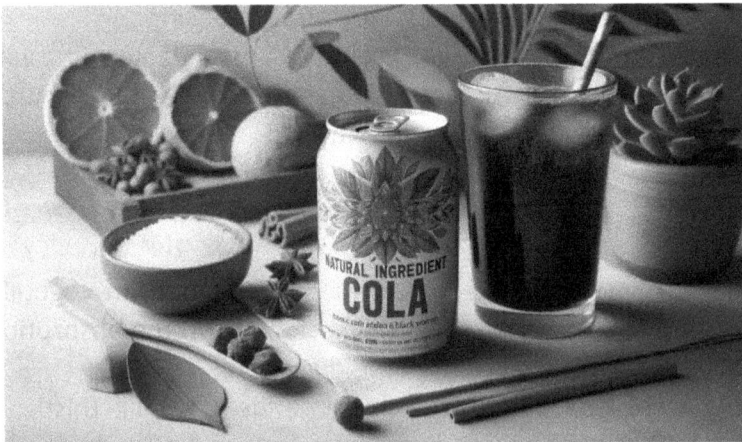

Natural Cola Recipe (Healthy Soda Dupe)

This recipe offers a healthier, natural version of popular cola sodas. The goal is to replicate the deep caramel flavor, sweetness, and refreshing fizz, but using natural ingredients that provide a similar taste without harmful chemicals, high-fructose corn syrup, or artificial flavors.

Ingredients Breakdown

Traditional Cola Flavor Profile: "Brand Name Sodas" contain caramel color, phosphoric acid, artificial flavors, and a high amount of refined sugar (often high-fructose corn syrup).

Natural Dupe: Instead of harmful additives, this natural soda recipe uses real herbs, spices, and sweeteners to recreate a rich and balanced flavor.

INGREDIENTS FOR NATURAL COLA DUPE

Sparkling Water (Carbonated Water): Provides the fizziness of soda without artificial carbonation or chemical preservatives.

Fresh Lemon or Lime Juice (Citrus): Adds the bright citrus notes found in cola, and replaces phosphoric acid, a chemical often found in sodas, with natural, vitamin-C rich citrus juice.

Coconut Sugar or Raw Honey (Sweetener): Coconut sugar is a low-glycemic sweetener that has a caramel-like flavor, mimicking the deep sweetness in cola. Raw honey can also be used as a more health-friendly alternative.

Molasses (Caramel-like Flavor): Molasses has a natural caramel flavor and is rich in minerals like iron and calcium, providing that rich, deep taste reminiscent of the caramel flavor in soda.

Vanilla Extract (Natural Flavor): Adds sweetness and richness to balance the citrus. This replaces the artificial "natural flavors" listed in cola recipes.

Cinnamon, Nutmeg, and Coriander (Spices): These spices add depth and complexity to the drink, similar to the spicy undertones found in traditional cola. You can experiment with amounts, but a small pinch of each is usually enough to get that subtle spice background.

Cola Nut (Optional): If you want to stay true to the original cola recipe, you can add a small amount of cola nut powder. Cola nuts are what gave Coca-Cola its original caffeine kick. However, this is optional and can be hard to find.

Maple Syrup (Additional Sweetness): Maple syrup adds an extra layer of sweetness and richness. It is healthier than HFCS and works well to balance the acidity.

Natural Caffeine (Optional): If you want the slight caffeine kick that cola gives, you can add a touch of natural caffeine in the form of **green tea extract** or **guarana** powder. These are natural stimulants, unlike synthetic caffeine found in sodas.

INSTRUCTIONS

In a small saucepan, heat 1 cup of water over medium heat. Add **2 tbsp of coconut sugar** (or raw honey) and **1 tsp of molasses**. Stir until dissolved.

Add a pinch of **cinnamon**, **nutmeg**, and **coriander** to the mixture, allowing the spices to steep for 5-10 minutes. This will help develop the rich and spicy undertones of traditional cola.

Stir in **1 tsp of vanilla extract** and the **juice of 1 lemon or lime** to give the mixture a tangy and sweet balance.

Remove from heat and allow the mixture to cool to room temperature.

Once cooled, mix the syrup with **sparkling water** in a 1:4 ratio (1 part syrup to 4 parts sparkling water) for the perfect fizz.

Taste test and adjust for sweetness by adding more maple syrup or lemon juice to suit your preference.

Serve over ice and enjoy!

FLAVOR NOTES

The *coconut sugar* and *molasses* combine to create a deep, caramel-like sweetness, mimicking the flavor found in *"Brand Name Sodas"*. The *citrus* adds the tanginess, replacing phosphoric acid with a natural, healthier acidity. The combination of *spices* provides a subtle complexity, replacing the chemical flavor agents. If you opt to use *cola nut* or *natural caffeine* like *green tea extract*, this will give the soda a subtle caffeine kick.

BENEFITS OF THE NATURAL INGREDIENTS

Coconut sugar is rich in minerals and has a lower glycemic index, making it a much better alternative to the high-fructose corn syrup found in commercial sodas. *Lemon juice* is packed with vitamin C, antioxidants, and helps detoxify the liver. *Molasses* contains essential minerals like iron, calcium, magnesium, and potassium, making it a health-boosting alternative to artificial caramel coloring. *Vanilla* is anti-inflammatory and can even have calming properties, making it an excellent natural flavor. *Spices like cinnamon and nutmeg* can help regulate blood sugar and have anti-inflammatory properties, unlike the synthetic flavors in regular soda.

Natural vs. Commercial Soda Comparison

Ingredient	Traditional Soda ("Brand Name Soda")	Natural Dupe
Sweetener	High-Fructose Corn Syrup	Coconut Sugar / Raw Honey / Maple Syrup
Acid	Phosphoric Acid	Fresh Lemon Juice / Lime Juice
Caramel Flavor	Artificial Caramel Color	Molasses
Flavors	Artificial "Natural Flavors"	Vanilla Extract + Spices
Caffeine Source	Synthetic Caffeine	Cola Nut / Green Tea Extract
Fizz	Artificial Carbonation	Sparkling Water

This natural cola dupe not only mimics the flavor of commercial sodas but also provides a healthier alternative that avoids the harmful effects of HFCS, artificial additives, and synthetic caffeine. Enjoy this refreshing and guilt-free drink with the added benefits of natural ingredients!

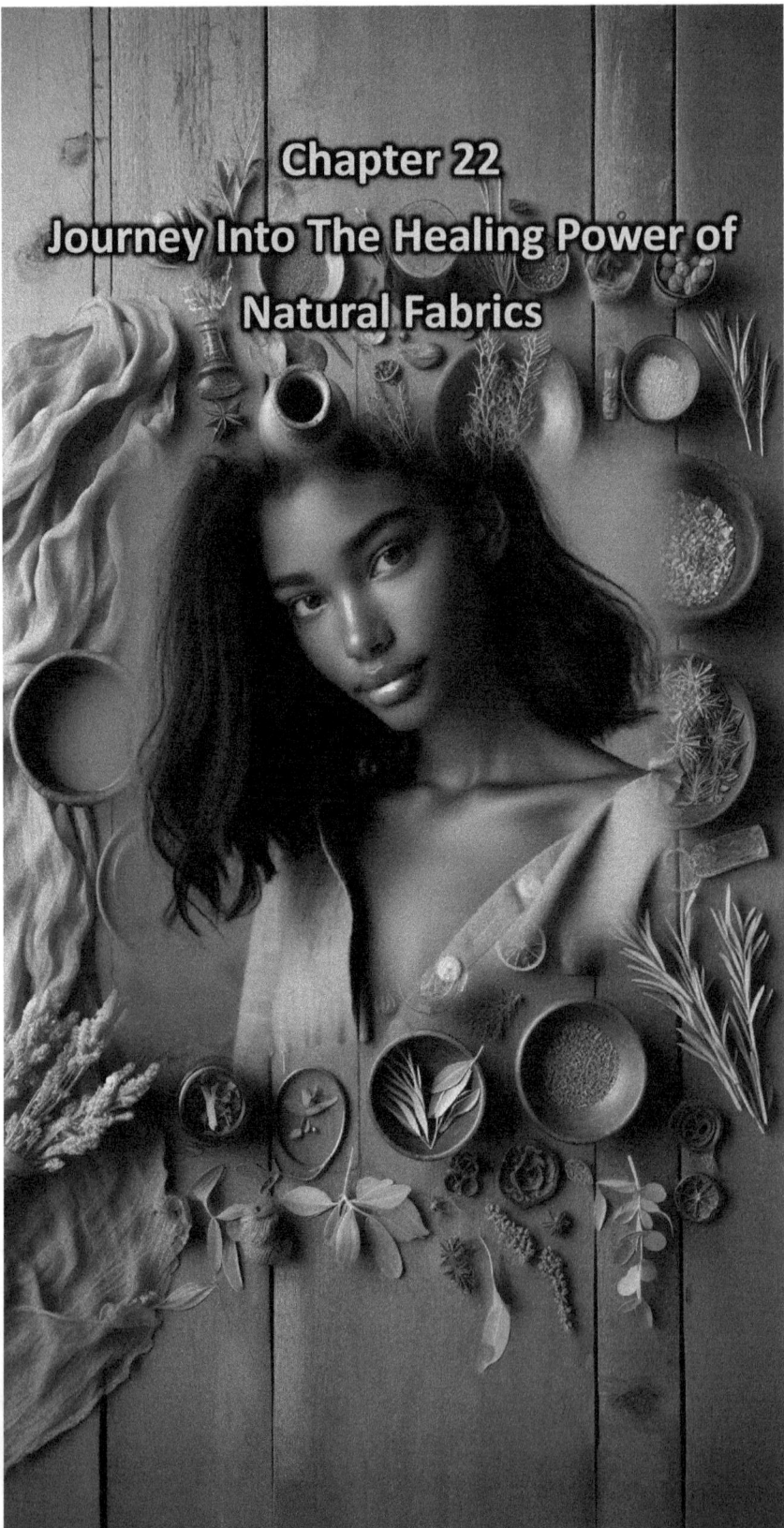

Chapter 22
Journey Into The Healing Power of Natural Fabrics

Healing encompasses the mind, body, and spirit, and the clothing we choose to wear plays a subtle yet profound role in this process. From ancient civilizations to modern-day wellness practices, natural fabrics like linen, cotton, wool, hemp, and silk have been recognized for their therapeutic properties. The fibers we place next to our skin can either support or hinder our body's natural rhythms, energy flow, and overall health. This section explores how linen and other natural fabrics impact holistic healing, the physiological and energetic responses they evoke, and how our choices from head to toe affect our body's wellness.

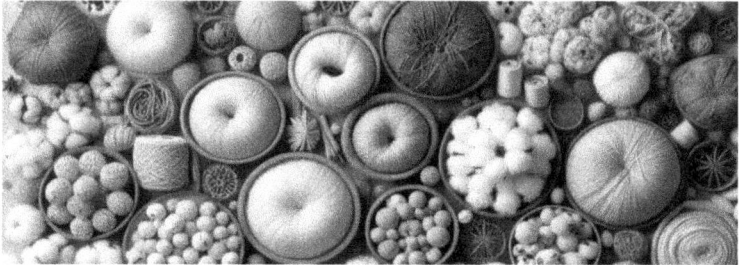

The Role of Fabrics in Healing

The skin is the largest organ of the human body and serves as a gateway between our internal environment and the world around us. What we wear can influence our body's ability to regulate temperature, energy, and even mood. Holistic healing recognizes the importance of living in harmony with nature, and natural fabrics, being derived from plants and animals, align with this principle. They allow the body to breathe, absorb, and release energy efficiently, promoting better physical and emotional well-being.

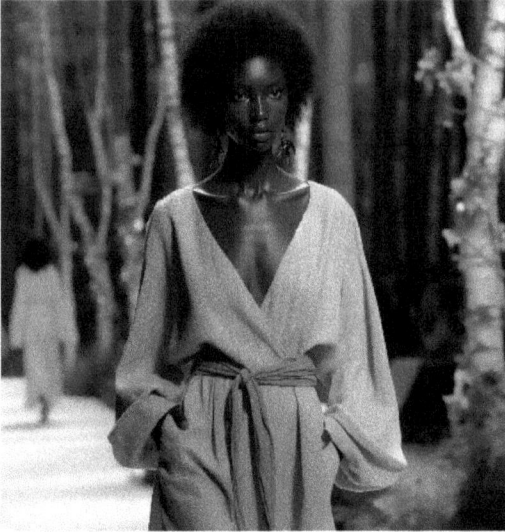

Linen: A Powerhouse

Linen, derived from the flax plant, has been revered for centuries for its healing properties. The structure of linen fibers promotes airflow, making it highly breathable and moisture-wicking. This fabric is particularly valuable in health for its ability to regulate body temperature, absorb sweat, and promote a feeling of calm and relaxation. Linen has also been noted for its natural frequency of 5,000 Hz, which is said to harmonize with the body's natural energy field.

Wearing linen can enhance bioelectric balance, promote restful sleep, and reduce the impact of environmental stressors on the body. Its antibacterial and hypoallergenic properties make it an excellent choice for sensitive skin or those dealing with allergies. Linen is a preferred fabric in many healing traditions due to its purported ability to increase the body's healing energy. Ancient Egyptians even wrapped their dead in linen to preserve their bodies because of the fabric's purity.

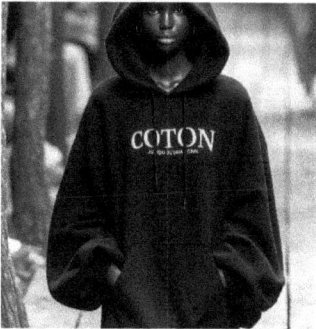

Cotton: The Everyday Healer

Cotton is one of the most widely used natural fabrics in the world. It is soft, breathable, and hypoallergenic, making it suitable for daily wear. Cotton allows the skin to "breathe," promoting sweat absorption and helping to prevent skin irritation. It's particularly beneficial for people with sensitive skin or those prone to rashes. In other terms, cotton is considered grounding. It helps to maintain the body's balance, supports comfort, and enhances relaxation.

The simplicity and purity of cotton, especially organic varieties, makes it a preferred fabric. Organic cotton retains its natural energy, free from the synthetic chemicals found in conventional cotton production, making it more aligned with the principles of health.

Wool: A Shield for the Body's Energy

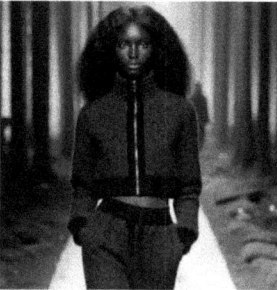

Wool is a natural fiber derived from sheep and other animals. It has insulating properties, making it ideal for cooler climates or winter months. Wool helps to regulate body temperature, keeping the wearer warm but not overheated. It can absorb a significant amount of moisture without feeling wet, allowing the skin to remain dry and comfortable.

Energetically, wool is considered protective. It acts as a shield, blocking negative or harmful energies while keeping the body's natural heat and energy within. Wool clothing is often recommended in holistic practices to enhance personal energy and well-being. Wool's lanolin content makes it naturally water-resistant, while its structure can protect against electromagnetic radiation.

Silk: The Spiritual Connector

Silk, produced by silkworms, has been valued for centuries as a luxurious, healing fabric. It has a naturally smooth texture, and its amino acids are believed to be beneficial to the skin, helping with anti-aging and preventing moisture loss. Silk's temperature-regulating properties also make it versatile for various climates, keeping the body cool in the summer and warm in the winter.

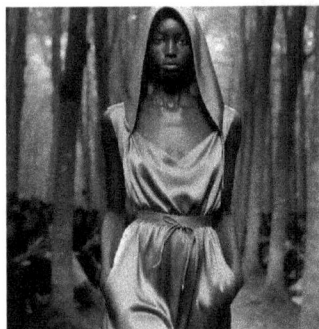

Spiritually, silk is considered a high-vibration fabric. In many Eastern traditions, silk is believed to help connect the wearer to higher spiritual frequencies and is often used in meditation garments and prayer shawls. It's soft, delicate energy complements practices that require mindfulness and focus. Silk is the only natural fabric produced by an insect and has been used in traditional Chinese medicine for centuries to balance the body's energy (Qi).

Hemp: The Eco-Friendly Healer

Hemp is a sustainable, eco-friendly fabric that is gaining popularity in the wellness community. Hemp fibers are strong, durable, and antimicrobial, which helps protect the skin from harmful bacteria. Hemp also has natural UV protection, making it a practical choice for outdoor wear. Hemp is associated with strength and balance.

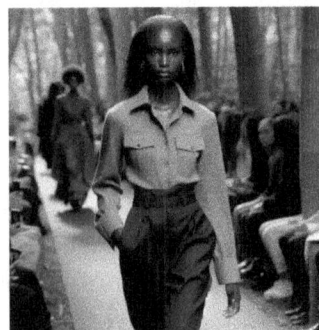

Its eco-conscious production methods and alignment with sustainable practices make it ideal for those seeking to live in harmony with the environment. Hemp fabric becomes softer and stronger with each wash, promoting both durability and comfort.

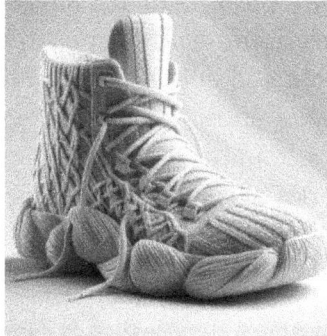

How Clothing from Head to Toe Affects the Body

The clothing we wear from head to toe impacts our body's energy flow, physical comfort, and mental state. Tight, synthetic clothing can restrict movement, trap sweat, and block natural energy pathways, leading to discomfort, irritation, or even fatigue. On the other hand, loose, breathable clothing made from natural fibers promotes circulation, energy flow, and a sense of freedom.

Headwear: Wearing natural fabrics like linen or cotton on the head helps maintain proper circulation and energy flow in the brain. Synthetic materials can create heat buildup, leading to headaches or discomfort.

Shirts and Dresses: Upper body clothing made from natural fibers supports breathability, allowing the skin to absorb oxygen and release toxins more effectively. This promotes better heart and lung function.

Pants and Skirts: Lower body clothing affects circulation to the legs and feet. Restrictive materials can impede blood flow and energy movement, while natural, loose fabrics support proper circulation and grounding.

Footwear: Shoes made from natural materials like leather or hemp allow the feet to "breathe" and maintain natural alignment. Barefoot grounding, or wearing shoes that allow for minimal foot restriction, connects the body directly to the Earth's energy.

The clothing we wear is more than just a fashion statement. It can influence our healing journey by supporting or disrupting the body's natural rhythms and energy flow. Linen, cotton, wool, silk, and hemp each offer unique healing properties, enhancing our physical comfort, emotional well-being, and spiritual connection. Choosing natural fabrics allows us to live in greater harmony with ourselves and the environment, promoting overall wellness from head to toe.

By becoming mindful of the fabrics we wear, we can make choices that not only support our body's needs but also align with the principles of holistic healing and sustainability. The synergy between natural fibers and the human body is a testament to the importance of integrating nature into every aspect of our lives— including our clothing.

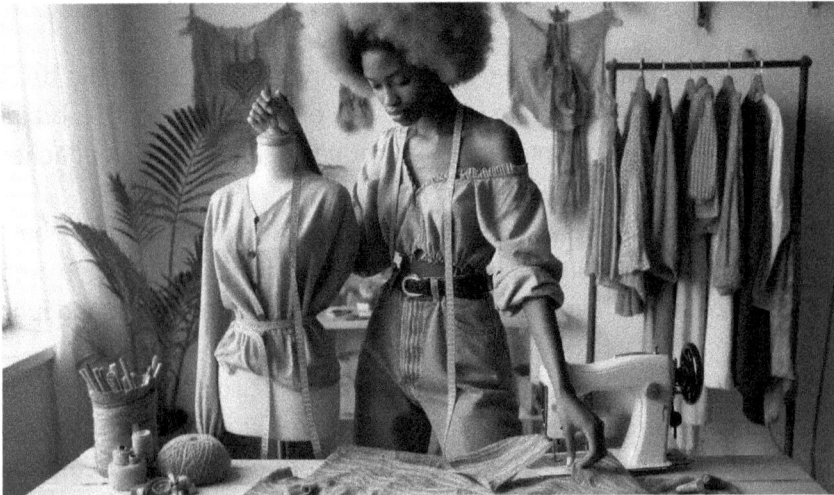

Fabric Chart: Holistic Impact of Natural Fabrics

LINEN

Healing Properties	Best Uses	Energy Alignment
Breathable, moisture-wicking, hypoallergenic, antibacterial, regulates body temperature	Summer clothing, bedding	High-frequency, aligns with bioelectric balance

COTTON

Healing Properties	Best Uses	Energy Alignment
Soft, hypoallergenic, absorbs moisture, breathable	Everyday wear, undergarments	Grounding, supportive of body balance

WOOL

Healing Properties	Best Uses	Energy Alignment
Insulates, moisture-wicking, protects from negative energy	Cold weather wear, blankets	Energy shield, protective

SILK

Healing Properties	Best Uses	Energy Alignment
Smooth, skin-nourishing, temperature regulating	Sleepwear, meditation garments	Spiritual connector, promotes higher frequency alignment

HEMP

Healing Properties	Best Uses	Energy Alignment
Durable, antimicrobial, UV-protective, eco-friendly	Outdoor wear, eco-conscious clothing	Strength, balance, environmentally harmonious

Impact of Synthetic Fabrics on Health and Symptoms

Fabric	Negative Effects on Health	Common Symptoms	Why It's Harmful
Polyester	Traps moisture, non-breathable, creates static electricity, can irritate skin	Skin irritation, sweating, rashes, body odor	Made from petroleum-based chemicals, non-absorbent, blocks airflow
Nylon	Non-breathable, retains odors, treated with harsh chemicals	Skin reactions, overheating, body odor	Often treated with formaldehyde and other chemicals, traps heat
Acrylic	Can cause skin allergies, traps heat, flammable	Itching, allergic reactions, sweating	Made from polyacrylonitrile, a carcinogenic chemical, non-breathable
Spandex Lycra	Restrictive, traps moisture, not breathable	Skin irritation, fungal infections, rashes	Tight-fitting, limits circulation, creates a breeding ground for bacteria
Rayon (Viscose)	Can cause skin irritation, absorbs moisture but doesn't wick it away	Skin irritation, sweating, bacterial growth	Chemically treated cellulose fiber, not eco-friendly, retains moisture

Fabric	Negative Effects on Health	Common Symptoms	Why It's Harmful
PVC (Polyvinyl Chloride)	Contains harmful chemicals like phthalates and dioxins	Headaches, dizziness, hormonal disruption, skin irritation	Releases toxic chemicals, potential endocrine disruptors, used in faux leather
Acrylic Wool	Contains harmful chemicals, traps moisture, irritating to sensitive skin	Rashes, allergies, skin irritation	Synthetic substitute for wool, often treated with formaldehyde
Acetate Triacetate	Non-breathable, retains static, treated with toxic chemicals	Allergic reactions, skin irritation, overheating	Chemically treated wood pulp, flammable, releases fumes when burned
Microfiber	Collects dust and bacteria, synthetic fibers can be harmful when inhaled	Respiratory issues, skin irritation	Made from plastics like polyester, can release microplastics into the environment
Polypropylene	Poor breathability, chemical additives	Sweating, irritation, discomfort	Used in thermal wear, non-biodegradable, can lead to skin irritation

Why These Fabrics Are Harmful

Non-breathability: Many synthetic fabrics trap moisture and heat, creating a breeding ground for bacteria and fungi, leading to rashes, body odor, and skin infections.

Chemical Treatment: Synthetics are often treated with formaldehyde, plasticizers, and other chemicals that can cause allergic reactions, respiratory issues, and even disrupt hormones.

Energy Imbalance: Synthetic fabrics block the body's natural energy flow and can build up static electricity, disrupting the body's electromagnetic field.

Environmental Toxins: Many synthetic fibers are derived from petroleum-based chemicals, contributing to pollution and releasing harmful microplastics into the environment.

Wearing synthetic fabrics can lead to a range of physical symptoms, including skin irritation, overheating, and more severe allergic reactions. Over time, continuous exposure to the chemicals in these materials may contribute to long-term health issues. Shifting toward natural fabrics not only improves personal health but also aligns with a more holistic and environmentally conscious lifestyle.

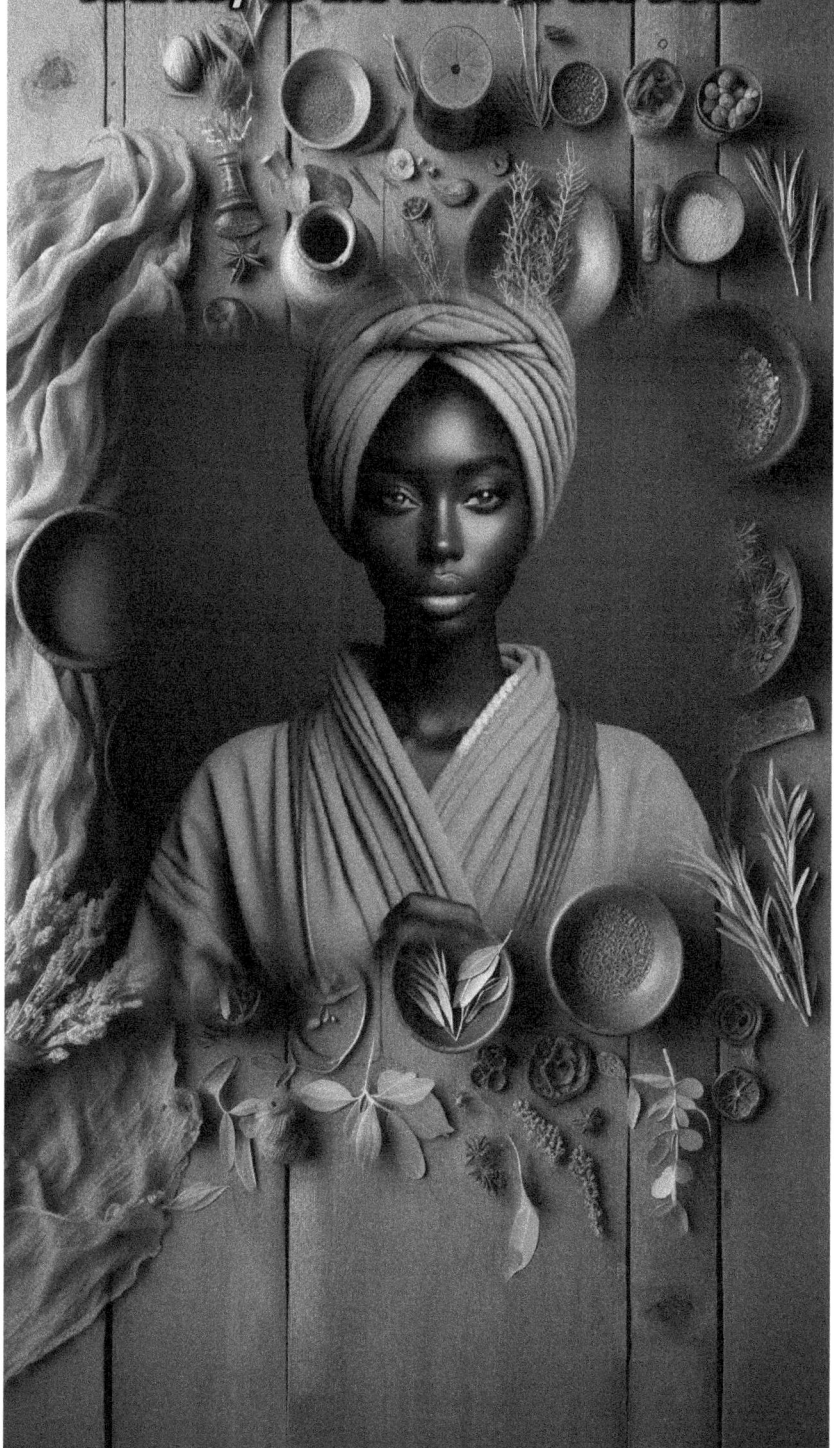

Journey to the back of the Book

Glossary

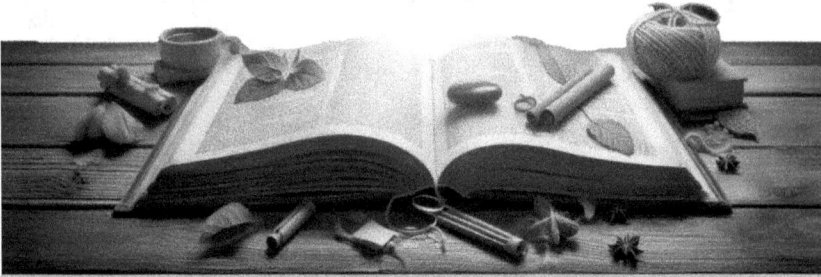

A

Adaptogen
Natural substances that help the body adapt to stress and restore balance.

Adaptogens
Herbs that are thought to help the body adapt to stress. The sources mention ashwagandha, Rhodiola, and holy basil as examples of adaptogens.

Adverse Reaction
An unwanted or harmful effect experienced after taking a medication or supplement.

Alkaline Diet
A way of eating that emphasizes consuming foods that have alkalizing effects on the body, such as fruits, vegetables, nuts, and seeds, while minimizing acidic foods like processed foods, animal products, and caffeine. It is thought to help balance the body's pH level.

Aloe Vera
A succulent plant known for its soothing and healing properties. Its gel is used topically to treat various skin conditions, such as burns, wounds, and dry skin. It is also thought to help with digestion.

Amino Acids
Building blocks of protein essential for muscle growth, repair, and immune function.

Antioxidant
A substance that prevents cell damage by neutralizing free radicals.

Anxiety

A mental health condition characterized by feelings of worry and fear that can affect daily functioning.

Aromatherapy

The use of essential oils from plants to enhance physical and psychological well-being.

Autism

A developmental disorder that affects social interaction, communication, and behavior.

Ayurveda

An ancient Indian system of medicine focusing on balance through diet, herbal treatments, and body care.

B

Bacteria

Microorganisms that exist naturally in the body and environment, some of which support health, while others can cause disease.

Balanced Diet

A diet that includes all essential nutrients in appropriate proportions to promote health and prevent disease.

Biotin

A B vitamin essential for healthy hair, skin, and nails.

Blood Sugar

The concentration of glucose in the blood, important for energy levels and diabetes management.

Blood Type

A classification based on the presence or absence of certain antigens in blood, affecting diet and health compatibility.

Blood Type Diet

A diet that recommends specific foods based on an individual's blood type. The sources mention that people with blood type O may benefit from a diet higher in protein and lower in grains, while people with blood type A may thrive on a more vegetarian diet.

Body Mass Index (BMI)

A measure of body fat based on height and weight.

Bone Density
A measure of the strength of bones, often decreased in conditions like osteoporosis.

Breathwork
A practice that involves controlled breathing exercises to improve mental and physical health.

Burdock Root
A herb traditionally used for its blood-purifying and detoxifying properties. It supports liver and skin health and promotes detoxification.

C

Candida Overgrowth
A condition that occurs when there is an overgrowth of the fungus Candida albicans in the body. This can lead to various health issues, including yeast infections, digestive problems, and skin rashes.

Cardiovascular Health
The health of the heart and blood vessels, crucial for overall well-being.

Cataracts
The clouding of the eye's lens, leading to blurred vision and potential vision loss.

Cell Regeneration
The natural process by which the body renews its cells, promoting healing.

Chakra
Energy centers in the body according to Eastern traditions, each linked to physical and emotional functions.

Chamomile
A herb known for its calming and soothing effects. It promotes relaxation, sleep, and digestive health.

Chronic Disease
A long-term health condition that may not be curable but is manageable.

Chronic Fatigue Syndrome (CFS)
A complex disorder characterized by extreme fatigue that is not relieved by rest and is often accompanied by other symptoms such as muscle and joint pain, cognitive difficulties, and sleep disturbances.

Chronic Obstructive Pulmonary Disease (COPD)
A group of lung diseases, including emphysema and chronic bronchitis, characterized by airflow obstruction and breathing-related problems.

Cleansing
The process of removing toxins from the body, often through diet and lifestyle changes.

Collagen
A protein that supports skin elasticity and joint health.

Complementary Medicine
Medical practices that are used alongside conventional treatments.

Copper
A mineral that plays a vital role in various bodily functions, including the production of red blood cells, iron absorption, and maintaining healthy nerves, bones, and connective tissues.

Cortisol
A stress hormone that regulates various bodily functions, including metabolism and immune response.

CROWN Act
A law that prohibits discrimination based on hair style and texture, primarily affecting Black people.

Cruciferous Vegetables
A family of vegetables, including broccoli and kale, that support detoxification and reduce cancer risk.

Cupping
An ancient therapy that involves placing cups on the skin to increase blood flow and reduce pain.

Curcumin
The active compound in turmeric, known for its potent anti-inflammatory and antioxidant properties.

Cytokines
Proteins involved in cell signaling that can impact inflammation and immunity.

D

Deglycyrrhizinated licorice (DGL)
A form of licorice root extract where glycyrrhizin, a compound that can cause side effects, has been removed. It is often used to soothe digestive discomfort.

Detoxification
The process of removing toxins and waste products from the body. The sources discuss various methods, including dietary changes, fasting, herbal remedies, and detoxification protocols for specific organs like the liver and kidneys.

Diabetes
A chronic metabolic disorder characterized by high blood sugar levels due to the body's inability to produce or effectively use insulin. The sources discuss the prevalence of diabetes in the Black community, the importance of blood sugar monitoring, and management strategies.

Dietary Fiber
A type of carbohydrate that the body can't digest, supporting digestive health and blood sugar balance.

Diuretic
A substance that promotes urination, often used to reduce water retention.

Dosha
In Ayurveda, a classification of physical and mental characteristics that guide personalized health approaches.

Doshas
In Ayurveda, the three fundamental energies that govern the body's functions

Dysautonomia
A condition affecting the autonomic nervous system, which controls involuntary body functions like heart rate, blood pressure, and digestion.

E

Echinacea
A herb commonly used to boost the immune system and fight off infections.

Electrolytes
Minerals that maintain fluid balance and nerve function in the body.

Electromagnetic Frequencies
Waves of energy that are present in the environment and can affect the human body. Examples include radio waves, microwaves, and visible light.

Endocrine System
A system of glands that produce hormones to regulate bodily functions.

Endometriosis
A condition where the tissue that normally lines the inside of the uterus grows outside of it, often causing pain and menstrual irregularities.

Enteric Nervous System (ENS)
A network of nerves in the digestive system that controls digestion. Sometimes referred to as the "second brain."

Epidermis
The outer layer of skin, providing a barrier against the environment.

Epsom Salt
Magnesium sulfate, a mineral compound often used in baths to relieve muscle soreness and promote relaxation.

Essential Oils
Concentrated plant extracts used for therapeutic benefits, especially in aromatherapy.

Ether

Often referred to as the "fifth element," it is a concept in ancient philosophy and traditional medicine that describes a subtle, energetic force that permeates the universe and connects all things.

Exfoliation

The process of removing dead skin cells to reveal smoother skin.

F

Fasting

Abstaining from food and/or drinks for a specific period. The sources discuss different types of fasting and their potential benefits for health and spiritual practice.

Fatty Acids

Essential fats, including omega-3 and omega-6, that support brain health and reduce inflammation.

Fenugreek

A herb that supports lactation in breastfeeding women and may help lower blood sugar levels in people with diabetes.

Fibromyalgia

A chronic condition characterized by widespread musculoskeletal pain, fatigue, and other symptoms like sleep disturbances, mood disorders, and cognitive difficulties.

Free Radicals

Molecules that can damage cells and contribute to aging and disease.

Frequencies

Vibrations or oscillations that occur at a specific rate. The sources discuss frequencies in relation to sound, light, and energy and their potential impact on health and well-being.

G

Gallbladder

A small organ that stores and releases bile, a fluid that helps digest fats.

Gastroesophageal Reflux Disease (GERD)
A condition where stomach acid flows back into the esophagus, causing heartburn and other uncomfortable symptoms.

Genetics
The study of genes and heredity, influencing individual health characteristics and responses to treatment.

Ginger
A rhizome known for its anti-inflammatory and digestive properties. It is often used to alleviate nausea, reduce inflammation, and aid digestion.

Ginseng
A herb believed to boost energy levels, support immune function, and improve cognitive performance.

Glaucoma
An eye condition that damages the optic nerve, leading to vision loss.

Glucose
A sugar that is a primary source of energy for the body's cells.

Goldenseal Root
A herb with antimicrobial properties, traditionally used for respiratory and digestive support, but prolonged use can be harmful to the liver.

Gotu Kola
A herb known for its cognitive-enhancing properties and is believed to improve memory, focus, and mental clarity.

Grounding
Connecting to the earth's energy by walking barefoot on natural surfaces like grass or soil. Grounding is thought to have various health benefits, including reducing inflammation and improving sleep.

Gut Microbiome
The community of microorganisms in the digestive tract that influences digestion, immunity, and mood.

Gut-Brain Axis
The bidirectional communication network between the gut and the brain, involving the nervous system, immune system, and gut microbiome.

H

Hawthorn Berry
A berry traditionally used to support heart health. It may help regulate blood pressure and improve circulation.

Health
An approach to health that considers the whole person—mind, body, and spirit—and emphasizes interconnectedness and balance.

Helicobacter pylori (HP)
A type of bacteria that can infect the stomach, potentially leading to ulcers.

Herbal Healing
A system of medicine that uses plants and their extracts to promote healing and well-being. The sources emphasize the historical and cultural significance of herbal healing in the Black community.

Hibiscus
A flowering plant known for its vibrant color and tart flavor. Its tea is thought to offer various health benefits, including lowering blood pressure and promoting heart health.

Holistic Health
An approach to wellness that considers the whole person, including physical, mental, and spiritual well-being.

Homeostasis
The body's ability to maintain a stable internal environment.

Hormones
Chemical messengers that regulate various bodily processes, including growth, metabolism, and mood.

Humming
The act of producing a continuous sound with the mouth closed. The sources suggest that humming can increase nitric oxide levels in the body, which has various health benefits.

Hydration

The process of providing adequate water to the body for optimal functioning.

Hydrogen Peroxide

A chemical compound (H_2O_2) with antiseptic and oxidizing properties. The sources caution against internal use but suggest it can be used topically for wound care, oral hygiene, and some other external applications.

Hyperpigmentation

A common skin concern characterized by the darkening of areas of the skin.

Hysterectomy

A surgical procedure to remove the uterus.

I

Immune System

The body's defense against infections and diseases.

Immunity

The body's ability to resist or recover from infections.

Inflammation

A response of the body's immune system to injury or infection, often causing redness and swelling.

Insulin

A hormone that helps regulate blood sugar levels.

Iron

A mineral crucial for the production of red blood cells, which carry oxygen throughout the body. Iron deficiency can lead to fatigue, weakness, and anemia.

Irritable Bowel Syndrome (IBS)

A common disorder that affects the large intestine and causes symptoms like abdominal pain, cramping, bloating, gas, diarrhea, and constipation.

J

Jimerito Honey
A type of honey, possibly sourced from the Dominican Republic, believed to have various health benefits, especially for the eyes. The sources highlight its antioxidant, anti-inflammatory, antibacterial, and moisturizing properties.

K

Keloids
Raised scars that grow larger than the original wound. They are more common in people with darker skin tones.

L

Lavender
A flowering plant known for its calming aroma and relaxing properties. Its essential oil is often used in aromatherapy to reduce stress and promote sleep.

Licorice Root
A herb known for its soothing properties and its ability to support the adrenal glands, which are involved in stress response. Deglycyrrhizinated licorice (DGL) is a form of licorice that is often used to treat digestive issues.

Lymphatic System
A network that helps remove toxins and waste from the body.

M

Magnesium
A mineral crucial for many bodily functions, including muscle and nerve function, blood sugar regulation, and blood pressure regulation. The sources emphasize the importance of magnesium for overall health and well-being.

Magnesium Oil
A topical solution of magnesium chloride flakes dissolved in water. It is applied to the skin and believed to be absorbed into the body, offering benefits like muscle relaxation and improved sleep.

Melanin
A pigment that provides color to the skin, hair, and eyes and protects against UV damage.

Menopause

The natural biological process that marks the end of a woman's menstrual cycles.

Menstrual Cycle

The monthly cycle of hormonal changes in a woman's body that prepares the uterus for pregnancy.

Metabolism

The body's process of converting food into energy.

Methylated Folate

A form of folate (vitamin B9) that is more easily absorbed and utilized by the body. Some people with autism spectrum disorder may have difficulty converting folic acid into its active form, so supplementing with methylated folate may be beneficial.

Microbiome

The community of microorganisms (bacteria, fungi, viruses) that live in a particular environment, such as the human gut. The gut microbiome plays a crucial role in digestion, immunity, and overall health.

Milk Thistle

A herb known for its liver-protective properties. It is thought to help detoxify the liver and protect it from damage.

Mindfulness

A mental state focused on awareness of the present moment, used to reduce stress and anxiety.

Minerals

Essential elements needed for various body functions, including calcium, magnesium, and iron.

Mucus-Free Diet

A dietary approach that aims to reduce mucus production in the body. It typically involves avoiding foods thought to be mucus-forming, such as dairy, wheat, and processed foods.

N

Neem
A tropical tree whose leaves, bark, and seeds are used for their Medicinal Properties , particularly in Ayurvedic and traditional medicine. It is known for its antibacterial, antiviral, antifungal, and anti-inflammatory properties.

Nervous System
The body's network for sending signals and coordinating actions, consisting of the brain, spinal cord, and nerves.

Nettle Leaf
A nutrient-rich herb known for its blood-cleansing and nourishing properties. It is often used to address anemia and support overall health.

Neurotransmitter
Chemicals that transmit signals across nerve cells, playing a role in mood and behavior.

Nitric Oxide (NO)
A molecule that plays a vital role in various bodily functions, including blood vessel dilation, blood pressure regulation, and immune response.

Nutrient Deficiency
A lack of essential nutrients that can lead to health issues.

O

Omega-3 Fatty Acids
Essential fats that support heart and brain health.

Oxidative Stress
An imbalance between free radicals and antioxidants that can lead to cell damage.

P

Panchakarma
A detoxification and rejuvenation therapy in Ayurveda that involves five procedures to cleanse the body of toxins.

Passionflower
A herb known for its calming and sleep-promoting effects. It is often used to alleviate anxiety and insomnia.

Pathogen
A microorganism that can cause disease, including bacteria, viruses, and fungi.

Peppermint
A herb renowned for its digestive benefits and its ability to relieve headaches, muscle pain, and respiratory issues.

Peripheral Nervous System (PNS)
The part of the nervous system that connects the central nervous system (brain and spinal cord) to the rest of the body, including the limbs and organs. It is responsible for transmitting sensory and motor information.

Phytochemicals
Plant compounds that have health benefits, often found in fruits and vegetables.

Polycystic Ovary Syndrome (PCOS)
A hormonal disorder common among women of reproductive age, characterized by irregular periods, cysts on the ovaries, and excess androgen hormones, which can lead to symptoms like acne and excess hair growth.

Polyphenols
Antioxidant compounds found in foods like tea, dark chocolate, and berries.

Probiotics
Live microorganisms that are beneficial to the digestive system and gut health. They can be found in fermented foods like yogurt and sauerkraut or taken as supplements.

Proteins
Nutrients essential for growth, repair, and immune function.

Q

Quercetin
A plant pigment with antioxidant and anti-inflammatory properties. It is often used to alleviate allergy symptoms.

R

Reiki

A form of energy healing that involves the practitioner channeling energy into the patient to promote healing and relaxation.

Respiratory System

The organs responsible for breathing, including the lungs and airways.

Rosemary Oil

An essential oil known for its stimulating and invigorating properties. It is often used to promote hair growth, improve memory, and relieve muscle pain.

S

Sarsaparilla

A herb traditionally used for its blood-purifying and detoxifying effects. It is thought to improve skin health and boost overall vitality.

Saturated Fat

A type of fat commonly found in animal products that can affect heart health.

Sea Moss

A type of red algae that is rich in nutrients and minerals, often consumed as a supplement for its potential health benefits, including digestive support and immune system boosting properties.

Self-Care

Intentional actions to care for physical, mental, and emotional well-being.

Serotonin

A neurotransmitter that regulates mood, sleep, and digestion.

Shea Butter

A fat extracted from the nut of the African shea tree. It is rich in fatty acids and vitamins and is commonly used as a moisturizer for skin and hair.

Sickle Cell Disease
A genetic disorder that affects red blood cells, causing them to become misshapen and leading to various health complications. It disproportionately affects people of African descent.

Skin Barrier
The outer layer of skin that protects against environmental damage.

Sleep Hygiene
Practices that promote restful and healthy sleep.

Slippery Elm
A tree whose inner bark is used for its soothing properties, particularly for the digestive tract. It helps relieve inflammation and irritation.

Stress Response
The body's reaction to stress, involving hormones like cortisol and adrenaline.

Superfoods
Nutrient-dense foods that provide health benefits, such as berries and leafy greens.

Systemic
Relating to or affecting the entire body.

T

Toxin
A harmful substance that can affect health, found in the environment, food, or medications.

Triglycerides
A type of fat in the blood that can contribute to heart disease if elevated.

Turmeric
A spice derived from the turmeric plant, known for its vibrant yellow color and potent anti-inflammatory and antioxidant properties.

U

UV Radiation
Ultraviolet radiation from the sun that can cause skin damage and increase cancer risk.

V

Valerian Root
A herb traditionally used to treat insomnia and anxiety due to its calming and sedative effects.

Vasovagal Syncope
A sudden drop in heart rate and blood pressure, leading to fainting.

Vata, Pitta, Kapha
The three doshas in Ayurveda representing body-mind types and guiding personalized health approaches.

Veganism
A lifestyle that avoids animal products, with benefits for health and the environment.

Vitamin D
A fat-soluble vitamin that is crucial for bone health, immune function, and overall well-being. The body produces vitamin D when exposed to sunlight, and it can also be obtained from certain foods and supplements.

Vitamins
Essential nutrients that support bodily functions and prevent deficiencies.

W

Water-Soluble Vitamins
Vitamins that dissolve in water and are not stored in the body, including B vitamins and vitamin C.

Wellness
A holistic state of well-being encompassing physical, mental, and spiritual health.

Y

Yellow Dock Root
A herb known for its blood-cleansing and detoxifying properties, often used to support liver health and address skin conditions.

Yoga

A practice that involves physical postures, breathing techniques, and meditation to improve physical and mental well-being.

Z

Zinc

A mineral that supports immune function, wound healing, and cell division.

H
$$\text{H} \diagdown \underset{\cdot\cdot}{\overset{\cdot\cdot}{O}} - \underset{\cdot\cdot}{\overset{\cdot\cdot}{O}} \diagdown \text{H}$$

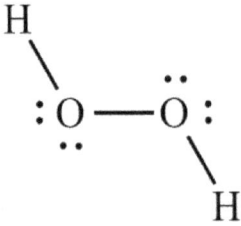

Hydrogen peroxide (H_2O_2) Health Effects

Hydrogen peroxide (H_2O_2) is a compound with a wide range of uses, from disinfecting wounds to household cleaning. It also has some health benefits when used correctly, but it must be handled with care due to its oxidative properties. Below are some of the detailed health benefits of hydrogen peroxide.

Antiseptic for Wounds

Hydrogen peroxide is commonly used as an antiseptic for cleaning wounds. It helps prevent infection by killing bacteria, fungi, and viruses on the skin. *How It Works:* When applied to a wound, hydrogen peroxide releases oxygen, which creates a bubbling action that helps to mechanically clean the wound by lifting dirt and debris. The oxygen also creates an environment that is hostile to anaerobic bacteria, which thrive in low-oxygen environments.

Oral Hygiene

Hydrogen peroxide can be used as a mouth rinse to whiten teeth, kill germs, and reduce gum inflammation. *How It Works:* The oxidative properties of hydrogen peroxide help to break down stains on teeth, making them appear whiter. Its antibacterial action also helps to reduce oral bacteria, which can prevent gum disease and bad breath. *Usage:* Dilute hydrogen peroxide (3% solution) with equal parts water and use it as a mouthwash. Swish for about 30 seconds and then spit it out. Avoid swallowing it, as hydrogen peroxide is not safe for ingestion.

Earwax Removal

Hydrogen peroxide can soften and remove earwax, which can relieve ear discomfort and improve hearing. *How It Works:* When hydrogen peroxide is applied to the ear canal, it breaks down the wax into smaller pieces, making it easier to remove. The bubbling action can also help to dislodge wax. *Usage:* Use a few drops of 3% hydrogen peroxide in the ear, let it sit for a few minutes, and then tilt the head to let the liquid drain out. This can be followed by gently flushing the ear with warm water.

Sinus Infection Relief

Hydrogen peroxide can be used to help clear sinus infections when used in a diluted form as a nasal rinse. *How It Works:* The antiseptic properties of hydrogen peroxide can help to kill pathogens in the nasal passages and sinuses, reducing infection and inflammation. *Usage:* Mix a few drops of 3% hydrogen peroxide with distilled water and use a neti pot or nasal spray bottle to rinse the nasal passages. This should be done cautiously and not too frequently to avoid irritation.

Foot and Nail Fungus Treatment

Hydrogen peroxide can treat fungal infections on the feet and nails, such as athlete's foot and toenail fungus. *How It Works:* The antifungal properties of hydrogen peroxide help to kill the fungus on the surface of the skin and nails. Regular use can reduce the severity of the infection and promote healing. *Usage:* Soak the affected area in a mixture of hydrogen peroxide (3%) and water for about 15-20 minutes daily until the infection clears up.

Hydrogen Peroxide in a Humidifier

Adding hydrogen peroxide to a humidifier can help purify the air, kill airborne pathogens, and reduce the risk of respiratory infections. *How It Works:* When hydrogen peroxide is added to the water in a humidifier, it releases oxygen, which can help to disinfect the air by killing bacteria, mold, and viruses. This can be particularly beneficial during cold and flu season. *Usage:* Add about 1-2 teaspoons of 3% hydrogen peroxide to a gallon of water in your humidifier's tank. This helps to keep the humidifier clean and ensures that the mist released into the air is less likely to carry harmful pathogens.

Disinfectant for Household Surfaces

Hydrogen peroxide is a natural disinfectant that can be used to clean and disinfect various surfaces in the home, helping to reduce the spread of germs and viruses. *How It Works:* The oxidizing properties of hydrogen peroxide effectively kill a wide range of microorganisms, including bacteria, viruses, and fungi, making it a good alternative to chemical disinfectants. *Usage:* Use a 3% hydrogen peroxide solution in a spray bottle to clean surfaces like countertops, doorknobs, and bathroom fixtures. Allow it to sit for a few minutes before wiping it down with a clean cloth.

Teeth Whitening

Hydrogen peroxide is often used in teeth whitening products because of its ability to remove stains and brighten the teeth. *How It Works:* The peroxide works as a bleaching agent by breaking down the stains on the surface of the teeth, making them appear whiter over time. *Usage:* You can create a homemade whitening paste by mixing hydrogen peroxide with baking soda and brushing your teeth with it. Do this sparingly, as overuse can damage tooth enamel.

Treating Minor Skin Infections

Hydrogen peroxide can be used to treat minor skin infections, such as cuts, scrapes, and pimples, due to its antibacterial properties. *How It Works:* By applying hydrogen peroxide to the affected area, the oxygen release helps to kill bacteria and dry out the infection, promoting faster healing. *Usage:* Dab a small amount of 3% hydrogen peroxide on the infection using a cotton swab. Do this once or twice a day until the infection clears up.

Important Considerations *Dilution: Always use hydrogen peroxide in its diluted form (3%) for health purposes. Higher concentrations can be harmful and cause irritation or burns.* **Avoid Ingestion:** *Hydrogen peroxide should not be ingested, as it can cause serious health issues if swallowed.*

Benefits and Health Facts of Tea Tree Oil

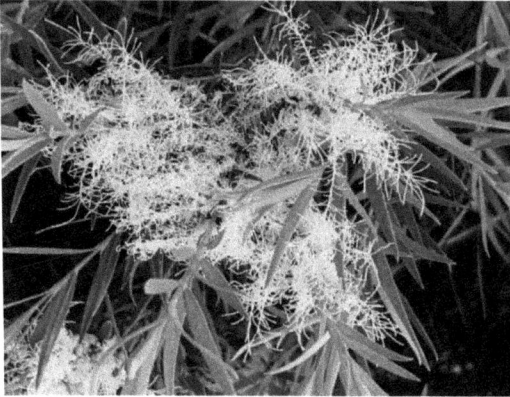

Tea tree oil, derived from the leaves of the *Melaleuca alternifolia* tree, is a powerful essential oil known for its wide range of medicinal properties. It has been used for centuries in traditional medicine and is particularly valued for its antiseptic, antifungal, and anti-inflammatory effects.

Where is Tea Tree Native To?

The tea tree is native to Australia, particularly the swampy, subtropical regions of the northeast coast, in New South Wales and Queensland. Aboriginal Australians have traditionally used tea tree leaves for medicinal purposes, including crushing them to extract the oil for treating wounds and infections.

Antiseptic and Disinfectant Properties

Tea tree oil is highly effective at killing bacteria, viruses, and fungi, making it a popular natural antiseptic. *Usage:* It can be applied topically to minor cuts, scrapes, and burns to prevent infection. Dilute with a carrier oil (like coconut or olive oil) before applying to the skin.

Acne Treatment

Tea tree oil is a well-known remedy for acne due to its ability to reduce inflammation and fight acne-causing bacteria. *Usage:* Apply a drop of diluted tea tree oil directly to pimples using a cotton swab. Regular use can reduce the severity and frequency of breakouts.

Antifungal Properties

Tea tree oil is effective against fungal infections, such as athlete's foot, nail fungus, and ringworm. *Usage:* For fungal infections, apply diluted tea tree oil to the affected area twice daily until the infection clears. For nail fungus, you can mix it with a carrier oil and apply it directly to the nails.

Anti-Inflammatory Effects

Tea tree oil can reduce inflammation, redness, and swelling, making it beneficial for conditions like eczema and psoriasis. *Usage:* Dilute tea tree oil in a carrier oil and apply it to inflamed or irritated skin to soothe symptoms.

Oral Health

Tea tree oil's antibacterial properties can help reduce plaque, prevent tooth decay, and treat bad breath. *Usage:* Add a few drops of tea tree oil to water and use it as a mouthwash. Do not swallow, as tea tree oil can be toxic if ingested.

Treating Dandruff and Scalp Health

Tea tree oil helps alleviate dandruff by reducing yeast overgrowth and soothing an itchy scalp. **Usage:** Add a few drops of tea tree oil to your shampoo and massage it into your scalp. Leave it on for a few minutes before rinsing.

Relief from Insect Bites and Stings

Tea tree oil's anti-inflammatory and antimicrobial properties can reduce itching, swelling, and the risk of infection from insect bites and stings. *Usage:* Apply a drop of diluted tea tree oil to the affected area for relief.

Respiratory Tract Infections

Inhalation of tea tree oil can help clear respiratory tract infections due to its antimicrobial and decongestant properties. *Usage:* Add a few drops of tea tree oil to a bowl of hot water and inhale the steam to relieve congestion. Alternatively, you can add it to a diffuser.

Natural Deodorant

Tea tree oil's antibacterial properties make it an effective natural deodorant by reducing the bacteria that cause body odor. *Usage:* Mix a few drops of tea tree oil with a carrier oil and apply it to your underarms as a natural deodorant.

Household Cleaner

Tea tree oil can be used as a natural disinfectant and cleaner around the home. *Usage:* Mix tea tree oil with water and vinegar to create a natural cleaning spray for surfaces in the kitchen and bathroom.

Important Considerations:

Dilution: Tea tree oil is potent and should always be diluted with a carrier oil (like coconut, almond, or olive oil) before applying to the skin to prevent irritation. *Patch Test:* Before using tea tree oil, perform a patch test on a small area of skin to ensure you don't have an allergic reaction. *Avoid Ingestion:* Tea tree oil should never be ingested, as it can be toxic when swallowed. *Sensitive Areas:* Avoid using tea tree oil on sensitive areas like the eyes, ears, and mucous membranes. Tea tree oil is a versatile and powerful natural remedy with numerous health benefits. When used properly, it can be an effective addition to your natural health and wellness routine.

Benefits of Celtic Sea Salt

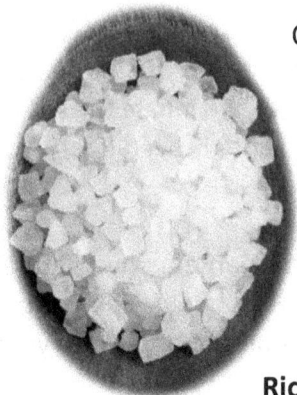

Celtic sea salt, a type of unrefined salt harvested from the coastal regions of France, is known for its natural mineral content and health benefits. For African Americans, who may face unique health challenges related to genetics, lifestyle, and environmental factors, Celtic salt can offer several natural benefits.

Rich in Essential Minerals

Celtic sea salt contains over 80 trace minerals, including magnesium, calcium, and potassium, which are vital for bodily functions. These minerals can help address common deficiencies in African Americans, such as magnesium, which is important for bone health, muscle function, and blood pressure regulation.

Electrolyte Balance and Hydration

The high mineral content helps balance electrolytes and maintain proper hydration. This is especially beneficial for African Americans who may have a genetic predisposition to high blood pressure (hypertension). The balanced electrolytes can aid in better hydration and heart health.

Improved Digestive Health

Celtic salt can help stimulate digestive enzymes, supporting better nutrient absorption. African American communities often face digestive issues like acid reflux or irritable bowel syndrome (IBS), and the use of Celtic salt can help promote healthy digestion and balance stomach acid levels.

Detoxification Support

Due to its unprocessed nature, Celtic salt can help the body eliminate toxins. African Americans may experience higher exposure to environmental toxins and pollutants, and incorporating Celtic salt can aid in the body's natural detoxification processes.

Supports Skin Health

Celtic salt, when used in baths or as a scrub, can help exfoliate the skin and draw out impurities. For melanin-rich skin, which can be prone to hyperpigmentation or eczema, the minerals in Celtic salt can help soothe inflammation, promote healing, and improve skin texture

.

Alkalizing Effects

Despite being a salt, Celtic sea salt has alkalizing properties due to its mineral content. It can help balance the body's pH, reducing acidity, which is beneficial for preventing chronic diseases that are more prevalent in African American communities, such as diabetes and gout.

How to Use Celtic Sea Salt:

In Cooking: Replace regular table salt with Celtic sea salt to boost mineral intake. **Salt Water Flush**: Drinking a warm glass of water with a pinch of Celtic salt in the morning can help with detoxification and digestive health. **Bath Soak**: Add a cup of Celtic sea salt to bath water for a relaxing and detoxifying soak, promoting joint health and skin healing. **Skin Scrub**: Mix Celtic salt with coconut oil for an exfoliating body scrub.

Incorporating Celtic sea salt into a holistic wellness routine can provide numerous health benefits, particularly for African Americans who may need additional support in areas such as hydration, detoxification, and mineral balance.

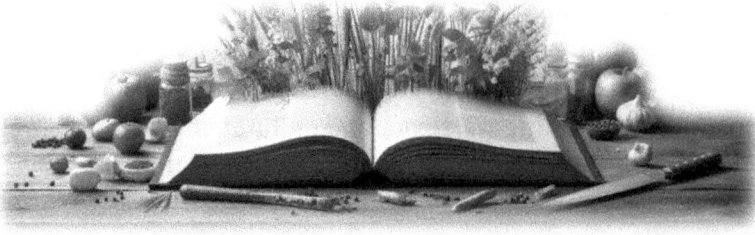

Herbal Reference Guide

A

Aloe Vera
Anti-inflammatory, wound healing **Usage** Topical, internal
Ashwagandha
Stress relief, adrenal support **Usage** Powder, capsule
Astragalus
Immune support, anti-inflammatory **Usage** Tea, supplement

B

Basil
Antibacterial, digestive aid **Usage** Culinary, tea
Bitter Melon
Blood sugar regulation, digestive aid **Usage** Culinary, supplement
Black Walnut
Antimicrobial, digestive aid **Usage** Tincture, supplement
Black Cohosh
Hormone balance, menopause symptoms **Usage** Capsule, tea
Blue Vervain
Nerve relaxant, digestive aid **Usage** Tea, tincture
Boneset
Immune support, fever reducer **Usage** Tea, tincture
Borage
Hormonal support, anti-inflammatory **Usage** Tea, oil
Boswellia
Anti-inflammatory, joint health **Usage** Supplement
Buchu
Urinary tract health, diuretic **Usage** Tea, supplement

Burdock Root

Blood purifier, liver support **Usage** Internal

C

Calendula

Anti-inflammatory, wound healing **Usage** Topical, tea

Caraway

Digestive aid, respiratory health **Usage** Culinary, tea

Cardamom

Digestive aid, respiratory health **Usage** Culinary, tea

Cascara Sagrada

Laxative, digestive aid **Usage** Supplement, tea

Catnip

Calming, digestive aid **Usage** Tea

Cayenne

Circulatory health, pain relief **Usage** Culinary, supplement

Chamomile

Calming, anti-inflammatory **Usage** Tea, topical

Chickweed

Skin health, anti-inflammatory **Usage** Tea, topical

Cilantro

Detoxification, digestive aid **Usage** Culinary, tea

Cinnamon

Blood sugar regulation, anti-inflammatory **Usage** Culinary, tea

Cleavers

Lymphatic support, diuretic **Usage** Tea, tincture

Clove   Antimicrobial, pain relief **Usage** Culinary, oil

Coltsfoot

Respiratory health, cough relief **Usage** Tea, tincture

Comfrey
Wound healing, anti-inflammatory
Usage Topical, tea
Coriander
Digestive aid, detoxification **Usage** Culinary, tea
Cornsilk
Urinary tract health, diuretic **Usage** Tea, supplement
Cramp Bark
Menstrual cramp relief, muscle relaxant **Usage** Tea, tincture

---

D

Damiana
Libido enhancement, mood support **Usage** Tea, supplement
Dandelion
Detoxifying, liver support **Usage** Tea, salad greens
Devil's Claw
Anti-inflammatory, pain relief **Usage** Supplement
Dong Quai
Hormonal balance, menstrual support **Usage** Tea, supplement

---

E

Echinacea
Immune-boosting, cold remedy **Usage** Tea, tincture
Elderberry
Immune-boosting, cold and flu prevention **Usage** Syrup, tincture
Eleuthero
Stress relief, energy boost **Usage** Supplement, tea
Eucalyptus
Respiratory health, antimicrobial **Usage** Aromatherapy, tea
Evening Primrose
Hormonal balance, skin health **Usage** Supplement, oil

F

False Unicorn
Hormonal balance, reproductive health **Usage** Tea, supplement
Fennel
Digestive aid, menstrual cramp relief **Usage** Culinary, tea
Fenugreek
Digestive aid, lactation support **Usage** Culinary, supplement
Feverfew
Migraine relief, anti-inflammatory **Usage** Tea, tincture

G

Garcinia Cambogia
Weight management, appetite suppressant **Usage** Supplement
Ginger
Digestive aid, anti-inflammatory **Usage** Culinary, tea
Ginkgo Biloba
Cognitive function, circulation support **Usage** Supplement, tea
Ginseng
Energy boost, stress relief **Usage** Supplement, tea
Goldenseal
Antimicrobial, digestive aid **Usage** Capsule, tea
Gokshura
Urinary tract health, libido enhancement **Usage** Supplement
Gotu Kola
Cognitive function, skin health **Usage** Tea, supplement
Gravel Root
Kidney health, diuretic **Usage** Tea, tincture

H

Hawthorn
Heart health, antioxidant **Usage** Tea, supplement
Hibiscus
Blood pressure regulation, antioxidant **Usage** Tea, syrup
Holy Basil
Stress relief, immune support **Usage** Tea, supplement

Hops
Sleep aid, calming **Usage** Tea, tincture
Horsetail
Bone health, diuretic **Usage** Tea, supplement
Hyssop
Respiratory health, digestive aid **Usage** Tea, tincture

J

Juniper
Urinary tract health, digestive aid **Usage** Tea, supplement

K

Kava Kava Root
Anxiety relief, muscle relaxant **Usage** Tea, supplement
Kudzu
Alcoholism support, anti-inflammatory **Usage** Tea, supplement

L

Lady's Mantle
Menstrual support, astringent **Usage** Tea, tincture
Lavender
Relaxant, sleep aid **Usage** Aromatherapy, tea
Lemon Balm
Anxiety relief, sleep aid **Usage** Tea, tincture
Lemongrass
Digestive aid, stress relief **Usage** Tea, oil
Linden Flower
Calming, respiratory health **Usage** Tea
Licorice Root
Soothing digestive aid, adrenal support **Usage** Tea, extract
Lobelia
Respiratory health, muscle relaxant **Usage** Tea, tincture

M

Maca
Energy boost, hormonal balance **Usage** Supplement, powder
Meadowsweet
Digestive aid, anti-inflammatory **Usage** Tea, tincture

Marjoram
Digestive aid, anti-inflammatory **Usage** Culinary, tea
Marshmallow Root
Soothing digestive and respiratory tract **Usage** Tea, poultice
Milk Thistle
Liver support, detoxification **Usage** Tea, supplement
Moringa
Nutrient-rich, antioxidant **Usage** Powder, tea
Motherwort
Hormone balance, heart health **Usage** Tea, tincture
Mugwort
Digestive aid, menstrual support **Usage** Tea, tincture
Mullein
Respiratory health, anti-inflammatory **Usage** Tea, tincture
Myrrh
Antimicrobial, wound healing **Usage** Tincture, oil

N

Nettle
Allergy relief, iron-rich **Usage** Tea, soup
Neem
Skin health, antimicrobial **Usage** Oil, supplement

O

Oregano
Antimicrobial, antioxidant **Usage** Culinary, oil

P

Parsley
Digestive aid, diuretic **Usage** Culinary, tea
Passionflower
Anxiety relief, sleep aid **Usage** Tea, tincture
Peppermint
Digestive aid, headache relief **Usage** Tea, aromatherapy
Plantain
Wound healing, digestive aid **Usage** Tea, topical

Q

Queen Anne's Lace
Hormonal balance, diuretic **Usage** Tea, tincture

R

Raspberry Leaf
Uterine health, menstrual support **Usage** Tea

Red Clover
Hormonal balance, skin health **Usage** Tea, tincture

Reishi Mushroom
Immune support, stress relief **Usage** Supplement, tea

Rhodiola
Stress relief, cognitive function **Usage** Supplement, tea

Rosehip
Vitamin C boost, immune support **Usage** Tea, syrup

Rosemary
Cognitive function, antioxidant **Usage** Culinary, tea

S

Saffron
Mood support, antioxidant **Usage** Culinary, tea

Sage
Antioxidant, antimicrobial **Usage** Culinary, tea

Sarsaparilla
Blood purifier, skin health **Usage** Tea, supplement

Saw Palmetto
Hormonal balance, prostate health **Usage** Supplement, tea

Schisandra
Stress relief, liver support **Usage** Supplement, tea

Sea Moss
Nutrient-rich, thyroid support **Usage** Supplement, powder

Senna
Laxative, digestive aid **Usage** Tea, supplement

Shepherd's Purse
Menstrual support, wound healing **Usage** Tea, tincture

Shatavari
Hormonal balance, reproductive health **Usage** Supplement, tea

Skullcap

Anxiety relief, sleep aid **Usage** Tea, tincture

Slippery Elm

Soothing digestive aid, throat relief **Usage** Tea, powder

Spearmint

Digestive aid, hormonal balance **Usage** Tea, culinary

Spirulina

Nutrient-rich, detoxification **Usage** Supplement, powder

Stevia

Natural sweetener, blood sugar regulation **Usage** Culinary, supplement

St. John's Wort

Mood support, anxiety relief **Usage** Tea, supplement

Stinging Nettle

Allergy relief, iron-rich **Usage** Tea, soup

T

Tarragon

Digestive aid, antibacterial **Usage** Culinary, tea

Thyme

Respiratory health, antibacterial **Usage** Culinary, tea

Tribulus

Libido enhancement, energy boost **Usage** Supplement

Tulsi (Holy Basil)

Stress relief, immune support **Usage** Tea, supplement

Turmeric

Anti-inflammatory, antioxidant **Usage** Culinary, tea

U

Usnea

Antimicrobial, respiratory health **Usage** Tincture, tea

Uva Ursi

Urinary tract health, antimicrobial **Usage** Tea, supplement

V

Valerian

Anxiety relief, sleep aid **Usage** Tincture, tea

W

Witch Hazel
Astringent, anti-inflammatory **Usage** Topical, tea
White Willow Bark
Pain relief, anti-inflammatory **Usage** Tea, supplement
Wormwood
Digestive aid, antiparasitic **Usage** Tea, tincture

Y

Yarrow
Fever reducer, wound healing **Usage** Tea, poultice
Yellow Dock
Liver support, blood purifier **Usage** Tea, supplement
Yerba Mate
Energy boost, antioxidant **Usage** Tea
Yohimbe
Energy boost, libido enhancement **Usage** Supplement

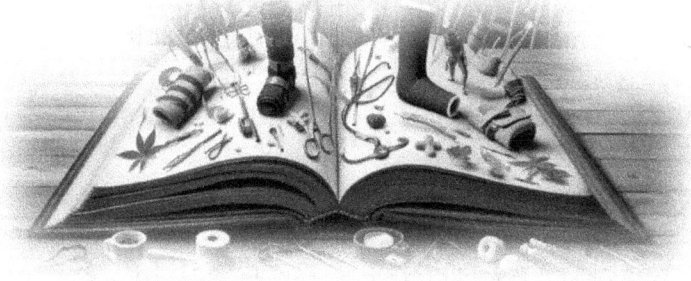

Common Aliments and Natural Remedies

A

Acid Reflux

Apple Cider Vinegar, Slippery Elm, Licorice

Usage Instructions

Dilute apple cider vinegar in water and drink before meals; take slippery elm supplements; chew deglycyrrhizinated licorice (DGL).

Acidity

Banana, Almonds, Licorice Root

Usage Instructions

Eat a ripe banana or a handful of almonds; chew a piece of licorice root slowly for relief.

Acne

Tea Tree Oil, Aloe Vera, Witch Hazel

Usage Instructions

Apply tea tree oil or witch hazel directly to affected areas. Use aloe vera gel as a soothing moisturizer.

Allergies

Local Honey, Quercetin, Nettle Leaf

Usage Instructions

Consume local honey regularly; take quercetin supplements; drink nettle leaf tea or use it in cooking.

Anemia

Iron-Rich Foods, Vitamin C, Beetroot Juice

Usage Instructions

Consume iron-rich foods like spinach and lentils; pair with foods high in vitamin C for better absorption; drink beetroot juice.

Anxiety

Chamomile Tea, Lavender, Valerian Root, Ashwagandha, Lavender Oil, Exercise

Usage Instructions

Drink chamomile tea before bed; use lavender essential oil in a diffuser or bath; take valerian root as directed. Take ashwagandha supplements as directed; inhale lavender oil or use in a diffuser; engage in regular exercise.

Arthritis

Turmeric, Ginger, Epsom Salt Baths

Usage Instructions

Add turmeric and ginger to cooking; soak in warm Epsom salt baths for relief.

Athlete's Foot

Tea Tree Oil, Garlic, Vinegar

Usage Instructions

Apply tea tree oil directly to affected areas; crush garlic and mix with coconut oil, apply; soak feet in diluted vinegar solution.

B

Bad Breath

Peppermint, Parsley, Oil Pulling

Usage Instructions

Chew fresh peppermint leaves or parsley; swish coconut or sesame oil in your mouth for 10-20 minutes.

Bloating

Peppermint Tea, Fennel Seeds, Exercise

Usage Instructions

Drink peppermint tea after meals; chew fennel seeds; engage in gentle exercise to aid digestion.

Bug Bites

Aloe Vera Gel, Lavender Oil, Oatmeal Bath

Usage Instructions

Apply aloe vera gel directly to the bite; apply diluted lavender oil to the affected area; take soothing oatmeal baths to relieve itching.

C

Cavities
Oil Pulling, Licorice Root, Neem
Usage Instructions
Swish coconut or sesame oil in your mouth for 10-20 minutes; chew deglycyrrhizinated licorice (DGL); use neem toothpaste or mouthwash.

Cellulite
Dry Brushing, Coffee Scrub, Massage
Usage Instructions
Use a dry brush on affected areas before showering; apply coffee grounds mixed with olive oil as a scrub; massage with firm pressure.

Chapped Lips
Honey, Coconut Oil, Aloe Vera
Usage Instructions
Apply honey directly to lips; use coconut oil as a moisturizer; apply aloe vera gel to soothe and hydrate.

Cold Sores
Lysine, Lemon Balm, Ice Packs
Usage Instructions
Take lysine supplements; apply lemon balm cream to affected areas; use ice packs to reduce swelling and pain.

Common Cold
Garlic, Ginger, Honey, Echinacea
Usage Instructions
Consume garlic and ginger in foods or teas; take honey alone or in tea; take echinacea supplements as directed.

Constipation
Fiber-Rich Foods, Prunes, Flaxseed
Usage Instructions
Eat plenty of fruits, vegetables, and whole grains; consume prunes or drink prune juice; add flaxseed to meals.

Cough
Honey, Ginger Tea, Thyme
Usage Instructions
Take honey alone or mix it with warm water or tea; drink ginger tea; brew thyme tea or use it in cooking.

Cramps
Ginger Tea, Heat Packs, Magnesium
Usage Instructions
Drink ginger tea; apply heat packs to the affected area; take magnesium supplements as directed.

D

Dandruff
Apple Cider Vinegar, Tea Tree Oil, Aloe Vera, BRAT Diet (Bananas, Rice, Toast), Probiotics
Usage Instructions
Rinse hair with diluted apple cider vinegar; apply diluted tea tree oil to the scalp; use aloe vera gel as a scalp treatment. Stick to the BRAT diet; consume probiotic-rich foods or supplements.

Dry Eyes
Omega-3 Fatty Acids, Flaxseed Oil, Blinking Exercises
Usage Instructions
Consume foods rich in omega-3s; take flaxseed oil supplements; perform blinking exercises regularly.

Dry Skin
Coconut Oil, Oatmeal Baths, Hydration
Usage Instructions
Apply coconut oil to damp skin after bathing; take soothing oatmeal baths; drink plenty of water to stay hydrated.

E

Ear Infection
Garlic Oil, Warm Compress, Breast Milk
Usage Instructions
Apply warmed garlic oil drops to the affected ear; apply a warm compress to relieve pain; apply a few drops of breast milk to the ear canal.

Earache
Warm Olive Oil, Garlic Oil, Mullein Oil
Usage Instructions
Warm olive oil and apply a few drops into the affected ear; use garlic or mullein oil drops as directed.

Eczema
Oatmeal Baths, Evening Primrose Oil, Probiotics
Usage Instructions
Take soothing oatmeal baths; apply evening primrose oil to affected areas; consume probiotics regularly.

F

Fatigue
Ginseng, Green Tea, B Vitamins
Usage Instructions
Take ginseng supplements; drink green tea; consume foods rich in B vitamins or take supplements as directed.

Fibromyalgia
Turmeric, Omega-3 Fatty Acids, Yoga
Usage Instructions
Incorporate turmeric into cooking; consume foods rich in omega-3s; practice gentle yoga for pain relief and relaxation.

Flatulence
Ginger, Activated Charcoal, Probiotics
Usage Instructions
Consume ginger tea or chew raw ginger; take activated charcoal supplements; consume probiotics regularly.

Food Poisoning
Ginger, Activated Charcoal, Peppermint Tea
Usage Instructions
Consume ginger tea or chew raw ginger; take activated charcoal supplements; drink peppermint tea for relief.
Foot Odor
Baking Soda, Black Tea, Epsom Salt
Usage Instructions
Sprinkle baking soda in shoes to absorb odor; soak feet in black tea or Epsom salt solution to kill bacteria and reduce odor.

G

Gas
Peppermint Tea, Chamomile Tea, Caraway Seeds
Usage Instructions
Drink peppermint or chamomile tea after meals; chew caraway seeds to reduce gas and bloating.
Gingivitis
Oil Pulling, Aloe Vera Gel, Turmeric Paste
Usage Instructions
Swish coconut or sesame oil in your mouth for 10-20 minutes; apply aloe vera gel to gums; make a paste of turmeric and water and apply to gums.
Gout
Tart Cherry Juice, Celery Seed Extract, Ginger
Usage Instructions
Drink tart cherry juice daily; take celery seed extract supplements; consume ginger in foods or teas.
Gum Disease
Oil Pulling, Saltwater Rinse, Vitamin C
Usage Instructions
Swish coconut or sesame oil in your mouth for 10-20 minutes; rinse with warm salt water; consume foods high in vitamin C.

H

Hair Loss
Rosemary Oil, Pumpkin Seed Oil, Scalp Massage
Usage Instructions
Dilute rosemary oil with a carrier oil and massage into the scalp; take pumpkin seed oil supplements; massage scalp regularly to improve circulation.

Halitosis (Bad Breath)
Mint Leaves, Fennel Seeds, Apple Cider Vinegar
Usage Instructions
Chew fresh mint leaves or fennel seeds; rinse mouth with diluted apple cider vinegar; drink plenty of water to stay hydrated.

Hangnails
Olive Oil, Vitamin E Oil, Moisturizer
Usage Instructions
Soak fingers in warm olive oil; apply vitamin E oil directly to hangnails; moisturize hands regularly.

Hangover
Coconut Water, Ginger, Lemon
Usage Instructions
Drink coconut water for hydration; consume ginger tea or chew raw ginger; squeeze lemon juice into water.

Headaches
Peppermint Oil, Lavender Oil, Feverfew
Usage Instructions
Apply diluted peppermint or lavender oil to temples; take feverfew supplements as directed.

Heartburn
Aloe Vera Juice, Ginger Tea, Slippery Elm, Licorice
Usage Instructions
Drink aloe vera juice; drink ginger tea; take slippery elm supplements as directed. chew deglycyrrhizinated licorice (DGL) tablets before meal

Hemorrhoids
Witch Hazel, Aloe Vera, Warm Baths
Usage Instructions
Apply witch hazel directly to affected area; apply aloe vera gel for soothing relief; soak in warm baths regularly.

Hiccups
Drinking Water, Holding Breath, Sugar
Usage Instructions
Drink a glass of water slowly; hold your breath for 10 seconds and repeat; swallow a teaspoon of sugar.

High Blood Pressure
Garlic, Hibiscus Tea, Hawthorn
Usage Instructions
Consume garlic in food or take supplements; drink hibiscus tea; take hawthorn supplements as directed.

High Cholesterol
Oats, Garlic, Plant Sterols
Usage Instructions
Incorporate oats into your diet; consume raw garlic or take garlic supplements; use spreads or supplements with plant sterols.

I

Impetigo
Tea Tree Oil, Manuka Honey, Colloidal Silver
Usage Instructions
Apply diluted tea tree oil to affected areas; apply manuka honey to affected areas; apply colloidal silver topically.

Indigestion
Peppermint Tea, Ginger Tea, Fennel Seeds, Apple Cider Vinegar, Ginger, Papaya
Usage Instructions
Drink peppermint or ginger tea; chew fennel seeds after meals. Dilute apple cider vinegar in water and drink before meals; drink ginger tea; eat fresh papaya or take papaya enzyme supplements.

Infections

Garlic, Echinacea, Goldenseal

Usage Instructions

Consume garlic in foods or take garlic supplements; take echinacea supplements as directed; take goldenseal supplements as directed.

Insomnia

Valerian Root, Chamomile Tea, Lavender

Usage Instructions

Take valerian root supplements as directed; drink chamomile tea before bed; use lavender essential oil in a diffuser.

Itchy Eyes

Cold Compress, Cucumber Slices, Tea Bags

Usage Instructions

Apply a cold compress over closed eyelids; place cucumber slices over eyes; use cooled tea bags as eye compresses.

Itchy Scalp

Apple Cider Vinegar, Tea Tree Oil, Baking Soda

Usage Instructions

Rinse scalp with diluted apple cider vinegar; apply diluted tea tree oil to the scalp; massage baking soda into damp hair before shampooing.

Itchy Skin

Oatmeal Baths, Coconut Oil, Calendula

Usage Instructions

Take soothing oatmeal baths; apply coconut oil directly to the skin; use calendula cream on affected areas.

J

Jet Lag

Melatonin, Hydration, Natural Light

Usage Instructions

Take melatonin supplements to regulate sleep; stay hydrated during travel; expose yourself to natural light to reset your internal clock.

Joint Pain

Turmeric, Cayenne Pepper, Massage Therapy

Usage Instructions

Incorporate turmeric into cooking; apply cayenne pepper cream topically; seek professional massage therapy.

K

Kidney Health

Dandelion Root Tea, Cranberry Juice, Water

Usage Instructions

Drink dandelion root tea regularly; consume unsweetened cranberry juice; stay hydrated by drinking plenty of water.

L

Liver Health

Milk Thistle, Dandelion Root, Turmeric

Usage Instructions

Take milk thistle supplements as directed; drink dandelion root tea regularly; incorporate turmeric into cooking.

M

Menstrual Bloating

Ginger Tea, Fennel Seeds, Magnesium

Usage Instructions

Drink ginger tea; chew fennel seeds; take magnesium supplements as directed.

Menstrual Cramps

Ginger Tea, Heat Packs, Chamomile Tea

Usage Instructions

Drink ginger or chamomile tea; apply heat packs to the lower abdomen.

Migraine
Magnesium, Feverfew, Peppermint Oil
Usage Instructions
Take magnesium supplements as directed; take feverfew supplements as directed; apply diluted peppermint oil to temples and forehead.
Morning Sickness
Ginger, Vitamin B6, Crackers
Usage Instructions
Chew raw ginger or drink ginger tea; take vitamin B6 supplements; nibble on crackers to settle the stomach.
Motion Sickness
Ginger, Peppermint, Acupressure
Usage Instructions
Consume ginger or peppermint in any form; apply pressure to the P6 acupressure point on the wrist.
Muscle Cramps
Magnesium, Hydration, Stretching
Usage Instructions
Take magnesium supplements as directed; stay hydrated; perform gentle stretching exercises regularly.
Muscle Strain
Epsom Salt Bath, Arnica Gel, Rest
Usage Instructions
Soak in a warm bath with Epsom salts; apply arnica gel to the affected area; rest and avoid strenuous activity.

N

Nail Fungus
Tea Tree Oil, Vinegar Soak, Coconut Oil
Usage Instructions
Apply diluted tea tree oil to affected nails; soak nails in a mixture of vinegar and water; apply coconut oil to moisturize and protect nails.

Nasal Congestion
Steam Inhalation, Eucalyptus Oil, Saline Spray
Usage Instructions
Inhale steam from a bowl of hot water; add a few drops of eucalyptus oil to the water; use a saline nasal spray.

Nausea
Ginger, Peppermint, Lemon
Usage Instructions
Chew raw ginger; drink peppermint or lemon tea; inhale the scent of lemon or peppermint essential oil.

P

Panic Attacks
Lavender Oil, Deep Breathing, Yoga
Usage Instructions
Inhale lavender oil or use in a diffuser during an attack; practice deep breathing exercises; engage in calming yoga poses.

Parasites
Garlic, Wormwood, Cloves
Usage Instructions
Consume raw garlic regularly; take wormwood supplements as directed; chew cloves daily.

Plantar Fasciitis
Epsom Salt Soak, Stretching, Ice Pack
Usage Instructions
Soak feet in warm Epsom salt water; perform stretching exercises for the calf and foot; apply ice pack to the affected area.
Usage Instructions

Plaque
Baking Soda, Oil Pulling, Vitamin D
Usage Instructions
Brush teeth with a paste of baking soda and water; swish coconut or sesame oil in your mouth for 10-20 minutes; ensure adequate vitamin D intake through diet or supplements.

Poison Ivy/Oak
Oatmeal Baths, Apple Cider Vinegar, Calamine Lotion,Baking Soda Paste, Jewelweed,
Usage Instructions
Take soothing oatmeal baths; apply diluted apple cider vinegar to affected areas; apply calamine lotion as needed. Make a paste of baking soda and water and apply to affected areas; apply crushed jewelweed leaves

Poor Digestion
Probiotics, Digestive Enzymes, Papaya
Usage Instructions
Consume probiotic-rich foods or supplements; take digestive enzyme supplements as directed; eat ripe papaya.

Poor Vision
Bilberry, Carrots, Eye Exercises
Usage Instructions
Take bilberry supplements as directed; eat carrots regularly; perform eye exercises to improve focus and flexibility.

R

Restless Legs
Iron Supplements, Stretching, Warm Bath, Massage
Usage Instructions
Take iron supplements if deficient; perform regular leg stretches; massage legs with gentle pressure.

S

Seasonal Flu
Elderberry, Chicken Soup, Rest
Usage Instructions
Take elderberry syrup or supplements; consume warm chicken soup; get plenty of rest and fluids.

Sinus Congestion
Eucalyptus Oil Steam, Neti Pot, Horseradish
Usage Instructions
Inhale steam with eucalyptus oil; use a neti pot with saline solution; consume horseradish in food.

Sinusitis
Neti Pot, Garlic, Spicy Foods
Usage Instructions
Rinse sinuses with a saline solution using a neti pot; consume garlic in food; eat spicy foods to help clear congestion.

Sinusitis
Steam Inhalation, Horseradish, Nasal Irrigation
Usage Instructions
Inhale steam from a bowl of hot water; consume horseradish to help clear congestion; use a saline solution in a neti pot to irrigate sinuses.

Skin Rash
Oatmeal Baths, Aloe Vera, Coconut Oil
Usage Instructions
Take soothing oatmeal baths to relieve itching and inflammation; apply aloe vera gel directly to the affected area to soothe and moisturize; apply coconut oil to moisturize and protect the skin.

Smelly Feet
Tea Soak, Cornstarch, Essential Oils
Usage Instructions
Soak feet in black tea to kill bacteria; sprinkle cornstarch in shoes to absorb moisture; apply tea tree or peppermint oil to feet.

Smokers Lung
Mullein, Lobelia, Peppermint
Usage Instructions
Drink mullein or lobelia tea; inhale peppermint oil vapor; practice deep breathing exercises regularly.

Sore Throat
Honey Lemon Tea, Salt Gargle, Sage Gargle
Usage Instructions
Drink honey lemon tea; gargle with warm salt water or sage tea.

Sore Throat
Honey Lemon Tea, Salt Gargle, Sage Gargle
Usage Instructions
Drink honey lemon tea; gargle with warm salt water or sage tea.

Stress
Ashwagandha, Rhodiola Rosea, Passionflower
Usage Instructions
Take ashwagandha or rhodiola supplements as directed; drink passionflower tea.

Stretch Marks
Cocoa Butter, Vitamin E Oil, Aloe Vera Gel
Usage Instructions
Massage cocoa butter or vitamin E oil into affected areas daily; apply aloe vera gel to keep skin hydrated and promote healing.

Sunburn
Aloe Vera Gel, Cool Compress, Coconut Oil
Usage Instructions
Apply aloe vera gel to sunburned skin; use cool compresses; apply coconut oil to moisturize and soothe.

Sunburn
Aloe Vera Gel, Cool Compress, Coconut Oil
Usage Instructions
Apply aloe vera gel to sunburned skin; use cool compresses; apply coconut oil to moisturize and soothe.

T

Thyroid Health
Seaweed, Brazil Nuts, Selenium Supplements
Usage Instructions
Incorporate seaweed into meals; consume Brazil nuts for selenium; take selenium supplements as directed.

Tinnitus
Ginkgo Biloba, Magnesium, White Noise
Usage Instructions

Take ginkgo biloba supplements as directed; take magnesium supplements if deficient; use a white noise machine to mask the ringing.

Tooth Decay
Fluoride Toothpaste, Xylitol, Green Tea
Usage Instructions
Brush teeth with fluoride toothpaste twice daily; chew xylitol gum or consume xylitol mints; drink green tea regularly.

Tooth Sensitivity
Clove Oil, Saltwater Rinse, Fluoride Toothpaste
Usage Instructions
Apply diluted clove oil to sensitive teeth and gums; rinse with warm salt water; use fluoride toothpaste for ongoing protection.

Toothache
Clove Oil, Saltwater Rinse, Peppermint Tea
Usage Instructions
Apply diluted clove oil to the affected tooth; rinse with warm salt water; drink peppermint tea for pain relief.

Toothache
Clove Oil, Saltwater Rinse, Peppermint Tea
Usage Instructions
Apply diluted clove oil to the affected tooth; rinse with warm salt water; drink peppermint tea for pain relief.

Travel Sickness
Ginger, Peppermint, Acupressure
Usage Instructions
Consume ginger or peppermint in any form; apply pressure to the P6 acupressure point on the wrist.

U

Urinary Tract Infection (UTI)
Cranberry Juice, D-Mannose, Probiotics, Hydration
Usage Instructions
Drink unsweetened cranberry juice; take D-Mannose supplements; consume probiotics to support urinary health. stay hydrated by drinking plenty of water.

V

Vaginal Odor
Yogurt, Tea Tree Oil, Baking Soda
Usage Instructions
Consume plain yogurt with live cultures; apply diluted tea tree oil to the external genital area; take baking soda baths.

Varicose Veins
Horse Chestnut, Compression Stockings, Exercise
Usage Instructions
Take horse chestnut supplements as directed; wear compression stockings; engage in regular low-impact exercise.

Vertigo
Ginger, Ginkgo Biloba, Epley Maneuver
Usage Instructions
Consume ginger in any form; take ginkgo biloba supplements as directed; perform the Epley Maneuver.

W

Warts
Tea Tree Oil, Duct Tape, Banana Peel
Usage Instructions
Apply tea tree oil directly to the wart; cover with duct tape; rub the wart with the inside of a banana peel.

Weight Loss
Green Tea, Apple Cider Vinegar, Fiber
Usage Instructions
Drink green tea regularly; consume diluted apple cider vinegar before meals; eat fiber-rich foods.

Wound Healing
Honey, Aloe Vera, Calendula Cream
Usage Instructions
Apply honey directly to the wound; apply aloe vera gel to the wound; use calendula cream on minor cuts and scrapes.

Y

Yeast Infection
Probiotics, Yogurt, Tea Tree Oil
Usage Instructions
Take probiotics orally or insert into the vagina; consume plain yogurt with live cultures; apply diluted tea tree oil to affected area.

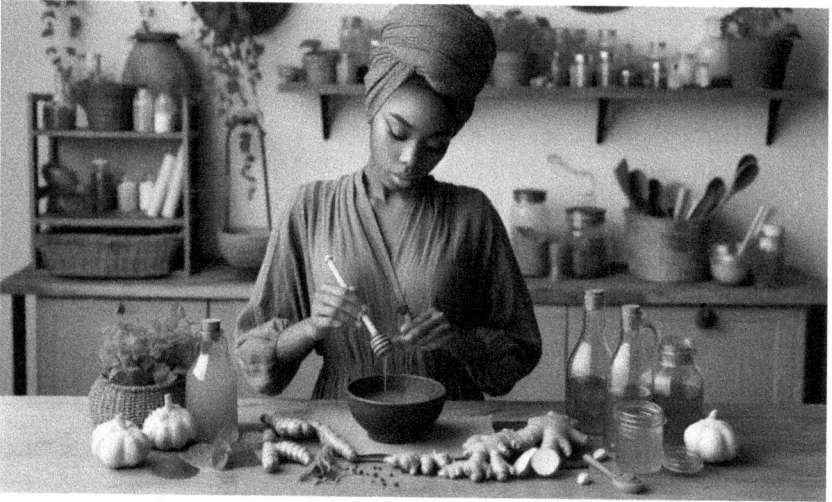

Natural Formulas Salves Elixirs Smoothies Teas Syrups Detoxes Sprays and Oils

Formula: Ginger and Lemon Tightening Skin Oil

Ingredients: 2 tablespoons of fresh ginger juice 2 tablespoons of fresh lemon juice 1/4 cup of coconut oil (or olive oil) 2 tablespoons of jojoba oil 1 tablespoon of vitamin E oil **Optional:** 10 drops of lavender essential oil (for soothing and additional skin benefits) **Instructions:** Prepare the Ginger Juice: Grate fresh ginger and extract its juice by squeezing it through a cheesecloth or fine strainer. Collect 2 tablespoons of fresh ginger juice. **Prepare the Lemon Juice:** Squeeze fresh lemons and strain the juice to remove any pulp. Collect 2 tablespoons of fresh lemon juice. **Mix the Ingredients:** In a small bowl, combine the ginger juice, lemon juice, coconut oil, jojoba oil, and vitamin E oil. Stir the mixture until all the oils and juices are well-blended.

Add Essential Oils (Optional): If you prefer a calming scent, add 10 drops of lavender essential oil to the mixture and stir. **Store the Oil:** Pour the mixture into a dark glass bottle with a tight-fitting lid to preserve its potency. Store the oil in a cool, dry place, away from direct sunlight. **Application:** To use, apply the oil to clean, dry skin, focusing on areas where you want to tighten the skin or reduce stretch marks. Massage the oil in circular motions for about 5-10 minutes to boost circulation and aid in absorption. For best results, apply the oil twice daily, morning and night.

Lion's Mane Elixir

Can be consumed daily to support cognitive health and overall well-being.

Ingredients: 1 cup of hot water 1 teaspoon of dried lion's mane mushroom powder 1 tablespoon of honey 1 teaspoon of lemon juice **Preparation:** Boil the water and pour it into a cup. Add the lion's mane mushroom powder and stir well. Mix in the honey and lemon juice.

Let the elixir steep for a few minutes before drinking.

Collagen-Boosting Smoothie

Ingredients: 1 cup mixed berries, 1 banana, 1 tablespoon chia seeds, 1 tablespoon flaxseed meal, 1 cup coconut water **Instructions:** Blend all ingredients until smooth. Drink daily to boost collagen production and support the health of connective tissues.

Anti-Inflammatory Joint Tea

Ingredients: 1 teaspoon turmeric powder, 1/2 teaspoon ginger powder, 1 teaspoon lemon juice, 1 teaspoon honey, 2 cups hot water **Instructions:** Mix turmeric and ginger powder in hot water. Add lemon juice and honey to taste.

Drink twice daily to reduce joint inflammation and support overall joint health.

Natural Anti-Inflammatory Cream for Joint Health

Ingredients: 1/2 cup coconut oil, 1/4 cup shea butter, 10 drops eucalyptus oil, 10 drops peppermint oil. **Instructions:** Melt coconut oil and shea butter, add essential oils, and let cool. Apply to joints to reduce inflammation and pain.

Herbal Bone Strengthening Tea

Ingredients: 1 tsp horsetail, 1 tsp nettle leaf, 1 tsp oat straw, 2 cups water. **Instructions:** Boil water and add herbs. Simmer for 10 minutes, strain, and drink twice daily to support bone density and joint health

Bone Strengthening Elixir

Ingredients: 1 cup almond milk, 1 tablespoon chia seeds, 1 tablespoon tahini, 1 teaspoon blackstrap molasses, 1/2 teaspoon cinnamon **Instructions:** Blend all ingredients until smooth. Drink daily to support bone health with a rich source of calcium and other essential nutrients

Natural Hair Growth Syrup

Ingredients: 1 cup nettle leaf (dried) 1 cup horsetail (dried) 1 cup fenugreek seeds 1 cup saw palmetto berries (dried) 1 cup burdock root (dried) 10 cups water 4 cups raw honey (or vegetable glycerin for a vegan option) **Instructions:** Prepare the Herbs: Lightly crush the dried herbs and fenugreek seeds to help release their beneficial compounds. **Directions:** In a large pot, add the nettle leaf, horsetail, fenugreek seeds, saw palmetto berries, and burdock root. Pour in 10 cups of water and bring to a boil. Reduce heat and let the mixture simmer for about 1-2 hours, until the liquid is reduced by half. **Strain the Herbs:** Remove the pot from heat and let it cool slightly. Strain the mixture through a fine-mesh sieve or cheesecloth into a clean container, ensuring to squeeze out as much liquid as possible from the herbs. Return the strained herbal decoction to the pot. Add 4 cups of raw honey (or vegetable glycerin for a vegan option). Gently heat the mixture on low, stirring continuously, until the honey (or glycerin) is fully dissolved and integrated with the herbal decoction. Do not boil. **Cool and Bottle:** Remove from heat and let the syrup cool to room temperature. Pour the syrup into sterilized glass bottles or jars, sealing them tightly.

Storage: Store the syrup in a cool, dry place. Refrigeration is recommended to extend shelf life. Use within 6 months. **Dosage:** Take 1 teaspoon (5 ml) twice daily, preferably with meals.

Hormone Balancing Herbal Tea

Anti-Inflammatory Turmeric Elixir

Ingredients: 1 cup almond milk, 1 teaspoon turmeric powder, 1/2 teaspoon cinnamon, 1/4 teaspoon ginger powder, 1 tablespoon maple syrup (optional). **Instructions:** Warm the almond milk and mix in the turmeric, cinnamon, ginger, and maple syrup. Drink this elixir to help reduce inflammation and support endocrine health.

Hormone Balancing Smoothie

Ingredients: 1 cup spinach, 1 banana, 1 tablespoon ground flaxseeds, 1 cup almond milk, 1/2 cup frozen berries, 1 teaspoon maca powder. **Instructions:** Blend all ingredients until smooth. Drink this smoothie daily to support hormonal balance

Hormone Balancing Herbal Tea

Ingredients: 1 teaspoon dried red clover, 1 teaspoon dried nettle leaf, 1 teaspoon dried dandelion root, 1 teaspoon dried licorice root. **Instructions:** Combine all ingredients in a teapot. Pour boiling water over the herbs and steep for 10-15 minutes. Strain and drink up to three cups a day to support hormonal balance.

Natural Remedies: Formulas for Powder, Salve, Syrup, and Pain Medicine

Always remember to use these remedies responsibly and consult with healthcare professionals when necessary.

Natural Antibiotic Powder (Comparable to Penicillin)

Ingredients: 1 tablespoon garlic powder 1 tablespoon turmeric powder 1 tablespoon echinacea powder 1 tablespoon goldenseal powder 1 tablespoon ginger powder **Instructions:** Mix all the powders together in a bowl. Store in an airtight container. **Usage:** Take 1 teaspoon of the powder mixed in warm water or juice 2-3 times daily for up to 10 days.

Natural Antifungal Salve

Ingredients: 1/4 cup coconut oil 2 tablespoons shea butter 2 tablespoons beeswax 10 drops tea tree oil 10 drops lavender oil 10 drops oregano oil **Instructions:** In a double boiler, melt the coconut oil, shea butter, and beeswax together. Remove from heat and stir in the essential oils. Pour into a clean container and let cool until solid. **Usage:** Apply to the affected area 2-3 times daily until the infection clears.

Natural Antiviral Syrup

Ingredients: 1 cup elderberries (fresh or dried) 4 cups water 1 cup raw honey 1 tablespoon grated ginger 1 cinnamon stick 5 cloves **Instructions:** In a pot, combine the elderberries, water, ginger, cinnamon stick, and cloves. Bring to a boil, then reduce heat and simmer for 45 minutes. Strain the mixture to remove the solids. Once the liquid has cooled to room temperature, stir in the honey. Pour into a glass jar and store in the refrigerator. **Usage:** Take 1 tablespoon daily for prevention, or 1 tablespoon every 3-4 hours if fighting an infection.

Natural Pain Reliever (Comparable to Vicodin)
Ingredients: 1 cup dried white willow bark 1 cup dried turmeric root 1 cup dried ginger root 1 cup dried devil's claw 1 cup dried cat's claw 1/2 cup black peppercorns (to enhance the bioavailability of curcumin in turmeric) **Instructions:** Grind all ingredients into a fine powder using a coffee grinder or blender. Mix the powders together thoroughly. Store in an airtight container. **Usage:** Take 1 teaspoon mixed in warm water or juice 2-3 times daily as needed for pain relief. Preparation and Storage Tips Quality **Ingredients:** Always use high-quality, organic herbs to ensure the best potency and efficacy. *Hygiene: Maintain cleanliness during preparation to avoid contamination. Storage: Store remedies in airtight containers, preferably in a cool, dark place to preserve their potency.* **Consultation and Caution** *Consult an Herbalist and or a Healthcare Professional: Before starting any new herbal regimen, consult with a healthcare professional, especially if you are pregnant, nursing, have a medical condition, or are taking other medications.* **Allergic Reactions:** *Test a small amount of the remedy first to check for any allergic reactions.*

Natural Remedies for Common Infections

Natural Remedy for Yeast Infections
Ingredients: 1 cup plain yogurt (with live active cultures) 2 tablespoons coconut oil 5 drops tea tree oil **Instructions:** Mix the yogurt and coconut oil together until smooth. Add the tea tree oil and mix well. Apply the mixture to the affected area 2-3 times daily until the infection clears.

Natural Remedy for Bacterial Vaginosis
Ingredients: 1 cup plain yogurt (with live active cultures) 1-2 garlic cloves, crushed **Instructions:** Mix the yogurt and crushed garlic together. Apply the mixture to the affected area or use as a vaginal suppository by placing it in a clean gauze or tampon applicator. Use once daily until symptoms improve.

Natural Remedy for UTIs
Ingredients: 1 cup cranberry juice (unsweetened) 1 cup water 1 teaspoon apple cider vinegar 1 tablespoon honey (optional) **Instructions:** Mix all ingredients together. Drink the mixture twice daily until symptoms improve.

Natural Remedy for Tooth Abscesses
Ingredients: 1 teaspoon clove oil 1 teaspoon coconut oil **Instructions:** Mix the clove oil and coconut oil together. Apply the mixture directly to the affected tooth and surrounding gums using a cotton swab. Use 2-3 times daily until the abscess improves.

Natural Remedy for Sinus Infections
Ingredients: 1 cup water 1 teaspoon sea salt 1/2 teaspoon baking soda 5 drops eucalyptus oil **Instructions:** Mix the water, sea salt, and baking soda together. Add the eucalyptus oil and mix well. Use a neti pot to irrigate the sinuses with the solution twice daily until the infection clears.

Natural Remedy for Sore Throat
Ingredients: 1 cup warm water 1 tablespoon honey 1 tablespoon apple cider vinegar 1/2 teaspoon cayenne pepper **Instructions:** Mix all ingredients together. Gargle with the mixture for 30 seconds and then spit it out. Repeat 2-3 times daily until symptoms improve.

Natural Remedy for Ear Infections
Ingredients: 1 tablespoon olive oil 3 drops tea tree oil 3 drops lavender oil **Instructions:** Warm the olive oil slightly (make sure it's not too hot). Add the tea tree oil and lavender oil to the olive oil and mix well. Using a dropper, place a few drops of the mixture into the affected ear. Let it sit for a few minutes, then tilt your head to let it drain out. Use 2-3 times daily until the infection improves. _Preparation and Storage Tips_ **Quality Ingredients:** *Always use high-quality, organic ingredients to ensure the best potency and efficacy.* **Hygiene:** *Maintain cleanliness during preparation to avoid contamination. Storage: Store remedies in airtight containers, preferably in a cool, dark place to preserve their potency.* **Consultation and Caution** *Consult a Healthcare Professional: Before starting any new herbal regimen, consult with a healthcare professional, especially if you are pregnant, nursing, have a medical condition, or are taking other medications.* **Allergic Reactions** *Test a small amount of the remedy first to check for any allergic reactions.*

Lung Detoxification for Heavy Smokers

Herbal Tea for Lung Detox
Ingredients: 1 tablespoon mullein leaf 1 tablespoon thyme 1 tablespoon eucalyptus leaf 1 tablespoon licorice root 4 cups water **Instructions:** Combine all the herbs in a pot. Add water and bring to a boil. Reduce heat and simmer for 15-20 minutes. Strain the mixture and let it cool. **Usage:** Drink 1-2 cups daily for up to two weeks.

Herbal Steam Inhalation
Ingredients: 1 tablespoon eucalyptus oil 1 tablespoon peppermint oil 1 liter boiling water **Instructions:** Add the oils to the boiling water. Place your face over the pot (keeping a safe distance) and cover your head with a towel to trap the steam. Inhale the steam deeply for 10-15 minutes. **Usage:** Repeat daily for one week.

Lung Detox Smoothie
Ingredients: 1 cup pineapple juice (contains bromelain, which helps reduce mucus) 1 tablespoon fresh ginger (anti-inflammatory) 1 tablespoon turmeric (antioxidant) 1 tablespoon raw honey 1/2 teaspoon cayenne pepper 1/2 cup water **Instructions:** Combine all ingredients in a blender. Blend until smooth. **Usage** Drink once daily for one week.

Herbal Kidney Cleanse Tea
Ingredients: 1 tablespoon dandelion root 1 tablespoon nettle leaf 1 tablespoon marshmallow root 1 tablespoon parsley 4 cups water **Instructions:** Combine all the herbs in a pot. Add water and bring to a boil. Reduce heat and simmer for 15-20 minutes. Strain the mixture and let it cool. **Usage:** Drink 1-2 cups daily for up to two weeks.

Kidney Detox Juice
Ingredients: 1 cucumber (hydrating and cleansing) 1 cup watermelon (diuretic properties) 1 lemon (alkalizing and cleansing) 1 tablespoon fresh ginger (anti-inflammatory) 1 tablespoon parsley (diuretic) **Instructions:** Combine all ingredients in a juicer. Juice until smooth. **Usage:** Drink once daily for one week.

Herbal Tincture for Kidney Health
Ingredients: 1 part juniper berry 1 part hydrangea root 1 part gravel root 80 proof alcohol (e.g., vodka) for extraction. **Instructions:** Place the herbs in a glass jar. Cover the herbs with alcohol, ensuring they are fully submerged. Seal the jar and store it in a dark place for 4-6 weeks, shaking it daily. Strain the mixture and store it in a dark glass bottle. **Usage:** Take 1-2 teaspoons daily for up to two weeks.

Herbal Blood Detox
Herbal Blood Cleanse Tea
Ingredients: 1 tablespoon burdock root 1 tablespoon dandelion root 1 tablespoon red clover 1 tablespoon nettle leaf 4 cups water **Instructions:** Combine all the herbs in a pot. Add water and bring to a boil. Reduce heat and simmer for 15-20 minutes. Strain the mixture and let it cool. **Usage:** Drink 1-2 cups daily for up to two weeks.

Blood Detox Juice
Ingredients: 1 beetroot (rich in antioxidants and supports liver health) 1 apple (contains pectin, which helps eliminate toxins) 1 carrot (high in beta-carotene and aids in detoxification) 1 lemon (alkalizing and cleansing) 1 tablespoon fresh ginger (anti-inflammatory) 1 cup water **Instructions:** Combine all ingredients in a juicer. Juice until smooth. **Usage:** Drink once daily for one week.

Herbal Tincture for Blood Health
Ingredients: 1 part echinacea 1 part yellow dock root 1 part cleavers 80 proof alcohol (e.g., vodka) for extraction **Instructions:** Place the herbs in a glass jar. Cover the herbs with alcohol, ensuring they are fully submerged. Seal the jar and store it in a dark place for 4-6 weeks, shaking it daily. Strain the mixture and store it in a dark glass bottle. **Usage** Take 1-2 teaspoons daily for up to two weeks.

Alkaline Herbal Blood Cleanse
Ingredients: 1 tablespoon sarsaparilla root 1 tablespoon burdock root 1 tablespoon yellow dock root 1 tablespoon elderberries 4 cups water **Instructions:** Combine all the herbs in a pot. Add water and bring to a boil. Reduce heat and simmer for 15-20 minutes. Strain the mixture and let it cool. **Usage:** Drink 1-2 cups daily for up to two weeks.

Natural Formula for Feminine Wash
Ingredients: 1 cup warm water, 1 tablespoon apple cider vinegar, 2-3 drops tea tree oil (optional) **Instructions:** Mix ingredients and use to gently rinse the vulva. Apple cider vinegar helps balance pH, while tea tree oil has mild antibacterial properties. Use once weekly.

Quick Formula for a Yoni Cleanser to Use During Menstruation
Ingredients: 1 cup distilled water 1 tablespoon apple cider vinegar (unfiltered, organic) 1-2 drops of tea tree or lavender essential oil (optional) **Instructions:** Mix all Ingredients in a clean bottle. Use to gently rinse the external area only, once a day during menstruation. Rinse with plain water afterward and pat dry.

Yoni Detox Bath Formula

Ingredients: 1 cup Epsom salt 1 tablespoon apple cider vinegar A few drops of lavender essential oil 1 tablespoon baking soda **Instructions:** Add all Ingredients to a warm bath. Soak for 20-30 minutes, allowing the Ingredients to help draw out impurities and soothe the skin. Rinse off with clean water and pat the skin dry.

Natural Deodorant Formula: Mix a few drops of tea tree oil with coconut oil for a natural deodorant that can help during menstruation. Apply gently to the outer area as needed.

Formula for Natural Cleansing Wipes

Ingredients: 1 cup distilled water, 1 tablespoon witch hazel, 2 drops lavender oil **Instructions:** Mix Ingredients and soak soft cotton pads or wipes in the solution. Use as needed for freshness.

Natural Formula for Under-Breast Deodorant

Ingredients: 1 tablespoon coconut oil, 1 teaspoon baking soda, 2 drops tea tree oil **Instructions:** Mix Ingredients and apply a small amount under each breast to reduce odor.

Herbal Yoni Cleanse

Ingredients: 2 tablespoons dried lavender, 2 tablespoons dried chamomile, 2 tablespoons dried calendula **Instructions:** Boil 4 cups of water and add the herbs. Let steep for 10 minutes, strain, and let cool. Use as a rinse.

Natural Feminine Deodorant

Ingredients: 1/4 cup coconut oil, 5 drops tea tree oil, 5 drops lavender oil **Instructions:** Mix Ingredients in a small jar. Apply a small amount to the external area after showering.

At-Home Yoni Wash Formula

Ingredients: 1 cup distilled or purified water 1 tablespoon apple cider vinegar (organic, raw, unfiltered) 2-3 drops tea tree oil (optional, for its antifungal and antibacterial properties) 1-2 drops lavender or chamomile essential oil (optional, for soothing effects) **Instructions:** Mix all Ingredients in a clean bottle. Use as a gentle wash for the external vaginal area only (never for internal use). Rinse thoroughly with water after application. *Note: Apple cider vinegar helps balance pH, while tea tree oil can offer antibacterial and antifungal benefits. Always do a patch test with essential oils to ensure there is no irritation.*

Natural Formula for Menstrual Cramp Relief Oil
Ingredients: 1 tablespoon coconut oil, 3 drops lavender oil, 2 drops clary sage oil **Instructions:** Mix and apply to the lower abdomen for relief.

Herbal Perineal Spray
Ingredients: 1 cup filtered water (boiled and cooled) 2 tablespoons witch hazel (alcohol-free) 1 tablespoon aloe vera gel (pure, no additives) 5 drops lavender essential oil (optional, for its antibacterial and calming properties) 5 drops tea tree essential oil (for its antifungal and antibacterial effects) **Instructions:** Combine all Ingredients in a small spray bottle. Shake well before each use. Spray directly onto the perineal area after using the bathroom or whenever you need relief. This can also be sprayed onto maternity pads for a cooling effect. **Tip:** Store the spray in the refrigerator for extra soothing relief.

Sitz Bath Healing Soak
Ingredients: ¼ cup Epsom salt (reduces swelling and promotes relaxation) 2 tablespoons baking soda (helps neutralize vaginal pH) 1 tablespoon dried calendula flowers (promotes healing) 1 tablespoon dried chamomile flowers (anti-inflammatory and calming) 1 tablespoon dried lavender (antibacterial and soothing) **Instructions:** Mix all the dry Ingredients together and store in an airtight container. When ready to use, add ¼ cup of the mixture to a sitz bath or shallow basin filled with warm, filtered water. Soak for 15-20 minutes, ensuring the perineal area is fully immersed. Gently pat dry with a soft towel after the bath. *Tip: For added healing benefits, brew the dried herbs in hot water first (like tea), strain, and add the herbal tea to your sitz bath.*

Soothing Postpartum Padsicles
Ingredients: Maternity pads (overnight size for better coverage) ¼ cup witch hazel (alcohol-free) 2 tablespoons aloe vera gel 5 drops lavender essential oil (optional) 5 drops peppermint essential oil (optional, for a cooling effect) **Instructions:** Lay the pads flat and apply a thin layer of aloe vera gel over the surface. Mix witch hazel with the essential oils (if using) and gently drizzle over the pads. Fold the pads back up, place them in a zip-lock bag, and freeze. When needed, take one out, allow it to thaw slightly, and place it in your underwear for soothing relief. *Tip: These are best used in the first week postpartum when swelling and discomfort are most intense.*

Gentle DIY Feminine Wash
Ingredients: 1 cup filtered water 2 tablespoons castile soap (unscented, gentle) 1 teaspoon apple cider vinegar (helps balance pH) 1 teaspoon aloe vera gel 3 drops lavender essential oil (optional) **Instructions:** Mix all Ingredients in a squeeze bottle. Use a small amount to gently wash the vaginal area while showering. Rinse thoroughly with filtered water. *Tip: This wash can be used in a peri bottle as well for gentle cleansing after using the toilet.*

Homemade Anti-Fungal Foot Balm
Ingredients: ¼ cup coconut oil (antifungal and moisturizing) 2 tablespoons shea butter (healing and moisturizing) 10 drops tea tree essential oil (antifungal) 10 drops eucalyptus essential oil (cooling and soothing) 5 drops peppermint essential oil (optional for a cooling sensation) **Instructions:** Melt the coconut oil and shea butter together in a double boiler. Remove from heat and stir in the essential oils. Pour into a small jar and let it cool until solid. Apply a thin layer to your feet, focusing on the heels and any affected areas, especially before bed. *Tip: For best results, apply the balm and wear cotton socks overnight to help the Ingredients penetrate the skin.* **Ingredients:** 1 probiotic capsule (***must contain Lactobacillus acidophilus***) 1 teaspoon coconut oil (antifungal and moisturizing) 1 drop lavender essential oil (optional, for soothing properties) **Instructions:** Mix the contents of the probiotic capsule with coconut oil and lavender oil. Shape the mixture into a small, bullet-sized suppository and place it on wax paper. Freeze for 10-15 minutes until solid. Insert gently into the vaginal canal before bedtime. Use once or twice a week as needed. ***Caution:*** *Always consult with a healthcare provider before using any vaginal suppository, especially if you have had any vaginal tearing or stitches.*

Hormone-Balancing Herbal Tea Formula:
Ingredients: 1 teaspoon red raspberry leaf (tones the uterus and supports hormone regulation) 1 teaspoon chamomile (calms the nervous system and promotes relaxation) 1 teaspoon nettles (rich in iron and supports postpartum recovery) 1 teaspoon fenugreek seeds (enhances milk supply) ½ teaspoon cinnamon (helps regulate blood sugar and supports hormonal balance) 1 cup boiled filtered water. **Instructions:** Mix all the herbs in a teapot or infuser. Pour boiled water over the herbs and steep for 10-15 minutes. Strain and enjoy warm, up to 2-3 cups per day. *Tip: Add a teaspoon of raw honey for additional soothing and immune-boosting benefits.*

Detoxifying Yoni Steam for Vaginal Health
Ingredients: 1 tablespoon dried mugwort (supports uterine health) 1 tablespoon dried rosemary (antibacterial and anti-inflammatory) 1 tablespoon dried lavender (calms and soothes the body) 1 tablespoon dried calendula (promotes healing of tissues) **Instructions:** Boil 4 cups of filtered water and add the herbs. Let the mixture steep for 10 minutes, then pour it into a large bowl. Position yourself over the bowl, sitting comfortably with a towel draped around your waist to trap the steam. Sit for 20-30 minutes. Relax and breathe deeply, focusing on your womb and pelvic area. *Caution: Avoid yoni steaming if you have stitches, open wounds, or any active infections.*

DIY Healing Perineal Balm
Ingredients: ¼ cup coconut oil ¼ cup shea butter 1 tablespoon beeswax (provides a protective barrier) 10 drops frankincense essential oil (anti-inflammatory and promotes healing) 10 drops myrrh essential oil (antimicrobial and soothing) **Instructions:** Melt the coconut oil, shea butter, and beeswax together in a double boiler. Remove from heat and stir in the essential oils. Pour into a small glass jar and allow it to cool until solid. Apply a small amount to the perineal area as needed. *Storage: Keep in a cool, dry place for up to 6 months.*

CHAPTER 5 JOURNEY INTO HERBS FOR SMOKING AND HEALING

Dear Melanin Gurlll,

As you reach the end of *Melanin Journey to Health and Wellness*, remember that this book is only the beginning of your own unique path to healing. In our melanin-rich bodies, we hold the power to connect deeply with nature, embracing earthly elements like natural herbs, healing waters, grounding crystals, and plant-based remedies. By surrounding ourselves with natural clothing, organic fabrics, and earth-toned garments, we're not just dressing our bodies; we're aligning ourselves with the energy of the earth to nurture and heal.

This journey is about reawakening the wisdom within us, honoring the rhythm of the seasons, and allowing nature to restore us—body, mind, and spirit. For Black women, this journey holds a sacred resilience, grounded in centuries of struggle, survival, and strength. From the brutal era of Colonial Slavery, when our ancestors endured unimaginable hardship, through the Revolutionary War and the false promise of "all men are created equal," to the deep scars of the Antebellum Era and the long road through the Civil War and Reconstruction, our history has forged a profound inner resilience. The Jim Crow Era and Civil Rights Movement showed us the determination to stand in our power, and now, in our present moment, we can draw upon the fortitude of those who came before us.

Black women have faced and overcome adversity across every period of history, emerging from each era with courage and wisdom that lives in us today. With these pages as a guide, take ownership of your journey—one that prioritizes your health, uplifts your spirit, and honors the power of melanin. Use this book as a resource to do your research and find what resonates with your unique journey. We are reclaiming our heritage, rebuilding our wellness, and reconnecting with our innate power as melanin-rich beings.

~ October Reign

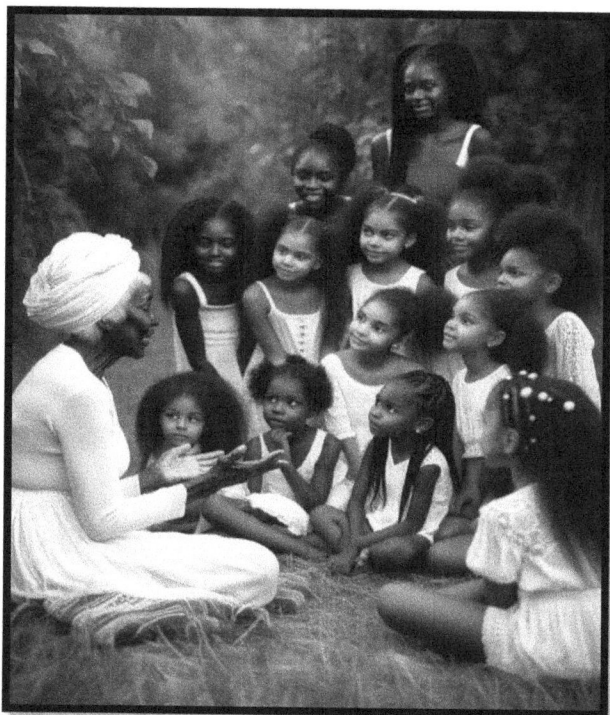

Your journey is a lifelong path; walk it with intention, grounded in the wisdom of nature. Move through your melanin journey with the resilience and strength of our ancestors. As we walk through this healing journey pass it along.

www.ingramcontent.com/pod-product-compliance
Lightning Source LLC
Chambersburg PA
CBHW071947270326
41928CB00009B/1373